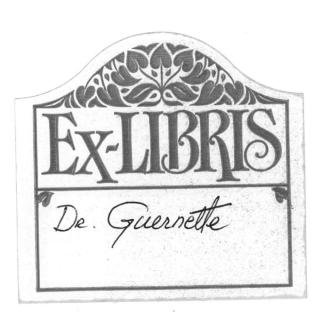

The Fate of Borderline Patients

DIAGNOSIS AND TREATMENT OF MENTAL DISORDERS
Allen Frances, MD, *Series Editor*

The Fate of Borderline Patients

SUCCESSFUL OUTCOME AND PSYCHIATRIC PRACTICE

Michael H. Stone, MD
Columbia College of Physicians and Surgeons

Foreword by Allen Frances, MD

THE GUILFORD PRESS
New York London

© 1990 The Guilford Press
A Division of Guilford Publications, Inc.
72 Spring Street, New York, NY 10012

Printed in the United States of America

This book is printed on acid-free paper.

Last digit is print number: 9 8 7 6 5 4 3 2 1

Library of Congress Cataloging-in-Publication Data

Stone, Michael H., 1933–
    The fate of borderline patients: successful outcome and
psychiatric practice / Michael H. Stone; foreword by Allen Frances.
        p.   cm. — (Diagnosis and treatment of mental disorders)
    Includes bibliographical references.
    ISBN 0-89862-399-5
    1. Borderline personality disorder—Treatment. 2. Borderline
personality disorder—Prognosis.   I. Title.   II. Series.
    [DNLM: 1. Borderline Personality Disorder. 2. Outcome and Process
Assessment (Health Care).   WM 190 S879f]
RC569.5.B67S76   1990
616.85′852—dc20
DNLM/DLC
for Library of Congress   90-3079
                                                                      CIP

For Dr. Lawrence C. Kolb

Foreword

This book describes a crucial study with an important and unexpected finding. Its implications should be widely disseminated and understood by patients with personality disorder, their families, and the clinicians who treat them. Stated simply, Dr. Stone has discovered that borderline patients tend to get better if only they live long enough. On long-term follow-up, approximately two-thirds of borderline patients who had once been quite severely impaired were functioning normally or with only minimal symptoms. This is surprising because such patients often spend long portions of their lives feeling utterly hopeless and also instilling a similar sense of hopelessness in their therapists and families. It is difficult for the patient or the clinician to believe that the current chaos and despair will ever abate, and all tend to assume the worst. This is particularly true for the staff of inpatient facilities who see these patients (and all others, for that matter) only at their very worst.

It provides great reassurance for us to learn that no matter how dreadful the current situation may seem, all is not lost. If the patient (and the clinician) can endure and survive the years of suffering and disappointment, there is likely to be a bright light at the end of the tunnel. It is important—sometimes lifesaving and often treatment saving—for the clinician to know this and to be able to impart a realistic optimism to the patient in a manner that does not diminish the empathic understanding of how terrible the patient's current experience is.

Such awareness broadens the clinician's and the patient's perspective about long-term prospects, reduces exaggerated demoralization in response to the inevitable setbacks that occur in life and in treatment, and helps to focus attention on the greatest risk in the management of such patients, namely, suicide. The suicide rate in borderline patients in appreciable, particularly when they also suffer from depression and substance abuse. Suicides occur fairly early in the course of the disorder and become even more tragic once we discover that long-term outcome is much better than anyone could have imagined. Knowledge about long-term outcome also makes suicide seem less necessary and inevitable and helps to alert the patient and clinician to be on guard against it. Based on Dr. Stone's work, we may conclude that one major goal in working with borderline patients is to keep them alive long enough for them to get better. In my own practice I try to enlist the patient's cooperation in learning techniques intended to reduce suicide risk.

It is natural to wonder why it is that borderline patients get better with time. Unfortunately, the naturalistic design of this study goes not allow us to draw any firm conclusions, although Dr. Stone does have some interesting hunches. Perhaps, most to the point, we cannot say with any degree of assurance whether treatment was beneficial (or harmful) to the patients in the study and how well or poorly they would have done without it. My own impression is that the treatment relationship is healing and indeed lifesaving for many borderline patients, that it is regressive and destructive for a few, and that it has little or no effect on some others. We have no definitive studies on this question and indeed this an especially difficult area of investigation. Certainly we cannot predict in advance who will benefit and who will not from treatment and it is usually wise to provide treatment to those who want it unless there is clear evidence that past treatment relationships have been consistently destructive and used in a regressive fashion.

We should also not underestimate the healing effects of time and maturation, perhaps especially for patients with borderline personality disorder. It has been well established for patients with antisocial personality (mostly males) that entry into the fourth decade of life, for those who make it that far, is often accompanied by a "burning out," or perhaps to put it in a better light, a "mellowing" with a reduction of impulsivity and antisocial behavior. It seems likely that the findings reported by Dr. Stone on patients with borderline personality disorder (mostly females) may be analogous to and perhaps a result of a similar process of maturation and reduced energy levels and impulsivity with aging. I like to tell patients that their current problems, however difficult, are likely to be no more than a stage in their lives—one that they will very likely outgrow. This puts borderline behavior into an easily understandable developmental context, normalizes it, and provides hope for its resolution.

As Dr. Stone himself indicates clearly, this is a study with many methodological limitations that might lead to bias. This is a naturalistic study which could only have been done in its current form by a nonblind rater who had known the patients during their early stages of illness. Original diagnoses were made retrospectively and also in a nonblind fashion. It is possible that Dr. Stone's knowledge of the patients, or their knowledge of him, might have influenced his ratings of the information provided to him by the patients and their families. Moreover, the data may be incomplete because most information was collected by telephone and without benefit of systematic interviewing instruments. My concern about the possible confounding is much reduced by the fact that three other long-term longitudinal studies of borderline personality disorder have reported findings and conclusions that very closely approximate those reported here. While each of the studies has its own limitations and possible confounds, the results converge strongly and are believable. This type of research is so difficult to conduct that it cannot be done at all without methodological shortcuts. We are lucky to have several studies all pointing in the same direction and providing a clear guide to prognosis and a clear call to patient psychoeducation.

Dr. Stone's case vignettes and appendices provide a rich evocation of patients that clinicians will find enjoying and insightful.

On a personal note, I have enjoyed a long and rewarding relationship to this study. Approximately 15 of the people described in the follow-up were my own patients, treated when I was a resident at the New York State Psychiatric Institute. I also got to know many of the others during my 18 months of training on the unit described in the book. Dr. Stone was an attending on that unit and became one of my most important teachers and mentors. Over the years I have maintained an intermittent contact with a number of the patients reported on in this book and have had a close relationship with Dr. Stone. It is, therefore, a special delight to learn more about how our patients have done and a relief to learn that so many have done so well. I feel a great gratitude to Dr. Stone and to the many wonderful, if once very unhappy, individuals he describes here. Their experience, and Dr. Stone's careful follow-up of it, provide a beacon of hope for many other such patients and their clinicians.

Allen Frances, MD

Acknowledgments

Among the many people who made this book possible, I owe the greatest debt of gratitude to the patients of the PI-500, to their relatives, and to their former therapists. I could not thank them all by name here, even if to do so were permissible—because they number more than 2,000. Those whom I can name include Dr. Richard Friedman, who read much of the manuscript and who offered many valuable criticisms and suggestions. Dr. Stephen Hurt gave unstintingly of his time and expertise, over a 2-year period, in the statistical analysis of the data. Dr. Hans Stassen and Dr. Jules Angst of the University Clinic (Bürghölzli) in Zürich carried out a multivariate analysis of various factors affecting outcome in the borderline patients, as well as the analysis of suicide risk within the major diagnostic groups. In the early stages of the study, even before the publication of his own seminal papers on the Chestnut Lodge follow-up project, Dr. Thomas McGlashan provided me with checklists to aid in the rediagnosis of the patients, and in the analysis of their work status and outcome patterns.

The guiding spirit behind this book was Dr. Lawrence Kolb. Throughout the years when the patients of the PI-500 were at the hospital and their therapists (including myself) were in training there, Dr. Kolb was chairman of the department of psychiatry. Dr. Kolb was, and remains to this day, a source of strength and clinical wisdom to all of us, and it is to him that I fondly dedicate this book.

Courtesy dictates that authors thank their spouses, whether they actually helped in the preparation or not. Thanking my wife for her help with this book is no mere courtesy. Her contributions were indispensable. Throughout 50 months, Beth uncomplainingly sustained me during the countless evenings that were lost to the follow-up study. She then edited the entire manuscript, polishing and clarifying the text in many places.

Special thanks are also due my elder son, David Stone. Once the chart materials were stripped of identifying information, David devoted all of two summers, and much of the time in between, to abstracting demographic and other key data from the records.

Finally, more thanks than can be put into words are due to the team of secretaries who set the final manuscript in type. The "team" consisted of one person, Ms. Ulrike Henderson, whose speed and accuracy with the text and whose artistic flair with the tables and figures made her the equal of three.

Preface

Professionals working in the exact sciences operate within systems that, at the macroscopic level, enjoy comfortable levels of predictability. This has led psychiatrists to turn their own phrase—"inferiority complex"—against themselves, as they embarrassedly admit how unpredictable are the "systems" they seek to measure, whether these be the efficacy of a treatment method or the long-term fate of an emotionally disturbed patient. Our work is thus very different from that of the artillery officer, whom the physicist can help predict the landing spot of a mortar shell—given only the angle of the mortar and the barometric and wind condition—to within a narrow circle some thousands of yards away. The most predictable *persons,* as to their long-term trajectory, are ironically the least interesting. Healthy children of normal intelligence, from nurturing families in tranquil environments, usually do well throughout life. Brain-damaged or chronically psychotic youngsters from abusive homes in a crushing environment usually do poorly. This much is common knowledge. What interests psychiatry, and what animated the present study, is the fate of persons in an *intermediate* range of emotional handicap. Here long-term predictability has thus far been of a low order. The situation is comparable to the artillery officer's firing the mortar straight up during a hurricane: Any particular shell could land at any point of the compass.

Actually, with careful regression analysis (as I hope to make clear in subsequent portions of the book), we can do a little better than the officer in the high wind. Within the domain of borderline patients, for example, we can explain 14–15% of the spread of outcomes. As Stassen (1988) informed me, this is the level of "explainability" one can anticipate in a long-term outcome study. Really, I think we should not be discouraged that the variables we choose for multivariate analysis can, however cleverly selected, account at best for a mere sixth of the variance. Our collective fates are, so to say, five-sixths in the hands of the gods. I take this as a sign that, except for a few unfortunate (and usually severely mistreated) persons, we are not robots going through the motions of some preprogrammed life, like the nameless humanoids of Zamyatin's *We*

(1924).[1] Although many of the patients of the PI-500 had had to cope with parental abusiveness, sexual molestation, humiliation, genetic liability, neglect, and the early death of loved ones, many surmounted such handicaps to become at once productive and contented members of society and living testimonials to the recuperative powers of the human organism.

The importance of the present study lay in its potential to enhance the predictive powers of clinicians who work with hospitalized psychiatric patients, especially with those exhibiting borderline personality disorder (BPD). Though we can in general account, as I mentioned above, only for a fraction of the variance in long-term outcome, there are many specific situations in everyday practice where, thanks to studies such as the present one, we can predict the fate of a patient with near certainty. Female BPD patients with concomitant major affective disorder and alcohol abuse, for example, have a 5-year survival rate barely in excess of 50%—unless they manage to curb their alcoholism. Borderline patients who have been the victims of parental abusiveness usually do less well than their nonvictimized counterparts. Those with mild obsessional traits tend to outperform those with other accompanying personality traits. These are some examples of what we might consider as entries in a clinical dictionary consisting of numerous combinations—graded from the prognostically most favorable to the least favorable. This book provides many such entries. Armed with such a dictionary, clinicians can situate patients with whom they are currently working along similar regions of the prognostic continuum embodied in this dictionary. The fate of the patient in question will, we would predict, closely resemble the fate of the traced patients described here whose clinical characteristics are the most similar.

[1]Zamyatin's book influenced Huxley and Orwell in their more popular novels about controlled human beings, *Brave New World* and *1984*.

ABBREVIATIONS AND EQUIVALENCES USED IN THE TEXT FOR MAJOR DIAGNOSTIC GROUPS AND DISORDERS

PTSD	Antisocial personality, as defined by DSM-III (1980)
BPD	Borderline personality disorder, as defined by Gunderson and Singer (1975) or by DSM-III
BPO	Borderline personality organization, as defined by Kernberg (1967)
D	Dysthymic (borderline); patients who had BPO and concomitant MAD, but who did not meet criteria for BPD
MAD	Major affective disorder, as defined by DSM-III
MDP	Manic–depressive psychosis, as defined by DSM-III
NPD	Narcissistic personality disorder, as defined by DSM-III
PMS	Premenstrual syndrome
PTSD	Posttraumatic stress disorder, as defined by DSM-III
SA	Schizoaffective psychosis, as defined by DSM-III
SF	Schizophreniform illness ("acute SZ-like reaction"), as defined by DSM-III
STP	Schizotypal personality disorder, as defined by DSM-III
SZ	Schizophrenia, as defined by DSM-III

Contents

Man is like a novel: one doesn't know until the very last page how the thing will end.
    —Yevgeny Zamyatin, *We* (1924)

The Fate of Borderline Patients

Introduction to the Study

THE UNIT

"PI-500" is a verbal shorthand, modeled after Tsuang's "Iowa 500" (Tsuang & Winokur, 1975), for the long-term follow-up study of consecutively admitted patients hospitalized during the years 1963 to 1976 on the General Clinical Service at the New York State Psychiatric Institute (PI). There were 550 patients in the study to begin with; of these, I succeeded in tracing 502. The unit, sometimes known as the "Long-Term Unit" because of the length of stay, specialized in the intensive, psychoanalytically oriented psychotherapy of adolescent and young adult patients. Until 1968 the unit consisted administratively of a male and a female section. The combined census was 60. During its last 8 years, the unit was under one administration. Because of governmental fiscal restraints, the census diminished in the mid-1970s to about 45 beds.

With few exceptions, the therapists were psychiatric residents who spent their entire second year on the unit. A caseload of four to six patients was the average. Most therapists saw their patients three times a week in sessions of 45 minutes. A quarter of the patients were adolescents, who received family therapy as well—at first under the supervision of Dr. Nathan Ackerman, later on of others who had trained at his institute. Almost every member of the staff had been in psychoanalytic therapy, as had nearly all of the residents. During the years of Dr. Otto Kernberg's directorship (1973–1976), many of the staff attended special group therapy exercises at one or another A. K. Rice Institute in the Northeast. The staff–patient ratio remained approximately 1:1 during all 14 cohorts of the study. Various forms of group therapy—some task-oriented, others more open-ended and analytic—were a part of every patient's treatment regimen. The great majority also received some form of pharmacotherapy, most often a neuroleptic or an antidepressant. Lithium became available in 1968–1969, for those manifesting symptoms that might be responsive to that drug.

The unit played an important role in the professional lives of the therapists, who saw the year-long rotation as a special opportunity to become grounded in analytic psychotherapy. Besides the residents, there were psychologists, senior social workers, and senior nurses who also carried out the role of primary therapist. About half the therapists were, or were about to be, in psychoanalytic training. The large cadre of supervisors were also analytically trained. Each therapist received supervision from four to six such supervisors, at least one of whom was a psychiatrist widely known for this type of therapy. This group included Drs. Philip Polatin, Alivin Mesnikoff, Lothar Gidro-Frank, Shervert Frazier, Lawrence Kolb, Nathan Ackerman, Harold Searles, and Otto Kernberg. A considerable *esprit de corps* animated the personnel throughout the years of the unit's existence. The unit served the entire state of New York and for the most part had permission to select, via an intake interview, those whom the staff felt would be amenable to the program of therapy offered. Patients who were convalescent by the time of the academic rotation on July 1 often continued with their original therapist; in other instances, transfer to a new therapist was necessary. Therapists who set up practice in the New York City area were able in some cases to continue working with their PI patients for 5, 10, and even 15 years.

The treatment philosophy of the unit was conservative. The unit was locked and maintained a graduated system of privileges in accordance with the patients' level of integration and trustworthiness with respect to self-destructive behavior. Suicide watch was sometimes excessively long; rarely was it too brief. The prevailing belief among the staff was that intensive psychotherapy would be instrumental in diminishing the vulnerability of the patients to the various life stresses that had overwhelmed them initially, and that it would confer benefits over and above what the milieu and the medications could achieve by themselves. This is not an easy determination to make under the best of circumstances, and staff members tended to be slow, when certain patients seemed not to improve, in shifting to other modalities of treatment or other plans of action. The psychiatric community considered the unit a court of last resort; therapists and the permanent staff were disposed to give the "old college try." Their efforts were made easier by the fact that the families paid nothing for those over the age of 21 and only nominal sums for their adolescent children. Allowing a patient to remain as long as might be necessary on the unit created no financial burden. For a few of the adolescent patients, the unit became an escape route between home and some safer environment (college, a shared apartment), in cases where the original home had been either inadequate or destructive.

INCLUSION CRITERIA

The follow-up study focused primarily on the natural history of the patients in their various diagnostic categories. In hopes that it might also be possible to assess the efficacy of the treatment program, the study concentrated on patients who had spent at least 3 months on the unit. This aspect of the design excluded only 17 patients. Also excluded were those over age 40 on admission or those with IQs under 90. There were only a few patients in either category.

DIAGNOSIS

Diagnostic standards in the United States a generation ago, especially before publication of the "Feighner criteria" (Feighner et al., 1972) or the *Diagnostic and Statistical Manual of Mental Disorders,* third edition (DSM-III, 1980), were less precise than they are at present. Ninety percent of the PI-500 patients received either of two diagnoses: "pseudoneurotic schizophrenia" or "chronic undifferentiated schizophrenia." These choices reflected in part the work of Dr. Philip Polatin, director of the unit in the 1940s and 1950s. With Dr. Paul Hoch, Polatin had coined the term "pseudoneurotic schizophrenia" as a label for less than full-blown cases of schizophrenia—cases with an abundance of "neurotic" (obsessive, phobic, depressive . . .) symptoms. For the diagnosis of schizophrenia itself, one relied on E. Bleuler's "four A's" (autism, ambivalence, affect incongruity, and associational loosening), not upon Kraepelinian concepts.

For the purposes of the follow-up study I reviewed each record and rediagnosed each case, using a checklist of signs and symptoms derived from DSM-III. The only other set of guidelines were those of Kernberg (1967) for the evaluation of borderline personality organization (BPO). Transcripts of taped admissions interviews were available for some 70 patients during the years 1969–1976. In choosing to rate the chart material myself, I had one major drawback and one major advantage. The drawback was in lack of blindness to the original diagnosis. The advantage lay in knowing nearly all the patients personally; this made it easier for me to sidestep the many verbal snares in the old records, where phrases such as "autistic thinking" or "tangentiality" became buzzwords for "schizophrenia." The patients had not always exhibited these signs. In many cases, the therapist responsible for the initial workup misconstrued some slight eccentricity of speech or verbal past-pointing as evidence of the above-mentioned "schizophrenic" signs, by way of justifying the seemingly inevitable conclusion of a schizophrenia diagnosis. I remembered most of the patients well enough not to be misled by this source of bias. Whether, on balance, I cured more bias than I succumbed to in adopting this method I cannot tell. I am fairly convinced, however, that blind rating of these records would have led to more diagnostic miscalls than someone might make who was able to recollect the patients and to view them anew through the lenses of DSM.

Table 1.1 shows the distribution of major diagnoses. The guidelines used were those of DSM-III except in the case of (1) the "dysthymics" (D), who represented the combination of major affective disorder (MAD; DSM-III) and BPO; and (2) the "other BPO patients"—a heterogeneous group with BPO but

TABLE 1.1.   Diagnostic Classifications after Chart Review

Category	Male	Female	Total
BPD	61	145	206
D borderlines	22	14	36
Other BPO patients	35	22	57
SZ	60	39	99
SA	23	41	64
MDP	24	15	39
SF	27	9	36
Delusional disorder	0	2	2
"Psychoneurotic" anxiety disorders	5	2	7
Undiagnosed; level indeterminate	4	0	4
Total	261	289	550

neither MAD nor borderline personality disorder (BPD; DSM-III). The latter compartment contained chiefly patients with anorexia nervosa/bulimia nervosa, schizotypal personality, antisocial personality, and alcoholism.

The main focus of the study was on the borderline patients and on those with DSM-III-defined schizophrenia (SZ), who comprised three-quarters of the entire series.

DEMOGRAPHIC CHARACTERISTICS

The typical patient of the PI-500 was just over 20 years of age and had completed 1 or 2 years of college, having dropped out of school because of emotional illness. Most came from families in New York State; some made New York their state of residence because of school, but came from families in the Midwest, the South, or foreign countries.

Age

The youngest patient was 13; the oldest, 39. Those under age 18 on admission constituted the adolescent group, numbering 143 over the 14 cohorts. The average admission age for all the patients was 22.

Gender

Numerically, there was near-parity between the sexes (261 males, 289 females). This was not so within the major diagnostic categories (see Table 1.1), where, for example, the female–male ratio was 2.5:1 in the borderline patients and nearly 2:1 among the schizoaffective (SA) patients. The schizophrenic and schizophreniform (SF) patients showed a male excess.

Socioeconomic Status

As interpreted by the guidelines of Hollingshead and Redlich (1958), the patients came predominantly from middle-class or upper-middle-class families. One in six came from an upper-class family; one in eight, from a lower-middle-class family. Only two came from families in Hollingshead and Redlich's category V. Table 1.2 shows the percentages in each category. The average rating was 2.48 on a scale of 1 (category I) to 5 (category V).

Marital Status

At the time of the index hospitalization, the patients were almost all single. Only 8.7% had ever married. As Table 1.2 shows, most of the latter no longer remained with their spouses, having either separated or divorced. Of those ever married, 12 had had at least one child, but only 8 were still actively involved in raising these children.

Religious Background

With respect to religious background, the families of the patients were not representative of the culture as a whole, nor even of New York State or New York City. Half the families were Jewish bilaterally; 40% were either Protestant or Catholic bilaterally. The remaining families were Eastern Orthodox or Buddhist, or, more often, of mixed background. Table 1.2 shows the percentage of patients from families of each religious background; it also provides the details on those from mixed backgrounds.

PRIOR HOSPITALIZATION

Information regarding the length of time spent in other hospitals before the index admission was available for all but 4 of the 550 patients. 140 were first admissions (25.7%); 254 (46.5%) had spent fewer than 3 months at other hospitals. A smaller number had spent 3–6 months (15.6%) or 6–9 months (3.1%) at other hospitals, often in two or three different facilities.

Only 50 patients (9.2%) had spent more than 9 months in hospitals before

TABLE 1.2. Socioeconomic Status, Marital Status, and Religious Background of the 550 Patients

	Socioeconomic status[a]	
	n	%
I	97	17.7
II	169	30.8
III	211	38.4
IV	70	12.7
V	2	0.4
?	1	—

Marital status on index admission				
	n			
	Males	Females	Total	%
Married	8	12	20	3.6
Separated	3	6	9	1.6
Divorced	6	13	19	3.5
Single	244	258	502	91.3

Religious background of families of origin[b]		
	n	%
Protestant	118	21.6
Catholic	99	18.0
Jewish	289	52.7
Greek Orthodox	6	1.1
Buddhist	1	0.2
Unknown	2	0.4
Mixed[c]	35	6.0

[a]The categories are those of Hollingshead and Redlich (1958).

[b]In the cases of adoptees, the religious backgrounds were those of the adoptive parents.

[c]21 with Jewish fathers (mothers: 10 Protestant, 9 Catholic, 1 mixed Protestant–Catholic, 1 Shinto); 2 with Greek Orthodox fathers (mothers: 1 Catholic, 1 Jewish); 6 with Protestant fathers (mothers: 4 Catholic, 2 Jewish); 5 with Catholic fathers and Jewish mothers; 1 with Jewish–Protestant father and Jewish mother; 1 with Russian Orthodox father and Lutheran mother.

coming to our unit. This usually included a hospitalization of a month or two before transfer to PI, plus one or two fairly lengthy stays within the 3 or 4 years that preceded the index admission.

The schizophrenic patients were more likely (16 of 99) to have spent 9 months or more in prior hospitalization than were the BPD patients (16 of 206), $\chi^2 = 5.02$, $p < .05$. The dysthymic and other BPO patients had rarely been in hospitals for as much as 9 months (5.6% and 3.5%, respectively). Differences between the SA, manic–depressive psychosis (MDP), and BPD patients in this regard were not significant.

The likelihood of suicide did appear greater in those with more than 9 months of prior hospitalization: 9 of 46 traced patients (19.6%), as against 8.6% suicides among those with no or briefer previous admissions, $\chi^2 = 5.86$, $p <$ .05. This correlation was more striking, if one compared the two extremes— those with *no* prior hospitalization (7 suicides out of 139 traced patients, or 5.0%) versus those with prior hospitalization of more than 9 months, $\chi^2 =$ 9.23, $p < .01$.

As for the Global Assessment Scale (GAS) scores at follow-up,[1] there were no marked differences within the major diagnostic groups between those with more than 9 months and those with less than 9 months of prior hospitalization. There was a trend, however, toward worse outcome in the BPD patients with lengthy prior hospitalizations: 6 of 14 (43%) had follow-up scores higher than 60, whereas about two-thirds of the BPD patients with no or brief prior admissions were in this good-to-recovered range at follow-up.

TRACING THE PATIENTS

Assembling the demographic data on the 550 patients of the study and rediagnosing their presenting traits and symptoms according to contemporary criteria were the first two steps in the follow-up process. Once these tasks were done, I was ready to trace the former patients. Because many had moved from their original homes, and because many of the parents had retired to different communities, I felt I could not rely upon questionnaires mailed to the old addresses. The telephone offered greater hope of reaching a high proportion of the patients or their families. The old records were rich in biographical material relating to the parents and the collaterals. This facilitated the tracing of at least some relatives who knew of the former patients' current whereabouts. Since I knew all the former therapists personally, as well as almost all the former patients and most of their parents, I was also able to locate some patients through my colleagues, a number of whom arranged to have their former patients call me.

I used a semistructured technic, whether on the phone or during a personal interview. I tailored the sequence of questions in accordance with the comfort of the respondents and the nature of the information they had begun to share with me. Personal interviews (carried out in some three dozen cases) usually

---

[1]The GAS (Endicott, Spitzer, Fleiss, & Cohen, 1967) is an anchored rating scale with endpoints of 0 (suicide) and 100 (perfect functioning in all spheres). Scores of 61 to 70 indicate good, almost asymptomatic functioning; scores above 70 indicate that a patient is recovered and asymptomatic. The GAS is discussed more fully in Chapter Three.

lasted an hour; phone interviews, from half an hour to an hour and a half. The material I sought concerned rehospitalization, subsequent therapy, work history, social network, avocational interests, marriage, and child-rearing. In addition, I gathered data on the life course of the parents and siblings. The time I devoted to tracing and interviewing was approximately 2 years; as noted earlier, I was able to trace 502 of the original 550 patients.

CHAPTER TWO

Borderline Patients: Definitions and Earlier Studies

DEFINITIONS

When the term "borderline" first became popular in psychiatry, it was a catchall for the most difficult and treatment-resistant patients in the psychoanalyst's caseload (Stern, 1938). These severely disturbed but nondelusional patients were "borderline" in the sense of being neither neurotic nor psychotic. Clinicians felt that these patients were on the border of one of the classical psychoses—namely, schizophrenia (Deutsch, 1942; Knight, 1953). The "schizophrenia" on whose border these cases were alleged to have settled was the broadly defined schizophrenia of E. Bleuler (1911). Given this lack of uniformity in the diagnosis, one would not anticipate great similarity in course or long-term outcome. Kernberg's (1967) redefinition provided a more sharply delineated boundary of what was still, by conventional diagnostic standards, a vast territory. Kernberg's definition of "borderline personality organization" (BPO) is useful as a descriptor of the habitual mental functioning of persons whom we might think of as occupying the space between one and two standard deviations below the norm in regard to mental health (the "outliers" being psychotics) (Stone, 1988a). This space contains dysthymics, agoraphobes, sociopaths, alcoholics, bulimics, and so on, alongside persons exemplifying "borderline personality disorder" (BPD) as currently understood. The coverage offered by this definition inevitably entails some loss in specificity. Therefore, this definition is of only limited use as a predictor of the life course, apart from the likelihood that, in general, "neurotics" would have a more favorable course than those with BPO and that "psychotics" would have a worse one.

The more recent definitions of a borderline disorder rely upon diagnostic features that are more amenable to consensual validation. These definitions represent improvements both in specificity and in reliability. Here one pays a price in reduced coverage and in a lessened degree of congruence with the earlier psychoanalytic literature (of which these definitions were intended to be refinements). Some patients diagnosed by the tighter criteria of Gunderson and

9

Singer (1975), for example, have rather different clinical features than some of the "borderline" cases of a generation earlier. The same is true of the equally objectifiable but less tight definition of BPD in DSM-III or its recent revision, DSM-III-R (1987). A certain proportion of the older "borderlines" really were in the penumbra of schizophrenia, as examples of "borderline schizophrenia" (Kety, Rosenthal, Wender, & Schulsinger, 1968) or of what would now be called "schizotypal personality" (STP; DSM-III). Many others showed a mixture of the traits and symptoms of STP and of BPD as currently defined (cf. Spitzer, Endicott, & Gibbon, 1979). The separation into categories is partly for didactic purposes and need not signify the coexistence of two truly separate conditions. The tendency during this decade to differentiate between BPD and STP has brought about a shift in the meaning of "borderline," in favor of cases exemplifying the items included in the Gunderson and Singer (1975) and DSM-III/III-R definitions.

In the sections that follow, I focus primarily on borderline patients meeting the DSM criteria for BPD. In some of the discussions, I describe the follow-up results in the entire borderline (BPO) domain. The patients with "borderline schizophrenia" (STP)—numerically a much smaller group in the PI-500, because they seldom required inpatient care—I discuss in Chapter Five.

Borderline Personality Disorder as a Construct

Despite the comparative tightness of the definition, one must still take into account its polythetic construction. Since only five items out of eight are required for the DSM-III or DSM-III-R diagnosis of BPD, 93 combinations are possible. Some combinations are admittedly rare; certain items are seldom absent (Frances, Clarkin, Gilmore, Hurt, & Brown, 1984). A patient showing impulsivity, self-damaging acts, and inordinate anger is nevertheless quite different from another BPD patient showing *only* the other 5 items. (The Gunderson schema, requiring a "1 +" or a "2 +" on at least four of its five broad subcategories [for a total score of 7 or more], admits of only six combinations and is thus a more cohesive definition than that of the DSM; Kolb & Gunderson, 1980.) In their preliminary analysis of 465 DSM-defined BPD cases, comprised of both ambulatory and hospitalized patients from several centers, Hurt et al. (1988) noted that the items tended to cluster along certain lines: (1) self-damaging acts and impulsivity; (2) anger, labile affect, and stormy relationships; and (3) identity disturbance, emptiness, and intolerance of being alone. Presumably, amenability to therapy and long-term course would not be the same for patients of these various subtypes. There is reason to regard the five items of the first and second subtypes as the most *typical* features of BPD and those that most successfully discriminate it from its conceptual neighbors, such as STP or narcissistic personality disorder (NPD).

The reader should be aware that the concept of BPD has hardly outlived its critics. Toffler and Modestin (1987), for example, who feel that "unstable relationships" is probably the key item in BPD, nevertheless contend that investigators have as yet to validate "borderline" as a diagnostic label. Like many European psychiatrists, these authors believe that the cases we now subsume under this heading fit fairly well in the territory represented by the *International Classification of Diseases,* ninth edition (ICD-9, 1977) personality disorders "hysterical" (301.5) and "sociopathic" (301.7). With respect to the present series, these objections are casuistical. The "borderline" label, if used in a consistent and reliable way, is useful in defining a special domain within the broad field of psychopathology—a domain many of whose features the ICD-9 system does not capture very well. I refer to the combination of impulsivity, hostility, moodiness, and turbulent interpersonal relationships that is central to the concept of BPD (in countries where the term is popular). The ICD-9 definitions do not "see" this combination except with peripheral vision. As I hope to make clear in Chapter Six, many borderlines have strong "hysterical" or "sociopathic" features, and the patients in these subgroups have rather different fates. I believe that patients with, for example, BPD *and* histrionic personality or antisocial personality (ASP) also have different fates, on average, from patients with histrionic personality or ASP who do *not* exhibit the traits of BPD. If I am correct in this, then "borderline" confers additional useful information concerning prognosis, as well as optimal treatment strategy.

Borderline Personality Disorder and Other Conditions

The relationship between BPD and other conditions that either overlap or hover near it conceptually is more easily visualized than described. Figure 2.1 portrays this relationship in connection with posttraumatic stress disorder (PTSD), premenstrual syndrome (PMS), and a dozen other conditions. The areas of conjunction should not be taken as an index of "percentage" of overlap—in most cases, this is not known—but as an illustration of the fact that the condition *does* overlap nosologically with BPD.

Schizophrenia (SZ) and schizoaffective psychosis (SA) do not overlap, for which reason I have drawn their circles at some distance from that of BPD. I have also purposely omitted multiple personality disorder because its proper position is unclear. Some regard this entity as a variant of BPD (where "splitting" is taken to its extreme)—that is, *within* BPD. Others regard it as usually external to the concept of BPD, especially when neither the main nor the alternate personalities, viewed separately, is "borderline."

Each of the conditions in Figure 2.1 is discussed in a relevant chapter or section of the book.

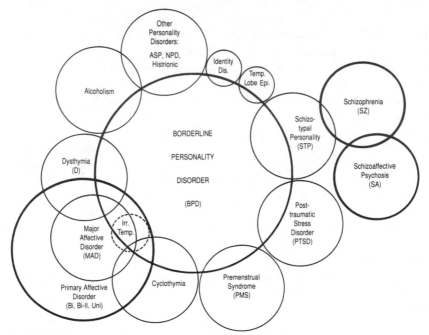

FIGURE 2.1. Borderline personality disorder and its diagnostic near neighbors.

Borderline Personality Disorder and Borderline Personality Organization

With Figure 2.2, I hope to clarify some of the confusion surrounding the distinction between BPD and Kernberg's BPO. Enmeshed in this area of confusion is another, having to do with the kinds of "borderline" case one finds in the writings of the important contributors to the literature on psychotherapy with borderlines. Abend, Bryce, Boyer, Buie and Adler, Chessick, Frosch, Grinker, Grotstein, Gunderson, Kernberg, Knight, Kohut, Little, Masterson, McGlashan, Meissner, Rinsley, Searles, Vanggaard, Volkan, Wallerstein, and Widiger are not all talking about the same kinds of patients. The whole domain of "borderline" in Figure 2.2 is coextensive with that of BPO. Within this broad definition are the smaller regions of BPD (the DSM region would be somewhat larger than that of Gunderson & Singer [1975]), whether "pure" BPD or BPD × major affective disorder (MAD). The latter regions would occupy more territory within the region of *ever-hospitalized* BPO patients (regions 1–4), whereas many *never-hospitalized* BPO patients (regions 5–8) show identity disorder, but little in the way of impulsivity or self-damaging acts. The BPO ×

MAD patients are the dysthymic (D) borderlines. The BPO-only group contains a variety of other types of patients, including substance abusers, sociopaths, some anorectics/bulimics, and so on. Some of the confusion among authors and disagreement about treatment recommendations dissipate when we take into consideration that the patients Kohut (1971), Masterson (1981), and Volkan (1987) are describing are mainly those in regions 5–8 (fewer of whom meet DSM criteria); those of Gunderson and colleagues (see below) and McGlashan (1985) are in regions 1 and 2; and those of Kernberg (1975) and Searles (1986) may be anywhere within the whole domain. The borderline patients of the PI-500, by virtue of their all having been hospitalized at least once, all belong in regions 1–4. Because Dr. Kernberg was director of the unit during the years 1973–1976 and participated in all the diagnostic interviews, the problem of reliability in the diagnosis of BPO does not arise for those cohorts.

PREVIOUS STUDIES

Follow-Up Studies in the Borderline Domain: A Cautionary Note

With respect to their usefulness, follow-up studies of borderline patients are in an ironical situation. The results of brief (2- to 5-year) studies are easier to relate to the original conditions. One can make more convincing statements about the

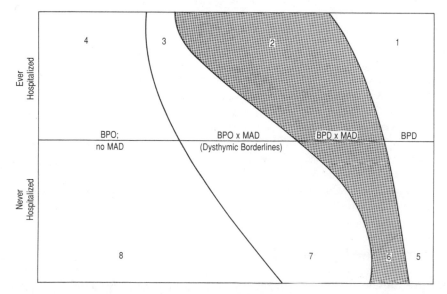

FIGURE 2.2. The borderline domain.

effectiveness of different treatment strategies, if, for example, significant differences emerge in an appropriately controlled study. Long-term studies must grapple with a host of intervening variables, especially non-treatment-related events that occur during the long interval; these make correlation between outcome and initial treatment hazardous, and "causal" statements even more hazardous. Yet the evidence thus far available suggests that improvement often occurs in borderline patients, but does *not* often do so until several years after initial consultation or hospitalization. Brief studies, though easier to handle scientifically (data analysis is more straightforward), tell less of what clinicians want to know about the life course of their borderline patients. Long-term studies give better answers about life course, but are not very illuminating about the connection (if any) between recent status and the therapeutic efforts of 15 or 20 years ago.

The more deeply we probe the matter of life trajectory, the more we will see that prognosis depends heavily upon factors regarded as unimportant at the outset, or upon factors overlooked entirely (e.g., traumatic events during childhood, likeableness of personality, etc.). Patient samples from different centers, carefully matched for age, sex, socioeconomic status, and the like, turn out to be woefully mismatched with respect to a factor not understood to be crucial when the study began. In a retrospective design, some factors known *currently* to be influential will not have been alluded to in the records of 20 or 30 years ago. A prospective design, no matter how thorough, will inevitably omit mention of data pertaining to factors that, 20 years hence, will be widely recognized as vital to the evaluation of prognosis and course.

In the absence of these hypothetically ideal studies where borderline personality is concerned, we must turn to a second-best line of inquiry involving data from outcome studies with varying intervals, based on roughly comparable patient samples. As an example, from five independent studies of similar patients conducted at 2, 5, 10, 15, and 20 years after initial symptoms, we could reconstruct a curve representing the typical life trajectory for the two decades after onset. Given the nonuniformity of outcome for most psychiatric conditions, including BPD, what we would actually establish would be a family of rough curves, reflecting a whole range of patterns, from most common to most unusual.

The section that follows examines these issues from the standpoint of some of the earlier reports (up to 1980), when diagnostic definitions were less comparable, the outcome intervals briefer, and the sample sizes generally smaller than are to be found in the more recent studies.

Earlier Follow-Up Studies

In a previous article (Stone, 1989a), I have reviewed the early follow-up studies of patients in the borderline domain. These studies included one by Hoch,

Cattrell, Strahl, and Pennes (1962) on 109 patients with "pseudoneurotic schizophrenia"; one by Gidro-Frank, Peretz, Spitzer, and Winikus (1967) on 24 hospitalized "pseudoneurotic schizophrenics"; and studies by Grinker, Werble, and Drye (1968), Grinker and Werble (1977), Werble (1970), and Masterson and Costello (1980). They also included two Scandinavian studies: those of Holm and Hundevadt (1976, 1981) and Nyman (1978). Because these early studies either were of small scale, did not rely upon standardized diagnostic instruments, or had low trace rates, they are not easy to bring in line with the more systematic studies of the past decade. Their value is largely anecdotal. Ironically, the study that was on firmest ground methodologically (Nyman's) focused on "borderline schizophrenics," whose overlap with "borderline" patients as the term is currently understood is slight. A special virtue of Nyman's monograph is the appendix in which she provides clinical sketches of all her 110 cases. From these, the reader can translate the data into the language of the DSM. The needs for confidentiality and for brevity of course make Nyman's approach difficult to emulate.

The first follow-up study using reliable diagnostic instruments is that of Gunderson, Carpenter, and Strauss (1975). Twenty-four hospitalized patients, selected according to the criteria for BPD outlined earlier that year by Gunderson and Singer (1975), were matched with 29 inpatients diagnosed as "schizophrenic" according to clinical, Schneiderian, and International Pilot Study of Schizophrenia (Carpenter, Strauss, & Bartko, 1973) criteria. Though the borderlines of this sample were, like Grinker's Type I patients, close to the psychotic border, they differed from schizophrenics symptomatically. Depression was a commonly encountered affective symptom in the borderline group. The two patient groups were closely matched at the outset with respect to prognostic variables (work history, previous hospitalizations, social contacts, and heterosexual relations). At a 2-year follow-up evaluation, their function in four major areas (hospitalization, social contacts, employment, and symptoms) was remarkably similar, both achieving near-identical scores (all in the range of moderate impairment) on the four subscales. In contrast to the schizophrenics, all but four of whom were still diagnosed as schizophrenic at follow-up, diagnostic changes seemed in order for 60% of the borderlines. The authors expressed puzzlement over the indistinguishable outcomes, despite the quite different arrays of initial symptoms.

In a later communication, these authors reported on the 5-year follow-up of this cohort (Carpenter, Gunderson, & Strauss, 1977), relying on data obtained from 14 of the 24 borderlines and from 20 of the 29 schizophrenics. At this stage some differences could be discerned. The borderlines were now showing better quality in the level of their social contacts. In the area of employment, the borderlines were showing a trend toward fuller and more steady work records than those achieved by the schizophrenics. A neurotic–depressive group also served as a comparison group. Gunderson (1977) reported that the borderlines showed more self-mutilative and suicidal behavior

TABLE 2.1.   Follow-Up Studies of Borderline Personality Disorder since 1980

Author (year)	Diagnostic method[a]	n[b]	Cohort years	Follow-up intervals	Patient source
		Short-term			
Akiskal (1981)	BPD-G BPD-D	100	1978–1980	0.5–3 years	Clinic
Wallerstein (1986)	Clinical	18	1954–1958	2–3 years or longer	Hospital (15); private practice (27)[c]
		Long-term			
Pope, Jonas, & Hudson (1983)	BPD-D (13) BPD × MAD (14)	27	1974–1977	4–7 years	Hospital
McGlashan (1985)	BPD-D BPD-G	81	1950–1975	2–32 years (average = 15)	Hospital (3 months or more)
Plakun, Burkhardt, & Muller (1985)	BPD-D (54) BPD × MAD (9)	63	1950–1976	13.6 years, average (± 6.6 SD)	Hospital (2 months or more)
Kroll, Carey, & Sines (1985)	BPD-G	13	1960–1968	20 years, average	Hospital (females)
Paris, Brown, & Nowlis (1987)	BPD-G	100	1958–1978	8–28 years (average = 15 years)	Hospital

[a]BPD-G, borderline by Gunderson criteria; BPD-D, borderline by DSM-III criteria; BPD × MAD, with concomitant MAD.

[b]Refers only to the number of *traced* borderline patients in the study.

[c]Of these 42 patients, 18 were probably cases of BPD.

than the neurotic–depressive groups, along with more drug abuse, more paranoid ideation, and more instability in interpersonal relations. There was a trend toward greater hostility in the borderlines; the neurotic–depressive patients had better initial work records. In other words, though discriminable from either group at the outset, the borderlines showed more commonality of features with (a more impaired subgroup of) neurotic–depressive patients than with schizophrenic patients.

Recent Follow-Up Studies

Studies pertaining to the follow-up and course of borderline conditions published since 1980 are almost all based on operational diagnostic criteria (those for BPD as set forth by Gunderson & Strauss [1975] and the DSM), and the majority cover intervals greater than 5 years. These reports are outlined in Table 2.1.

Short-Term Studies

Akiskal (1981) and his colleagues at the Mood Clinic of the University of Tennessee College of Medicine carried out a short-term follow-up of 100 patients who met the Gunderson and Strauss (1975) criteria for BPD. Having been conducted with a clinic population, their study complements the others cited in Table 2.1, which, apart from a few of the private-practice patients in Wallerstein's (1986) study, represent only hospital-based samples. This series contained a large group of patients with concomitant affective disorder (recurrent depression, 6; dysthymic, 14; cyclothymic, 7; and bipolar II "atypical," 17). There were smaller proportions with severe "neuroses" (phobias, 10; obsessive–compulsive disorder, 8); sociopathy/somatization disorder (21); STP (9); organic disorders (grand mal epilepsy, temporal lobe epilepsy, attention deficit disorder—1 each); and a residual group of patients with chronic identity disorder (4). Substance (including alcohol) abuse was common (57 instances). Regarding affective disorders, 37 had already experienced 52 episodes in one form or another, 2 or 3 years later. Four had already committed suicide. Only one patient evolved in an unmistakably schizophrenic direction; those with any traits suggestive of even the "borderline" (attenuated) forms of schizophrenia (viz., STP) were very much in the minority. Akiskal understands the high frequency of movement toward affective disorders as a consequence of the high concentration of affective traits already apparent in his borderline population—a coincidence that is not surprising in view of the DSM-III definition of BPD, which contains many affectively colored items (Akiskal, 1981, p. 37). Even a trait such as identity disturbance, which is central to the psychoanalytic definitions of "borderline" but not customarily associated with affective illness, can arise as a function of wide mood swings that bring about an unstable and ever-shifting self (Akiskal, 1981, p. 44).

The richly detailed monograph of Wallerstein (1986) on the results of the Menninger Foundation study of psychotherapy and psychoanalysis describes 42 patients treated by the Menninger Clinic staff beginning in the mid-1950s. The focus of the study was on the effects of analytically oriented and of supportive therapies, as well as of psychoanalysis, on a group of patients with fairly severe emotional disorders. Though the participants also aimed at following up their patients (at least at a 2- to 3-year posttreatment interval, if not beyond), theirs was not an outcome or natural-history study in the usual sense. They did not limit their observations to distinct diagnostic subgroups or utilize operational diagnostic criteria. In my reconstruction of the cases, 24 of the patients were "neurotic" and 18 were "borderline" by the clinical measure of the time. The borderlines were more likely to have been hospitalized (12 of 18) than the neurotic patients (3 of 24). Wallerstein used a 4-point scale for outcome. Collapse of the scale to "good" versus "bad" for statistical purposes yields a 2 × 2 table: outcomes in the neurotic patients, 19 "good" versus 5 "bad" (including 1 suicide); in the borderlines, 6 "good" versus 12 "bad" (including

5 suicides). Anecdotal material was available on many of the patients 10–20 or more years later, although the design called for only short-term follow-up. The results are not easy to compare with studies using standardized outcome measures (see below). The relatively poor outcomes in the borderlines may be partly a reflection of the brief follow-up intervals in some cases and of the high proportion of alcoholics in the series as a whole (19 of 42). In other respects, the demographic characteristics resemble those of McGlashan's Chestnut Lodge series (see below). The high suicide rate in the borderlines (5 of 18, or 28%) is not unlike that of the BPD alcoholics in the PI-500 (see Chapters Four and Nine); 4 of the 5 Menninger borderline suicides abused substances (alcohol in 3 cases).

Long-Term Studies

Pope, Jonas, and Hudson (1983) reported on the 4- to 7-year follow-up of 33 young adult patients at the McLean Hospital who fulfilled DSM criteria for BPD, as well as the less stringent Gunderson criteria for BPD (cutoff score of 6 instead of 7 on the Diagnostic Interview for Borderline Patients). The sample was preponderantly female (27 females, 6 males). Seventeen had concomitant MAD. The authors were able to trace 27 (82%) of their sample. None had gone on to develop DSM-defined SZ. The BPD × MAD patients showed a greater tendency to exhibit affective symptoms (i.e., persistence of MAD) at follow-up (10 of 14, or 71%) than did the "pure"-BPD patients (3 of 13, or 23%). Yet the symptoms of 3 of the BPD × MAD patients had remitted entirely. Interestingly, these patients outperformed the pure-BPD group, as well as a schizophrenic comparison group, on the outcome scales pertaining to social function and residual symptoms. Nearly half the BPD × MAD patients no longer fulfilled BPD diagnostic criteria at follow-up, though most of them, along with the pure-BPD group, did show signs of other personality disorders (chiefly, histrionic personality, NPD, and ASP). A bipolar–manic comparison group did significantly better even than the BPD × MAD patients, demonstrating, as the authors mention, "the serious morbidity of the B.P.D. diagnosis with or without concurrent M.A.D." (Pope et al., 1983, p. 29). The patients comorbid for MAD seemed to respond more favorably to antidepressants or lithium than did the pure-BPD patients, raising the question whether this drug responsivity contributed to the more favorable course. Two patients (one with MAD)—that is, 6% of the traced sample—had committed suicide during the follow-up interval.

McGlashan (1985) has reported extensively on his long-term, large-scale follow-up study of hospitalized patients. The BPD patients—rediagnosed by both the Gunderson and the DSM criteria—had been treated from 2 to 32 years earlier, in an average hospital stay of 2 years, at Chestnut Lodge in Maryland. Having traced 86% of the pure-BPD group (81 of 94), McGlashan gathered information concerning 38 outcome dimensions. Chief comparison groups were the 44 traced unipolar depressives and the 163 traced schizophrenics. The typical BPD patient was female, had become symptomatic at age 20, had been hospitalized elsewhere at 25, and had been transferred to Chestnut Lodge at 27. A fair proportion eventually signed out against advice; only a few were sent directly to other facilities. In contrast to the schizophrenics, the BPD patients were rehospitalized *after* Chestnut Lodge less frequently (one or two times) and more briefly. Of the 81 BPD patients who were traced, 70 were still alive at follow-up. Two of the 11 who died were suicides.

Intensive (three to four sessions/week) psychotherapy had been the mainstay of treatment for these borderline patients; only a fourth had received psychotropic medications. At follow-up, half were still in some form of therapy. Two-thirds were working full-time—a record similar to that of the unipolars, and much better than that of the schizophrenics. The BPD patients had either married or found a steady sexual partner, or else lived alone in "studious avoidance of relationships" (McGlashan, 1985, p. 29). Whereas the schizophrenic and unipolar patients' functioning at follow-up was about the same as at discharge from Chestnut Lodge years earlier, the BPD patients followed a more complex course. If they became symptomatic again, the symptoms were usually those reminiscent of BPD in general: substance abuse or other manifestations of impulsivity. Suicidal thoughts were still common; one in five had continued on occasion to make suicidal gestures. The average Health–Sickness Rating Scale (HSRS; Luborsky, 1963) score at follow-up was 64 (the maximum score being 100) for the BPD group, as against 37 for the SZ group (but 60 for the unipolars).

Looking at average outcome scores at ex-patients in different age brackets, McGlashan was able to reconstruct a typical BPD life trajectory. This consisted of continuing poor adaptation through the 20s and into the early 30s, followed by good functioning during the 40s. Some patients, especially after the dissolution (through death, divorce, rejection) of a close relationship, suffered another downturn during their late 40s or early 50s. McGlashan noted that the patients who most closely resembled Pope et al.'s (1983) "BPD × MAD" group—namely, the "BPD × unipolar" patients—usually exhibited lower scores on the key outcome variables than did Pope et al.'s group (whose BPD × MAD patients outperformed the pure BPDs).

Elsewhere, McGlashan (1987) noted that the rate of completed suicide was highest in the comorbid BPD × unipolar group (16%), intermediate in the pure unipolars (8%), and lowest in the BPD-only group (2%). Though all three types of patients had been about equally given to suicidal gestures and the like at index admission, they pursued divergent courses over time with respect to suicide risk. As McGlashan observed, "It appears that mixing affective dysregulation with action-oriented personality style constitutes a particularly lethal combination" (1987, p. 471). Alcohol abuse was quite common in the comorbid patients. Since long-term follow-up demonstrated "changes" in both directions in a proportion of patients (BPD to unipolar, but also unipolar to BPD), McGlashan cautions that "we are dealing with highly fluid and heterogenous entities among which we must also include the more 'classical' affective disorders" (1987, p. 473). The life course of patients with BPD appears to depend upon the varying degrees of "admixture" of affective and impulsive tendencies, of autoplastic and alloplastic defenses, inchoate or already manifest in any given patient. This is as yet a difficult determination, especially since BPD is often a diagnosis of young persons; we as clinicians perceive such patients' condition during their late teens or early 20s only in a not yet fully developed form.

McGlashan (1986c) also studied the long-term outcome in the Chestnut Lodge patients with STP. Global outcome measures could be aligned within a "spectrum." At one end were either patients with DSM-defined SZ only or patients with SZ who also manifested the STP profile; both usually functioned only marginally (HSRS values in the mid-30s). Patients with STP alone or those with SZ × STP × BPD were less impaired (HSRS values in the mid-40s). At the opposite end, patients with STP × BPD did as well (average HSRS = 68) or slightly better than the pure-BPD group (average HSRS = 64). The STP patients were generally loners, less flamboyant and self-destructive (and less often hospitalized) than the BPD patients. The latter, however, were "object-seeking" (1986, p. 333) and more successful at establishing love relationships as well as friendships, whereas the STP patients tended to have friends but not lovers. As in most American (by contrast with Scandinavian) studies, STP was uncommon in the Chestnut Lodge hospital setting, and the n's were comparatively small (for the STP group, $n = 10$; for STP × BPD, $n = 18$). Whereas the pure-STP patients seemed symptomatically as well as genetically closer to SZ, the STP × BPD group appeared closer to the affective pole symptomatically and often had both MAD and a family history of affective illness.

Plakun, Burkhardt, and Muller (1985) followed up 878 patients hospitalized for at least 2 months at Austin Riggs Center between 1950 and 1976. The authors used a mailed-questionnaire/informed-consent method and elicited 237 (27%) positive responses. Of the remainder, 94 had died; others refused or else could not be contacted. Retrospective DSM-III diagnoses were made by two raters blind to the chart diagnoses. The main diagnostic groups within the traced patients consisted of SZ ($n = 19$), MAD ($n = 24$), STP ($n = 13$), BPD ($n = 63$), and schizoid personality ($n = 19$). Among the borderlines, there were 9 with concomitant MAD, 43 with BPD alone, 6 with BPD × STP, and five with BPD × schizoid personality. The mean Global Assessment Scale (GAS) levels in the Plakun et al. study are all actually quite similar, ranging from that for the SZ group (59.3) to that for the small BPD × STP group (72). Their results differed from those of Pope et al. (1983) in that their BPD × MAD group did worse than their pure BPDs (mean GAS = 67) and did not differ significantly in outcome from the SZs. The authors did not claim to assess treatment effects, but felt that "there is no reason to assume that treatment has no effect and that we are dealing with the natural history of B.P.D." (Plakun et al., 1985, p. 453).

In 1985, Kroll, Carey, and Sines reported on their follow-up study of 15 patients, hospitalized up to 20 years earlier and meeting Gunderson's criteria for BPD as determined by scores on the Diagnostic Interview for Borderline Patients. They were able to trace all but two of these patients. Two had committed suicide (within 3 years of discharge); two others had died of natural causes. Of the remaining nine, three were now well and working at responsible jobs, four were functioning marginally, and two were unemployed, receiving public assistance. Of the latter, one showed a schizoaffective evolution. This Minneapolis-based study, though small in scale, is comparable in its distribution of outcomes to the other studies mentioned here that were based on larger samples.

The most recent of the large-*n*, long-term studies is that of Paris, Brown, and Nowlis (1987), who traced and interviewed 100 of 322 patients diagnosed as borderline by the Gunderson criteria (256 females, 66 males) and admitted to Jewish General Hospital, Montreal, between 1958 and 1978. HSRS scores averaged 63.2 (*SD* = 11), indicating good general functioning with some mild symptoms and some meaningful interpersonal relationships. The suicide rate thus far was 8.5%. Many of the patients in the Montreal study came from lower-middle-class homes; half had never completed high school. The study thus complements McGlashan's series and the PI-500, suggesting, given the similarity of results, a wider applicability across the whole socioeconomic spectrum to the findings reported in the other studies. This homogeneity of outcome in the different studies lends support to Paris et al.'s claim that the interviewed patients were representative of the sample as a whole. Although it would be hard to substantiate this claim with respect to certain variables (were there more sociopathic males in the untraced than in the traced groups, for example?), it is nevertheless true that patients of lower socioeconomic status are difficult to trace even after a few years (they may lack phones or live as lodgers, using a phone listed under a landlord's name). For this reason, Paris et al.'s trace rate is very respectable, and their findings are of considerable value.

TABLE 3.2.   Homogeneity of Follow-Up GAS Scores in Various Diagnostic Groups

| Diagnostic group | % in GAS range | | |
	Lowest	Median ± 15	Highest
SZ	14	66	20
SA	31	34	35
MDP	24	47	29
SF	28	56	16
BPD males	26	48	26
BPD females	21	70	9
D	15	76	9

Note. "Lowest" signifies the group with follow-up GAS scores less than the (median − 15). "Highest" signifies the group with follow-up GAS scores greater than the (median + 15).

"homogeneity." Patients with scores outside this band, we may consider as "outliers" with respect to the central tendency for their subgroup.

Table 3.2 shows the degree of homogeneity of GAS scores in the major diagnostic groups, with the exception of the "other BPO" patients. The latter group, composed of patients with eating disorders, antisocial personality (ASP), alcoholism, schizotypal personality, and other personality disorders, is too heterogeneous etiologically to permit generalizations about outcome comparable to those for the other seven groups. The most homogeneous groups with respect to global function are the D patients, the BPD females, and the SZ patients: Two-thirds of the patients in each group had follow-up GAS scores within a range of ± 15 of the median. The SA patients showed the most diversity, followed by the MDP group and the BPD males. Angst, Felder, and Lohmeyer (1980) have noted a similar flattening of the outcome curves in SA and MDP patients; that is, their outcomes were distributed more evenly in the successive ranges of possible functioning. The SA patients with one or more manic episodes before the index hospitalization were too few in number to permit assessment of whether their long-term course was better than that of SA patients with only depressive episodes.[1]

REINSTITUTIONALIZATION

For most patients who required some form of institutional care at any point following their release from the index hospitalization at PI, this care came in the form of another hospital stay. A few spent time only in a sheltered residential center with some psychiatric supervision, short of a full-service hospital. A small

[1]Angst, to whom a larger series of SA patients was available for follow-up, has suggested to me (Angst, 1988) that those with manic episodes tended to fare better.

TABLE 3.3. Rehospitalization and Reinstitutionalization

Diagnostic category	Never rehospitalized	Rehospitalized			Jailed > 3 months	Other sheltered facilities	Total reinstitutionalized	% ever reinstitutionalized	Difference from SZ by χ^2
		Once	Twice	Three or more times					
All borderlines	202	30	11	17	3	0	61	23.2	$p < .0001$
BPD	131	23	11	15	3	0	52	28.4	$p < .0001$
D	27	4	0	1	0	0	5	15.6	$p < .0001$
Other BPO	44	3	0	1	0	0	4	8.3	$p < .0001$
SZ	19	17	6	36	1	4	64	77.1	—
SA	14	18	3	15	0	1	37	72.5	N.S.
MDP	14	8	3	10	0	0	21	60.0	$.05 < p < .10$
SF	18	6	4	3	0	0	13	41.9	$p < .01$

number of the patients, though not rehospitalized, spent long periods of time in prison.

Table 3.3 shows the numbers of patients from the major diagnostic categories who returned to a hospital once, twice, or three or more times, or who spent time either in a residential facility or in prison. Roughly one in four of all borderlines required reinstitutionalization, whereas about three out of four schizophrenic or schizoaffective patients required such care at some point during the follow-up period. Of the schizophrenic patients, 24% spent the entire time since leaving PI in either chronic care hospitals, sheltered facilities, or (in two cases) prison. None of the borderlines spent the entire postdischarge time in hospital, though a small number required multiple rehospitalizations. One borderline man had been in prison for 15 years at the time of follow-up. The tendency in schizophrenia is toward *multiple* rehospitalizations; in the other groups, toward no more than one rehospitalization.

OUTCOME ON IMPORTANT LIFE VARIABLES

The remainder of this chapter focuses on long-term outcome for the PI-500 patients in two significant aspects of life: (1) work, and (2) marriage and fertility.

Work

As an outcome variable, work has the advantage of being more easily measurable than satisfaction with life, quality of friendships, success of intimate relationships, or the like. Work is also a key variable, insofar as it divides groups of people into those capable of autonomy and those who require varying degrees of public or family assistance. Independently wealthy persons, for whom the correlation between not working and not having a good outcome is irrelevant, are exceptions. In the PI-500, independent wealth was not an important factor: Only five patients (one borderline, one manic–depressive, one schizophreniform, and two schizophrenic) had trust funds ample enough to take care of all their needs.

Work status affects patients in another way, not directly related to survival and autonomy, insofar as society reacts differently to working-age people who work than it does to those who do not. The assumption people tend to make about unfamiliar persons (from the middle and upper classes, especially) who are not working or managing a household is that they are "ill"—if not physically, then emotionally. As our former patients tried to re-establish themselves after leaving the hospital, those who were unable to work or could work only at levels beneath their "capacity" (as judged by acquaintances before they were ill) often suffered a certain stigmatization, over and above the more obvious effects of their disability. Entrée into certain social circles, including those in which they had once been welcome, was also difficult for many of the unemployed and underemployed former patients. The patients who could work blended in with these around them and were accepted, even if their private lives were meager or in disarray. As one of the former patients put it, "Work is the best cure."

In evaluating the work history of the PI-500 patients, I used the scales McGlashan (1984a) developed for the Chestnut Lodge follow-up. McGlashan rated, on 5-point scales, (1) percentage of time worked since discharge; (2) percentage of time worked during the past year; (3) level of complexity; (4) competence; and (5) satisfaction with the work. With regard to the PI-500, I placed more reliance on data concerning the first three of those variables. Information about competence and satisfaction was harder to obtain. I was not always able to speak with both the former patients *and* their parents; even when I could, their impressions did not always agree.

Percentage of Time Worked

The borderline and the schizophrenic patients provide the greatest contrast in their postdischarge work histories. At the time of follow-up, most of the borderline patients had gone back to complete schooling, managed a household, held a job, or pursued a career more than half the time since leaving the hospital. Only a handful of schizophrenic patients had succeeded in any of these work-related areas to that degree. Among the borderlines as a whole, the never-worked group contains most of the 19 borderline suicides plus the small minority of still-alive borderlines who had never worked (29 of 251, or 11.6%). Of the 56 schizophrenics who had never worked (31 males and 25 females), 7 were suicides. Suicides accounted for 37% (17 of 46) of the never-worked borderlines, but only 12% (7 of 56) of the never-worked schizophrenics.

For purposes of simplicity, we may telescope McGlashan's (1984a) five time levels (0 = never worked; 1 = worked about 25% of the time since discharge; 2 = worked about 50% of the time since discharge; 3 = worked about 75% of the time since discharge; 4 = worked all the time since discharge) into three: never or rarely (0–25%); approximately 50%; and 75–100%. Table 3.4 shows the percentages of patients within each of the major diagnostic groups, by gender, whose work histories at follow-up corresponded to these three categories. The few patients supported by trust funds are not included in these figures.

All the borderline groups had been able to work more than half the time, except for the BPD males without concomitant major affective disorder (MAD). This group contains a larger proportion of patients with ASP comorbidity than do the other BPD groups. The patients functioning at the borderline level but *not* showing the BPD characteristics (i.e., the nonpsychotic personality-disordered and eating-disordered patients) had worked about three-quarters of the time.

TABLE 3.4. Percentage of Time Worked since Leaving Hospital

Diagnostic group	% of group working at each time level		
	0–25%	Approx. 50%	75–100%
Borderlines			
BPD males	50	17	33
BPD females	27	14	59
BPD × MAD males	33	11	54
BPD × MAD females	26	18	56
D males	5	25	70
D females	8	8	84
Other BPO males	8	15	77
Other BPO females	5	24	71
Psychotics			
SZ males	73	11	16
SZ females	91	3	6
SA males	62	5	33
SA females	60	18	22
MDP males	31	13	56
MDP females	40	20	40
SF males	32	18	50
SF females	43	29	28

As Table 3.4 indicates, the most handicapped groups were the schizophrenics of both sexes and the schizoaffective females.

Almost all the borderline patients who had ever worked were doing so at follow-up. The exceptions were a few patients who had sustained serious injuries, and several patients with MAD who had relapsed during the year prior to follow-up. The schizophrenic patients who had ever worked often did so sporadically, in between periods of rehospitalization.

Level of Complexity

In McGlashan's scale of work complexity, level 1 corresponds to the simplest tasks; level 5, to the most complex and demanding. Complexity provides a better index of achievement than income, since many types of work earn similar wages but differ widely in complexity, necessary training, and the like. In aligning the patients' work with the various levels, I took into consideration the nature of the work as they or their relatives described it to me, rather than the mere label. Thus a laboratory technician just starting out after graduating from college, and carrying out relatively simple tasks, would represent level 3; a senior

TABLE 3.5.　Levels of Work Complexity

| Diagnostic group | n | % of group working at each complexity level | | | | | Averge level per group |
		1	2	3	4	5	
Borderlines							
BPD males	16	6	25	19	19	31	3.4
BPD females	29	0	10	48	31	11	3.4
BPD × MAD males	22	5	9	18	27	41	3.8
BPD × MAD females	83	5	10	37	26	22	3.5
D males	20	0	15	35	25	25	3.6
D females	13	0	0	38	54	8	3.7
Other BPO males	24	0	17	42	29	12	3.4
Other BPO females	20	0	10	20	55	15	3.7
Psychotics							
SZ males	26	23	35	15	23	4	2.5
SZ females	12	25	25	42	8	0	2.3
SA males	14	21	7	29	29	14	3.1
SA females	22	5	27	32	27	9	3.1
MDP males	20	5	10	30	40	15	3.5
MDP females	12	0	8	58	8	26	3.5
SF males	19	16	11	11	37	25	3.4
SF females	7	0	29	29	42	0	3.1

technician/supervisor in charge of a chemistry lab might represent level 4 or 5. An impaired physician (of which there were several in the study) might be functioning currently at level 2 instead of 5. The five levels correspond roughly to the descriptors "unskilled" (1), "semiskilled" (2), "requiring high school diploma plus some training" (3), "requiring a master's degree and/or considerable training" (4), and "requiring doctoral-level education" (5). But this would not give an altogether accurate picture, since some level 5 achievers were entrepreneurs with perhaps a bachelor's degree but were running large corporations; others were concert artists with a musical training that does not translate easily into the usual yardsticks of educational level.

Table 3.5 shows the percentages of patients within each of the major diagnostic groups, by gender, who had worked at the various levels of complexity. Since patients who had never worked are not included, the total n is only 359. The average or "typical" levels for each group, apart from the schizophrenics, are quite consistent (3.45 ± 0.35). The schizophrenic patients who had ever worked did so, on average, at a lower level of complexity (2.4 ± 0.1).

The complexity levels of the nonschizophrenic patients, particularly of the borderline patients, mirror those of their original families. The socioeconomic status of the families was predominantly middle- to upper-middle-class; the fathers and mothers of these patients also worked for the most part at complexity levels 3 or 4. The borderline patients who remained impaired were "under-achievers" with respect to their parents' occupational levels, but these cases were counterbalanced by other borderlines who achieved distinctly higher levels of work complexity than anyone else in their families.

Short-term (3- to 5-year) follow-up of our borderline patients would seldom have reflected the heights of work complexity they would eventually attain. Few were on the "fast track." One who *was* on the fast track made a spectacular financial success while still in his 20s, within a few years of leaving the unit. He is one of a dozen former borderlines whose successful stories can scarcely be hinted at, lest their identities be revealed. Other financial successes included a manufacturer, the chairman of a large corporation, three high-level corporate executives, the head of an accounting firm, a computer expert, and the director of a philanthropic organization. One of the schizophreniform patients, who had been uninterruptedly well for 23 years at the time of follow-up, made a considerable success in the media and publishing. Many of the patients at follow-up were accomplishing in their 30s what their high school classmates were able to complete in their 20s, making up (usually at a gradual pace) for the lost time of their illness and school interruption. Not surprisingly, the mental health professions attracted the interest of quite a few former patients: 10 former borderlines became PhD-level psychologists. Several others became social workers, alcohol rehabilitation counselors, counselors for disturbed adolescents, or nurses in mental health facilities. Among the other borderlines at complexity levels 4 and 5 at follow-up were 6 lawyers; 5 physicians; 3 members of the clergy; 10 teachers; and 4 each of editors, accountants, and musicians. Twenty others were now managing stores, restaurants, or laboratories, or were middle-level executives in large corporations.

Hidden behind the aggregate values for the more easily measurable variables are the subtleties of the patients' satisfaction with life, their sense of fulfillment, and so on. The men and women in the various diagnostic categories worked at similar levels of complexity. The female patients, however, had open to them an option not available to the males—namely, that of managing a household and raising a family. Some of the women pursued this traditional (and no less demanding) role. Others chose careers. Several excelled at both, such as the former borderline woman who worked for several years as a highly successful model and then married a man in comfortable circumstances. Some of the women would have preferred to marry and raise a family; having failed to find suitable partners, they pursued a career *faute de mieux*. But many of the borderline women did not wish to have children by preference and pursued fulfilling careers (e.g., law, office management, editing, psychology) that also served well to bolster self-esteem.

Among patients who showed antisocial tendencies during adolescence, the females did better at follow-up than the males. The female borderlines, for example, whose antisocial behavior seldom went beyond shoplifting or truancy, had settled into conventional lives as they entered their 30s. This was also true of about half the antisocial male borderlines; however, the remainder, especially those with pronounced tendencies to violence, were still distinctly antisocial— usually unemployed or involved in shady activities and otherwise unrecovered— when traced 10 to 20 years later.

Some of the schizophrenic patients with fairly consistent work records (75–100% of the time since discharge) were also working at levels in keeping with the expectations they and their parents originally entertained as they were growing up. One became a lawyer; another, an accountant; the two most successful, a store manager and a contractor. The majority, however, had uneven work records, and their jobs represented a "downward drift" from their supposed ceiling of potential before they became ill. Thus, one schizophrenic man graduated *summa cum laude* from college and was a chauffeur at the time of follow-up; another equally bright man found contentment when he shifted from emotionally taxing to less pressured jobs, and at follow-up was handling the filing at a law firm. Another became a housepainter. Several worked as post office clerks. A few of the schizophrenic women gravitated toward artistic careers, especially those permitting most of the work to be done at home, with little need to interact with the public. Two became artists; another a (published) poet.

The schizoaffective group had the flattest curve of outcome distribution; the nonuniformity showed up in their work histories as well. Some maintained good positions over long periods of time in the face of residual symptoms. One man, married and with two children at follow-up, had worked for years in the computer industry, despite lingering irritability and suspiciousness. The schizoaffective man with the highest recent GAS score (81) had been self-supporting and asymptomatic ever since leaving the hospital: He worked in the civil service, had completed college, had recently become engaged, had a large circle of friends, and no longer saw a therapist or required medication. Among the recovered or minimally symptomatic female schizoaffectives were a novelist, a nurse, an actress, a lawyer, and a tutor. One of the most remarkable patients was a once desperately ill, impulsive schizoaffective woman who, over the 10 years prior to follow-up, became self-supporting as a secretary. At follow-up, in her early 40s, she had recently settled into a satisfying long-term relationship and had mended fences with her family.

The manic–depressive patients—those who already showed a recognizable clinical picture on entering the hospital—had work histories similar to that of the borderline (BPD) patients with concomitant MAD. The manic–depressive males included a free-lance writer, a teacher, a journalist, a psychologist, a computer programmer/analyst, and an administrative assistant of an opera company. The females, a numerically small group, included a teacher of handicapped children, the vice-president of a marketing firm, the director of a radio station, a real estate agent, and a salesperson in a large jewelry concern. Another, originally carried along under the diagnosis of "schizophrenia" and rehospitalized several times until lithium became available, had been stable for 10 years at follow-up; she was working as a court stenographer.

With few exceptions, the schizophreniform patients were male adolescents who suffered acute schizophrenia-like episodes following abuse of psychotomimetic drugs. At the time of their admission to the unit, we were rarely able to distinguish their reactions from "idiopathic schizophrenia." Time, we assumed, would aid us in making the distinction. Even at follow-up, results were hard to interpret. I cannot be altogether sure that I have escaped circularity in designating certain patients as "schizophreniform" on the basis of their drug history, even though rediagnosis for the study antedated the tracing of the patients. A few "schizophrenics," for example, had similar drug histories but had been psychotic a year or so before they aggravated their conditions with hallucinogens. Taking the two groups together, I estimate a zone of confusion affecting 5–10% of the patients, consisting of some "schizophrenics" whom other investigators might call "schizophreniform" and vice versa. One of the patients I continue to list with the schizophreniforms, for example, was almost uninterruptedly ill for 22 years after hospitalization with a paranoid form of schizophrenia, though he had not abused drugs for many years. This man worked sporadically and briefly, though (as a systems analyst) at the highest level of complexity.

In general, the schizophreniform patients did well. Most have ceased to use illicit drugs. Many showed no signs of illness at follow-up, and thus resemble, in their life course, the recovered borderlines. One man became an engineer; another, an accountant; a third, a moderately successful real estate broker. One of the patients with a GAS score in the 90s was a physician; another, with one of the highest outcome GAS scores in the PI-500 (96), was a successful author and media executive. A patient who developed neuroleptic malignant syndrome (see Appendix A) in response to the chlorpromazine he received on our unit looked like a "back-ward case" even when the neuroleptic was discontinued. This syndrome had yet to be identified as a clinical entity in those years. His life trajectory has shown a totally unexpected upturn: At follow-up, he was married with children and working as an executive in advertising. In fact, he was now outperforming even the other members of his highly successful family.

One of the schizophreniform female patients has become a testimonial to the human spirit. Comatose for weeks following a near-fatal injury shortly after she left the unit, she slowly recovered (with some residual disability), completed college, and took advanced work; at the time of follow-up, she was married, working part-time, and deriving great pleasure from caring for her two children. Religion played an important part in her recovery. For a time she fell under the influence of an unscrupulous cult leader who absconded with his followers' funds (see Appendix B); later, she found solace in a more conventional denomination. Maintaining a sunny disposition in the face of every adversity, this woman is also a testimonial to the positive impact of likeableness—the key factor in her much-better-than-expected outcome. Also important in her recovery was the fact that both her parents had been warmly supportive throughout her life. In designing studies of the efficacy of therapy, we tend to rely on "matched patients." Future studies should also control for the quality of parenting, lest we attribute certain successes to "good therapy" where more might be owed to good parents.

Marriage and Fertility

As several of the former patients mentioned at the time of follow-up, marriage and fertility cannot be considered reliable indices of mental health or happiness. Still, the accuracy with which these variables can be measured make them attractive, as a first step in the evaluation of interpersonal relations—of the *Liebe* of Freud's famous *Liebe und Arbeit*. With some of the former patients, love, marriage, and children were intermingled in a harmonious way. With others, marriage or fertility occurred in ways quite dissociated from love.

Most of the patients (and many of the readers of this book) belong to a generation in which marriage and child-rearing have become much less central to the lives of women—especially highly educated, urban women—than was so even a generation earlier. Marriage is no longer the near-exclusive context within which emotional health can be found. The percentage of the PI-500 who have created "nuclear families," though of interest, is no longer a strong correlate of their interpersonal success.

As we examine the marriage statistics, we should be mindful of the importance of other living arrangements: unmarried couples living as *de facto* husband and wife, short-term relationships, homosexual partnerships, and so on.

Marriage

The average age of the PI-500 at the time of writing is 38½. The likelihood of ever having been married for people of their generation is, in our country, approximately 94% for women and 89% for men. These figures would have to be modified in accordance with other factors, such as locale, level of education, religious/ethnic subgroup, and so forth. Nevertheless, these percentages provide a range permitting one to detect wide deviations from the expected. The marriage rates at follow-up in all diagnostic subgroups of the PI-500 were markedly lower than the population averages. The only group where this rate exceeded 50% was that of the D females: 9 of 13 (69%) had been married at some point. Table 3.6 shows the percentages in this and in the remaining diagnostic subgroups. Not particularized in the table are any distinctions relative

TABLE 3.6. Number and Percentage of Patients Ever Married among the Major Diagnostic Groups

Diagnostic group	*n* ever married/*n* traced	% ever married
Borderlines		
BPD females	69/134	51.5
BPD males	15/52	28.9
D females	9/13	69.2
D males	8/21	38.1
Other BPO females	9/21	42.9
Other BPO males	12/27	44.4
Psychotics		
SZ females	7/38	18.4
SZ males	5/58	8.6
SA females	11/40	27.5
SA males	8/21	38.1
MDP females	7/15	46.7
MDP males	8/23	34.7
SF females	2/8	25.0
SF males	11/24	45.8

to MAD comorbidity in the BPD patients. In the BPD females, the percentages were the same (50%) whether MAD coexisted or not. BPD males *without* MAD had a lower marriage rate (17%) than those with MAD (37%). This may be a reflection of the high proportion of patients with coexisting ASP in the former subgroup.

Borderline females were, in general, more likely to have married than the males, except in the group satisfying neither BPD nor MAD criteria (i.e., the patients who were borderline only by broad criteria, or "other BPO"). In this group, the females often had anorexia nervosa and/or bulimia nervosa when first admitted. These women tended to avoid or postpone marriage to an extent greater than that shown by their counterparts with BPD or MAD. The males in this group exhibited a variety of personality disorders, most prominently ASP. But unlike the BPD × ASP males (few of whom ever married), the ASP-only males whom I managed to trace were less angry and irritable than the BPD × ASP males; they may have had fewer impediments to the formation of stable relationships. Several of the ASP males remain untraced, however; they happened to be among the more hostile and dyssocial of the entire ASP group and may well have remained unable to form lasting relationships of any sort.

Among the patients with an initial psychosis, the marriage rate was also well below population norms—either to levels resembling those for some of the borderline subgroups or, in the case of SZ, to extremely low levels (see Table

3.6). If we look at the marriage rate in whole groups, not divided as to gender, a graded series emerges: MDP (43%) > SA (31%) > SZ (13%). This is in line with clinical impressions. Patients with MDP tend to turn toward others; those with SZ tend to turn away from others. The difference in rates between males and females in the SF group may be an artifact of the small number of females in this group.

The marriage rates indicated above are lower by about 10% than the "true" rates (the percentage ever married, once the youngest patient passed the age where marrying for the first time was no longer likely). The youngest patient in the PI-500 is 27 at this writing; the oldest is 62. Several of those in their early 30s were engaged to be married at the time of follow-up. Social class may be a relevant factor in certain diagnostic groups. As difficult as intimacy and sustained relationships are for schizophrenic patients in general (especially those with prominent "negative signs"; see Chapter Twelve), they may be even more problematical for schizophrenic males from affluent homes. Their ability to earn may be well below that of their original families, making it more difficult for them to feel confident in the role of breadwinner. If the job a schizophrenic male is able to perform successfully happens to be similar to the jobs held by his father and by other wage earners in his family, the sense of disparity—and the potential for humiliation—will be correspondingly less. As in McGlashan's Chestnut Lodge series, the contrasts in schizophrenic patients were often overpowering. Less than 1 in 10 of the males had married by the time of follow-up; of the five who did marry, four of the marriages had lasted. One cannot base generalizations on such a small sample, but, interestingly, three came from families in average circumstances. Several of the male schizophrenics from wealthy or prominent families committed suicide (see Chapter Four).

Fertility

The former patients of the PI-500, of either gender, were less likely to have children than would be true of similar-age persons in the general population. This finding cuts across all diagnostic groups, but is especially striking in relation to the schizophrenic and schizoaffective patients. The top half of Table 3.7 shows the percentage of women in each of the major categories who had had one or more children by the time of follow-up. The BPD females appeared to be more fertile than their schizophrenic counterparts, though the difference was just short of statistical significance, $\chi^2 = 3.64, p \cong .07$. The dysthymic women also appeared more likely than the schizophrenic women to have become mothers, $\chi^2 = 4.98, p < .05$. The dysthymic women, at this writing, are at an average age of 44 (range 33–62)—5 years older than the nonsuicide BPD group (average age now 39; range 27–55), and 7 years older than the BPO borderlines without MAD or BPD (average age 37; range 27–52). One of the latter had her first child, at age 38, as I was writing this section. In 8 years' time, 22 more (i.e.,

TABLE 3.7.   Fertility in PI-500 Patients

| Diagnostic group | n traced | Patients with one or more children | | Number of children | |
		n	%	Total	Per patient
		Females			
BPD	141	36	25.5[a]	69	0.49
D	13	5	38.4	10	0.77
Other BPO	21	5	23.8[b]	8	0.38
SZ	38	4[c]	10.5	7	0.18
SA	40	5[d]	12.5	7	0.18
MDP	15	3[e]	20.0	6	0.4
SF	8	2	25.0	3	0.38
Totals	276	60	21.8	110	0.4
		Males			
BPD	52	8	15.4	15	0.29
D	21	3	14.3	6	0.29
Other BPO	27	5	18.5	7	0.26
SZ	58	2	3.4	7	0.12
SA	21	4	19.0	7	0.33
MDP	23	2	8.7	2	0.09
SF	24	10	41.7	15	0.63
Totals	226	33	14.6	59	0.26

[a]If suicides are excluded, 36/131 = 27.5%.
[b]If suicides are excluded, 5/20 = 25%.
[c]Includes one mother who gave her child up for adoption.
[d]Consists of two mothers raising their children, one who lost her child at birth, and two who gave their children up for adoption.

all but 3) of the BPD females will have passed beyond the usual age for child-bearing, whereas the dysthymic patients are already nearer this point. Subsequent follow-up may thus reveal smaller intergroup differences within the borderline domain.

Women with anorexia or bulimia often express a disinclination to become mothers; some anorectics fast with the conscious intention of suppressing their menses and of avoiding pregnancy (see Jeammet, Jayle, Terrase-Brechon, & Gorge, 1984). Each borderline subgroup contained some women with eating disorders: BPD, 19 of 145; dysthymics, 3 of 14; and other BPO patients, 11 of 22. One (BPD) patient committed suicide while still hospitalized; one remains untraced. Of the remainder, the percentage with at least one child at follow-up was 22.6% (7 of 31). This is in the same range as shown by the whole borderline group. Furthermore, 14 of the eating-disordered patients are aged 36 or less as of this writing; several may become mothers within the next 5 or 10 years. Although it may be true that women hospitalized with eating disorders during late adolescence or early adult life are less apt to produce children than their non-eating-disordered peers, they do not seem less fertile than hospitalized borderline women. (The eating disorders are discussed further in Chapter Eight.)

All this stands in contrast to the women in the combined schizophrenic and schizoaffective groups, only 9 (out of 77) of whom had given birth at follow-up and only 5 of whom (6.5%) were involved in the raising of their children. To some extent, this low birth rate may be a function of social class (see Erlenmeyer-Kimling, 1966), though the relatively lower rate compared with that of the borderlines appears to be a valid observation, since there are no socioeconomic status differences across diagnostic groups in the PI-500.

As Table 3.7 also shows, the total number of children born to the PI-500 women thus far is 110, or 0.4 per woman—about a fourth the number expected of their age mates in the general population.

The issue of paternity is always more problematical than that of maternity, since women always know when they have become mothers, but some men sire children without realizing it. I have, of course, no idea how often this may have happened with the former male patients in the PI-500. Some of the schizophrenic and schizoaffective women who gave children up for adoption had become pregnant by male fellow-patients during hospitalizations that followed their stay on our unit. The one borderline woman who had a child by a fellow-patient from our unit knew, as did her partner, who the father was.

The bottom half of Table 3.7 reflects the percentages of men in the major diagnostic groups who are known to have become fathers by the time of follow-up, and the total number of children they have thus far sired. All but one child (belonging to one of the schizophreniform men) was born in wedlock. The former male patients were less likely to have become fathers than were the female patients to become mothers, in all categories except SA and SF. Many of the SF patients were, underneath the psychosis they had often induced in themselves through substance abuse, less impaired than the patients with a "classical" psychosis or even than many of the borderlines. This may help to account for the surprisingly high percentage of SF males who went on, after conquering their drug problem, to lead fairly normal and conventional lives.

CHAPTER FOUR

Suicide and Suicidal Behavior

COMPLETED SUICIDES

The all-or-none quality of suicide—attempters emerge either alive or dead—lends an air of authenticity to the statistics. In contrast to such baseline variables as likeableness or outcome variables such as satisfaction with work, suicide figures are "hard data." Even these data, however, contain an element of "softness," since a few patients who tried desperately to die survived. Of these, some are now grateful to have survived; others are merely marking time till the end finally comes. I describe these patients in greater detail in the section "Almost-Suicides," below. Included there are a small number who nearly died inadvertently from drug overdoses, not having consciously willed their deaths at the time.

With 93% of the PI-500 now traced,[1] I have established that there were 49 suicides. Table 4.1 shows the percentage of suicides in each diagnostic group. The resulting figures may be compared with the overall suicide rate for the entire PI-500, which stands at the present writing, with an average postdischarge interval of 16½ years, at 9.4%. I cannot say with confidence that any of the 49 who died did so through "miscalculation." Half chose methods not consistent with lack of resolve: shooting, jumping, hanging. The remainder died of overdoses, gas, drowning, or walking in front of oncoming traffic—any of which permits some chance of rescue.

Borderline Patients

Among the borderlines, the risk of suicide was significantly higher in those meeting DSM criteria for borderline personality disorder (BPD). These criteria include self-damaging acts, impulsivity, and inordinate anger, all of which are associated with heightened suicidality. The risk was particularly high in males with concomitant major affective disorder (MAD). In general, however, males

[1]When this chapter was written several additional patients were traced, bringing the total to 511, or 93%.

40

TABLE 4.1. Completed Suicides in the PI-500, by Diagnostic Group

Diagnostic category	n	Traced		Suicides	
		n	%	n	%
Borderlines					
BPD	206	192	93	17	8.9
Males	61	52	85	7	13.2
With MAD	34	28	83	5	17.9
No MAD	27	24	89	2	8.3
Females	145	141	97	10	7.1
With MAD	104	101	97	8	7.9
No MAD	41	39	95	2	5.1
D					
Males	22	21	95	0	0
Females	14	13	93	0	0
Other BPO					
Males	35	27	77	1	3.6
Females	22	21	95	1	5.0
Unclassified	4	1	25	0	0
Psychotics					
SZ	99	96	97.0	9	9.4
Males	60	58	96.7	6	10.3
Females	39	37	94.9	3	8.1
SA	64	61	95.3	14	23.0
Males	23	21	91.3	5	23.8
Females	41	40	97.6	9	22.5
MDP	39	38	97.4	4	10.5
Males	24	23	95.8	2	8.7
Females	15	15	100.0	2	13.3
SF	36	32	88.9	2	6.3
Males	27	24	88.9	2	8.3
Females	9	8	88.9	0	0
Neurotics	7	7	100.0	1	14
Other	6	4	67	0	0

with BPD were not at greater risk than their female counterparts. Fewer males than females with BPD showed MAD comorbidity (Table 4.1). If one begins with the broad Kernberg criteria and then narrows the sample down to those with BPD, the suicide risk turns out to be concentrated almost entirely in the BPD group: 17 suicides in 193 traced BPDs (8.9%), compared with 2 suicides in 83 traced non-BPD borderlines (2.4%), $\chi^2 = 3.78$; $p \leq .05$. These last 2, as noted in Table 4.2, consisted of an alcoholic male and a woman with schizotypal features.

History of substance abuse	Incest history	Relevant family history
Alcohol	(Eroticized relationship with father)	—
—	—	Father, ECT for depression; aunt, suicide attempts
Alcohol, marijuana, LSD	—	(Adoptee)
—	(Eroticized relationship with father)	—
—	—	—
Alcohol	(Eroticized relationship with father)	Father, violent and abusive
—	Probable molestation by father	Father, major depressive episodes
—	—	Father and mother, alcoholic suicides
Alcohol	—	(Raised as "adoptee but "adoptive father" was real father; biological mother unknown; stepmother schizophrenic)
—	—	Maternal aunt, MDP
Alcohol, marijuana, LSD, cocaine, heroin, barbiturates	Incest with father, brother	Father, hospitalized for depression; two brothers, committed suicide
Alcohol, marijuana, LSD, peyote	—	—
—	—	—
—	Incest with mother	Mother committed suicide 6 months before patient was hospitalized
Alcohol	Incest with brother	Mother and father, alcoholic
Marijuana, amphetamines, LSD	Incest with adoptive mother	(Adoptee)
Marijuana	—	Mother and father, alcoholic
Alcohol	—	—
—	—	—

The borderlines *least* likely to commit suicide were those with MAD who did not meet DSM criteria for BPD. This was essentially the dysthymic (D) group: patients with dysphoria, but relatively little impulsivity, hostility, or aggressivity. Thus far, their suicide rate is 0, with 94% traced. One of the two still-untraced D patients is a likely candidate for suicide: His mother killed herself when he was 7, shortly after his abusive and schizophrenic father was released from a mental hospital. Thereafter, this man lived in a succession of foster homes.

Table 4.1 shows the similarity in suicide rate between the BPD group and the schizophrenic (SZ), manic–depressive psychosis (MDP), and schizophreniform (SF) patients. The risk was appreciably higher only in the schizoaffective (SA) group.

As noted in many compilations of young suicides, the 19 borderline suicides (average age 26; range 15–40) were almost all single. One killed herself shortly after her wedding and two shortly after their husbands left them; the others had never married. Only five had ever worked (two, sporadically). In comparison with the large remainder of borderlines, those who eventually committed suicide were more marginal in their adaptation up till the time of death, and had meager support systems. Sometimes there was *no* support system, as in the case of the woman who killed herself while on a pass from the hospital during the Christmas season: Both parents had recently committed suicide (one through alcoholic debauch), and she had no friends.

Three-fourths of the suicides had concomitant affective illness, almost always depressive in nature, but in two instances with bipolar evolution a few years after their release from the hospital.

With respect to genetic and environmental liability, six of the suicides had at least one first-degree relative with major depressive illness; three had experienced the suicide of one or more of these close relatives. Another three were adoptees. Although information is lacking about their biological antecedents, they had to grapple with the psychosocial stresses of adoption, which in their cases, happened to be severe. One of the adolescent males, hyperactive from birth, broke down after learning he was adopted and began thereafter to abuse drugs, set fires, and assault his family. The other adolescent male was seduced by his alcoholic adoptive mother. The female adoptee had the ill luck to have a violent, schizophrenic adoptive mother. Rather late in the day, the courts interceded on the patient's behalf, but she was already a crushed human being—alcoholic, truant, promiscuous, and self-mutilative.

Three of the borderline suicides came from families where *both* parents were chronically alcoholic and abusive; another, from a family where the father was grossly seductive and where she was forced to have sex with several of her brothers. Altogether, only two nonadopted borderline suicides had *neither* MAD comorbidity nor a family history of affective illness or of alcoholism in a first-degree relative. Both came from families characterized by chronic bickering and criticism (the "high expressed emotion" of Leff & Vaughn, 1980). One had been an effeminate adolescent, ridiculed at camp and treated seductively by his mother in order to "correct" his homosexual tendencies.

In some of the homes of the psychotic patients who committed suicide (see below), the family environment had been benign and nurturing; constitutional rather than environmental factors appeared to play the major role in the suicidal dénouement. The borderline suicides all came from difficult environments, which interacted synergistically with hereditary/familial predisposition in at least half the cases. It may be mere coincidence, but, ironically, two of the suicides (one a borderline, the other a schizoaffective) had been named after grand-mothers who had committed suicide years earlier.

Two of the female (BPD) borderlines exhibited severe premenstrual syndrome (PMS), with rage outbursts and occasional suicide gestures a day or so before the menses. One later developed bipolar illness. It is not known whether their suicides occurred during this phase of their cycle. Another borderline woman, one of the almost-suicides, made half a dozen serious suicide attempts premenstrually before she was admitted to our unit; while there, she once hanged herself premenstrually but was rescued at the last minute by the nursing staff. (For further discussion of PMS, see Chapter Eight.)

Although the DSM and Gunderson systems emphasize manipulative suicide gestures as important diagnostic items for BPD, the fatal attempts of the 19 borderlines who died by their own hand often had manipulative overtones as well. These acts were less often the expression simply of despair and lifelong ineffectiveness, as one found in the histories of some of the schizophrenic and schizoaffective suicides. One of the borderlines, for example, killed himself after his birthday party, leaving a note guaranteed to have maximal traumatic impact upon the surviving family members. Here the desire was more to wound than to manipulate for any specific purpose. Likewise, the borderline woman who killed herself shortly after her marriage broke up meant more to wound than to get the husband back; about the latter she had abandoned hope—and *hopelessness* was what probably pushed her to a fatal rather than to a milder and more obviously exploitative act. The message might have been "*après moi le déluge.*" (This may also have been the message the borderline adolescent who swallowed thumbtacks had wished to convey, except that he survived.)

The borderline subgroup whose suicide risk was the highest consisted of females with BPD, concomitant MAD, and alcohol abuse. Alcohol figured prominently in the histories of seven borderline suicides, polydrug abuse in two others. But what drew my attention to the BPD × MAD × alcoholism combination was that I could identify only 13 female patients with all three—and 5 have thus far committed suicide (38%). I was not able to establish just when these patients first became seriously alcoholic, but, as a group, their 5-year survival rate after release from our unit was only 58%. Of the five who died, four came from particularly traumatic environments (incest, physical abuse, parental alcoholism, etc.); perhaps they were too shattered and impulsive to have stayed with and been salvaged by Alcoholics Anonymous.

TABLE 4.3. Suicide Gestures and Attempts in Borderlines Who Eventually Committed Suicide

Patient no.	Previous suicide attempts	Previous suicide gestures	Comments
1	0	2	Hypnotics
2	1	1	Hypnotics
3	0	3	Seconal®; Valium®
4	2	1	Doriden® (2); aspirin
5	0	0	—
6	>3	>3	Hypnotics
7	0	0	—
8	>3	>3	Hypnotics
9	1	1	Hypnotics
10	0	0	—
11	Many	Many	Various drugs; set fire to room
12	0	0	—
13	>3	>3	Hypnotics; cut self with glass
14	1	0	Hypnotics
15	1	1	Carbon monoxide; pills
16	1	0	Barbiturates
17	1	1	Aspirin
18	0	0	—
19	0	Many	Self-mutilation with razor

Suicide gestures or attempts were common in the borderline patients, especially in the BPD group (whose illness was in part defined by the history of manipulative suicide gestures, as noted above). Whereas half the BPD patients had this history, three-fourths of those who eventually committed suicide had made one or more gestures only ($n = 3$) or attempt(s) only ($n = 2$) or both ($n = 9$). Almost all of these suicidal acts were overdoses (hypnotics, aspirin, Valium®); a few had cut themselves with glass or inhaled carbon monoxide. Only one patient had indulged in frequent superficial self-mutilation with razors. The suicidal acts in the borderline suicides are summarized in Table 4.3.

A number of authors have stressed the significance of *repeated* suicide attempts as an indicator of eventual suicide. Kurz et al. (1987) showed, for example, that in a consecutive series of suicide completers, those with a history of frequent attempts were more likely to have died than were those hospitalized because of a first attempt. Similarly, Kotila and Lönnqvist (1987), in their study of 406 adolescent suicide attempters, found that 5 years later 4% of the repeated attempters were dead, but only 1% of the first-time attempters. Pallis, Barraclough, Levey, Jenkins, and Sainsbury (1982) noted that attempters in general died at about a rate of 1% per year.

In the PI-500, I could identify altogether 49 patients who had made one suicide attempt before index hospitalization, and 22 who had made two or more serious attempts. Borderlines were overrepresented in *both* groups: They constituted 32 of the 49 first-time attempters, $\chi^2 = 20.5$, $p < .01$, and 17 of the 22 repeat attempters, $\chi^2 = 15.5$, $p < .01$. *All* of these borderlines (32 + 17) met criteria for BPD. In the PI-500 series, both situations were fairly strong predictors of suicide, but those making repeated attempts were not more likely to have completed suicide. The rates in the group as a whole (9 suicides in 49 first-time attempters, or 18.3%; 4 suicides in 22 among the repeaters, or 18.2%) were identical. Within the BPD group the rates were similar (first-time attempters, 5 of 32, or 16%; repeaters, 2 of 17, or 12%). I do not believe that these figures permit me to challenge the findings of Kurz et al. (1987) and of Kotila and Lönnqvist (1987). Repeat attempters probably are at greater risk for suicide. Peculiarities of the sample may account for the absence of this correlation in the PI-500 series. The *overall* suicide rate thus far in the PI-500 patients with BPD (8.9%) is close to that observed during similar time frames by Paris, Brown, and Nowlis (1987) (8.5% over the period 1958–1978) and in a Swedish series (12%), though in the latter study (spanning 1961–1980) the number of original BPD patients (16) was small (Kullgren, Renberg, & Jacobsson, 1986). Kullgren et al. speculated that the fairly high suicide rate in BPD might relate in part to a cohort effect—namely, the fact that treatment philosophy underwent appreciable changes during the 1970s. Hospital units became less hierarchical, more likely to be "open-door," and less structured. These changes might be too permissive and not sufficiently limit-setting for the average BPD patient. Kullgren et al.'s observation is true of many hospital units both in America and in Europe. Their remarks apply only in part to the PI-500, however; our unit became less hierarchical in the early 1970s, yet remained locked, conservative, and highly structured.[2]

Another group of Swedish investigators (B. Jacobson et al., 1987) felt that they could often correlate the mode of suicide with certain perinatal difficulties. For example, they stated that suicides involving asphyxiation were more apt to have been preceded by perinatal hypoxia, and that suicide by violent mechanical means was associated with birth trauma. In the absence of detailed obstetrical records, I could hazard no guesses about possible antecedent factors that may have inclined the borderline patients (one of whom suffocated after placing a plastic bag over her head) toward any particular method of taking their lives.

Steer, Beck, Garrison, and Lester (1988) recently drew attention to the unexpectedly high suicide rate (15%) at a 7-year follow-up of 41 patients hospitalized because of an *interrupted* suicide attempt (i.e., someone on the scene interfered with the attempter's act), compared with the rate in noninterrupted attempters (5% of 458 patients). Steer et al. felt that those who appeared to be

---

[2]Compare Robins's (1989) caveat: "It is probable that the only generally effective means of reducing the suicide rate is to hospitalize suicidal patients in *closed wards*" (p. 130; italics in original).

"crying for help" may have had as much lethal intent as those who hid these acts more successfully, but were merely expressing this intent more obviously (1987, p. 126). Because of the unevenness of the old records, I was not able to reconstruct precise percentages within the PI-500 of suicide rates in interrupted versus noninterrupted attempters. In the largest subgroup—BPD females—those who had made one or more (foiled or otherwise) were about four times as likely to commit suicide eventually as were those who, before index hospitalization, had made only a gesture (18% as against 4%). This difference did not hold up among the BPD males (see "Parasuicide," below). In general, the findings among the BPD suicides in the present study corroborate the impressions of Robins (1989) and of Hirschfeld and Davidson (1988) that affective disorder and alcoholism are common antecedents in the histories of completed suicides.

Schizophrenic Patients

Although the suicide rate thus far in the schizophrenics is approximately the same as that in the BPD patients, the apparent suicidality in the two groups looked different at the outset. If we take a propensity toward suicide gestures and attempts as a prognostic indicator of eventual suicide, the ranks of the borderlines seem filled with "false positives" who have not (as yet) gone on to commit suicide; by contrast, the schizophrenics have included many "false negatives," who one day suddenly killed themselves after giving little or no warning. One cannot generalize much in a series of only nine suicides, but only three of the nine schizophrenics who committed suicide had a history of suicidal acts before coming to the hospital. One of the males had threatened to kill his father and then himself during an argument, but had never acted aggressively toward himself or others until his own suicide 2 years after leaving the unit. Another male, beset with fears of being homosexual, sought to prove himself by provoking fights with larger men; however, apart from this dangerous habit, he never acted in an outright suicidal manner until he drowned himself several years after he left the unit. A schizophrenic man who was so uncommunicative that his therapist imagined she meant nothing to him at all shot himself the day her tour of duty ended on the unit. He had never behaved self-destructively before, though it is probably meaningful that his grandmother killed herself and his mother nearly did.

For many of these schizophrenic patients, what released the trigger to a lone but definitive suicidal act was an ever-intensifying sense of hopelessness about being able to compete successfully in the outside world. They misinterpreted their inability to make even minimal contact with members of the opposite sex (let alone achieve intimacy) as proof of "homosexuality"; humiliation eventually passed some threshold of intolerability and led to the suicide. For others, it was occupational rather than sexual defeat that precipitated the final act. Their failure was all the more poignant for their having been unusually intelligent. The average IQ of both the borderline and the schizophrenic suicides was 123—slightly above the mean (119) for the PI-500 as a whole. Whereas we originally imagined that their extraordinary endowment would save our schizophrenic patients, allowing them to recover—in a way that the less intelligent schizophrenics of the May (1968) study did not—the reverse seemed to be true. Since their brightness was apparent long before their illness, they were raised in an atmosphere of high expectations. This only served to aggravate their problems with self-esteem as their illness manifested itself during adolescence. Many of their parents and siblings had achieved high status; the latter served inevitably as the yardsticks by which they were to measure themselves. This factor may help account for the discrepancy between the fate of the PI-500 (or of the Chestnut Lodge) schizophrenics and that of the group followed by Harding and Strauss (1985) in their Vermont study. I believe that the world around them expected a good deal less from the rural patients of average mental endowment in the Vermont sample than it demanded of the schizophrenics in our series and in McGlashan's. We failed to appreciate the severity and tenacity of their illness; perhaps retreat from the competitive world into a humane and unstressful setting could have spared them more of the illness's worst effects than relentlessly pushing them into that world did. Instead of offering these fragile young people sanctuary, sheltered work settings, and dignity, we offered brief hospitalizations, crash courses, and shabby "single-room occupancy" living quarters—splintered crutches that could support them only momentarily. Perhaps many schizophrenics have less biochemical predisposition to suicide than do certain affectively ill patients (cf. Siever & Coursey, 1985); this may permit the majority of schizophrenics, even under less than ideal treatment conditions and in the face of constricted lives, to avoid suicide, while a number of seemingly "better off" manic–depressives nevertheless go on to suicide.

Schizoaffective Patients

The suicide rate among the schizoaffective patients was 23%. Although a few variables predicted even higher rates (ever in jail, 33%; alcoholic women with BPD × MAD, 38%), the schizoaffectives constituted the most suicide-prone diagnostic group. Both sexes appeared equally at risk. Other investigators, including Tsuang and Dempsey (1979), have commented on the high suicide risk in patients with "atypical psychosis" or with the nosologically similar SA. The magnitude of the risk is not always easy to gauge from the literature, owing to the controversy surrounding the diagnosis itself. Space does not permit a detailed review of this controversy, many facets of which others have examined at some length (Angst, Felder, & Lohmeyer, 1979; Angst, Scharfetter, & Stassen, 1983; Brockington & Meltzer, 1983; Pope, Lipinski, Cohen, &

Axelrod, 1980; Scharfetter & Nusperli, 1980; Strauss, 1983). Suffice it to say that a number of investigators define "schizoaffective" in a manner more closely akin to the definitions of "schizophrenia" (Welner, Fishman, & Robins, 1977); others define it in a way overlapping more closely with concepts of "affective psychosis" (Clayton, Rodin, & Winokur, 1968). Differences of this kind could explain some of the disparity in the published suicide statistics, despite general agreement that the risk is high. How might we account for this risk?

According to commonly held clinical opinion, schizoaffectives, in comparison to "process schizophrenics," have certain advantages and certain disadvantages. Kasanin (1933), who first described the condition, underlined its *reactive* and often abrupt (as opposed to insidious) onset. He also spoke of the schizoaffective's greater tendency to recover. But with respect to *suicide*, schizoaffective patients seem doubly cursed: They seem more susceptible to depression and hopelessness; they often have a greater awareness of illness (in effect, better reality-testing) than do many "process schizophrenic" patients. Some clinicians speculate that this awareness serves paradoxically to intensify the anguish that certain schizoaffectives experience, inclining them even more strongly to suicide than is the case with psychologically more impaired schizophrenics (some of whom act as though blithely unaware of their handicaps).

Explanations that confine themselves to the realm of psychology alone cannot, I believe, resolve the paradoxical outcomes in the SA group (any more than they can for other patients manifesting destructiveness toward self or others). Dynamic interpretations about internalized rage or about the interplay between aggressivity and suicidality are in many ways correct, but do not cast a wide enough net to capture all that is of etiological significance. Evidence is beginning to accumulate to the effect that innate factors are important determinants of aggressive, impulsive, and suicidal behavior in those with affective disorders, and also in those (viz., hostile and impulsive non-MAD borderlines) with only the aggressivity and impulsivity (see Åsberg, Nordström, & Traskman-Bendz, 1989). Brown et al. (1982), for example, found alterations in serotonin metabolism in (aggressive) male borderlines without concomitant MAD: The central nervous system (CNS) levels of 5-hydroxyindoleacetic acid (5-HIAA) were significantly lower in the subjects with a history of suicidal behavior than in those who had not been suicidal. Kety (1979, 1989) has pointed to the likelihood of a genetic factor in suicidal behavior. This factor is associated with affective disorder, rather than with SZ as stringently defined (e.g., by DSM-III). The PI-500 can shed no light on the possible biochemical underpinnings of suicidality, because it considerably antedates all but the earliest of the studies concerning either suicide and neurotransmitters (see Åsberg, Traskman, & Thorén, 1976) or the effects of lithium on impulsive/aggressive behavior (Sheard, Marini, Bridges, & Wagner, 1976). The suicide rate in the PI-500 was, however, concentrated in patients with concomitant affective illness—those with BPD × MAD as opposed to BPD alone; the schizoaffectives more so than the schizophrenics. The high suicidality of the schizoaffectives may relate in part to their painful "double awareness," but almost surely is a reflexion of innate biochemical CNS abnormalities that render them more suicide-prone than schizophrenics who are not affectively ill. A few of the schizoaffective suicides were young women who had been incest victims (two instances). But 10 others who had incest experiences have not committed suicide.

In the PI-500, one in four female schizoaffectives with a prior history of suicidal acts went on to a complete suicide by the time of follow-up; one in six of those with no such history ultimately committed suicide. This does not allow the clinician much comfort even when confronted with a schizoaffective woman who has not made previous gestures. With the *male* schizoaffectives, I could find not even the semblance of a linkage between prior acts and eventual suicide: Of the five who have thus far taken their lives, only one made prior gestures. He was, in fact, the *only* male schizoaffective out of 23 to have made either a gesture or an attempt before the index admission. If there is a clinical lesson here, it would be that schizoaffectives are a worrisome group because they often kill themselves (males and females alike), having given either "warnings" that are hard to interpret (the females) or no warnings at all (the males).

A final sad comment on the PI-500 schizoaffectives concerns the 1976 cohort. The 26 patients of this cohort were the last to be admitted to the unit before it closed at the end of the academic year (June 1977). In the ensuing upheaval (change of personnel, altered discharge plans, a sense of diminished support), four of the patients, aged 16, 17, 18, and 19, took their lives within a few months of leaving the unit. The contagion-like quality of this outbreak was reminiscent of the waves of suicides among certain groups of adolescents that have recently captured the public's attention. Of these four patients, one was borderline; three were schizoaffective.

The deaths of several of the other schizoaffectives who committed suicide coincided with the loss of a therapist or of the hospital's supportive milieu. As alert as our staff members were to such patients' exquisite sensitivity to loss, we still at times misread or underestimated their reactions. Often enough, they gave us very few clues about their suicidal intentions. Perhaps simply knowing that a patient is schizoaffective—and therefore at "high risk" both for recovery and for suicide—may help psychiatric personnel henceforth to redouble their efforts to safeguard these patients at critical junctures in the course of their treatment, so that in the future more are enabled to partake of their good potential for recovery.

General Comments

The completed suicides in the PI-500 chose violent methods more often than overdoses. As in most studies, this tendency was more apparent in the males.

Their preferred method was jumping off buildings (half the male suicides). Only one-sixth died of overdoses; the remainder shot themselves, drowned, or threw themselves in front of cars. From the standpoint of Linehan's (1986) Lethality Scale, most of these patients showed high "intensity" of suicidality, as measured by their lethality of method, nonrescuability, and planfulness. Half the female suicides, by contrast, chose overdose. In the other half, jumping accounted for most of the deaths, shooting and hanging for the remainder.

Many of the high-risk factors noted by Rosen (1976) were present in the completed suicides of either sex and of all diagnostic categories: living alone (only one was currently married; one lived with a roommate); unemployed-ment; psychosis (in 29 of the 49); alcohol or drug abuse; sudden life changes (divorce, loss of therapist [5 cases], death of a parent); and past suicide attempts. Similarly, six of the patients had a family history of suicide. These included the two women who were named after grandmothers who had committed suicide; in effect, these women were *branded* as suicides from the day of their birth. The mother of a seventh patient was an almost-suicide, having recovered fortuitously from a highly lethal and not ordinarily rescuable attempt.

Mann's (1987) point that suicide is more a form of violence than a manifestation of depression seems pertinent to many of the PI-500 suicides, particularly to those whose suicide followed closely on the heels of a violent outburst against a family member. One schizophrenic woman, for example, tried (unsuccessfully) to kill her mother, and then killed herself. The age span in which most of the suicides occurred was, for the most part, the third decade of life: 70% of those committing suicide were between 18 and 30; only 20% were over 30. This decade is also associated with high rates of homicide (Wilson & Herrnstein, 1985).

Among the PI-500 alcoholics who were suicides, violence-proneness and depression were often commingled. This is true in the general alcohol-abusing population as well—15% of alcoholics eventually commit suicide—but the timing of the act more often coincides with a recent loss than is the case with depressives (26–32% of alcoholic suicides had a recent loss, as compared with approximately 3% of depressives who committed suicide; Hawton, 1987).

Angst and Clayton (1986), using the Freiburg Personality Inventory, found that aggression scores were high in persons who died either by suicide or by accidents; they were also high in those who had made suicide *attempts,* compared with those who had only manifested suicidal ideation.

The likelihood of suicide depends upon the interplay of innate and environmental factors. Innate factors include both specific biochemical abnor-malities (e.g., deviations in the availability of serotinin, dopamine, or norepinephrine along certain CNS pathways) and nonspecific abnormalities of temperament (e.g., depressive/irritable). The latter may themselves represent the phenotypic expression of neurotransmitter or other biochemical abnormalities. One may view psychosis as another nonspecific and often hereditary/familial

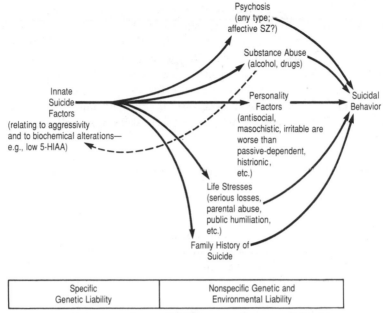

FIGURE 4.1. Factors thought to contribute to suicide risk.

factor—"nonspecific," to the extent that suicide risk is heightened not just in MDP but in SZ.

Interacting with these factors are a number of psychosocial stressors, such as substance abuse (especially abuse of alcohol, which, besides its other effects, acts as a serotonin "poison"); a family history of suicide; and a number of other stresses, both distal and current (death of a parent, divorce or other serious loss, a history of parental abusiveness, public humiliation, etc.). As we have seen, many of the PI-500 suicides labored under a multiplicity of these adverse factors. The suicide of one borderline woman, in particular, resulted from the fatal synergism of family history of MDP death of two siblings via suicide, severe alcohol and drug abuse, parental exploitativeness and molestation, scandal, and an explosive temperament.

Figure 4.1 provides a schema of the factors contributing additively to suicide risk. These factors are quite similar to the five broad and intersecting areas outlined by Blumenthal and Kupfer (1986, p. 329) in their "*overlap*" model of suicide risk: biological factors, psychiatric disorder, family history and genetics, personality traits, and a fifth factor related to life events and any pre-existing chronic medical illness.

In general, the PI-500 suicide completers, in contrast to those who made gestures or attempts but are still alive, showed many of the characteristics Pallis et al. (1982) noted in their analysis of 75 suicides and 146 attempted suicides. Higher risk in their sample was associated with being male, being under 45, being in socioeconomic status category I or II, being unemployed, living alone, being depressed, abusing alcohol, and speaking to someone about suicidal intentions. In addition, the completed suicides were often divorced or widowed—an attribute not as pertinent to the PI-500, who were a young group and, at the time of their index hospitalization, almost all single. The bulk of the suicides occurred before age 30 (when most were still single, and none had been widowed).

ALMOST-SUICIDES

As awesome as the actual suicide rate was in the PI-500—so far, nearly 10% of the entire group—the figures would have been even more dismal if certain patients had had their way. There were 10 whose suicide attempts were so serious that death would unquestionably have resulted, had not they been rescued by sheer luck or the wizardry of medical technology. Three of these patients, dead stethoscopically but not electroencephalographically, were defibrillated in the emergency room, following lethal overdoses of barbiturates or heroin. They were literally seconds away from death. Two others nearly hanged themselves (in the bathroom shower of the hospital unit), and were found and cut down less than a minute before brain death would have resulted. Two jumped in front of trains: In one instance, the patient was knocked to the side and temporarily pinioned between the onrushing train and the wall, without sustaining much injury; in the other, the patient fell beneath the wheels, and the whole train passed over him with no effect other than to have mussed his hair. Another became the only survivor of those who leaped from one of New York City's taller bridges. All bones having been broken except those of the inner ear, this patient was in a body spica for 6 months before coming back, as a kind of ghost or revenant, to our unit. Another took a lethal overdose just before her roommate left for work, only to be rescued when the roommate, having forgotten an important document, returned unexpectedly to their flat an hour later. Still another set off an explosion causing a great blast and fire; ironically, however, the blast ejected him from the room, which was otherwise destroyed by the fire.

Every one of these patients was chastened by the near-death experience. Some, their "statement" of revenge or despair having clearly registered, felt they had more or less accomplished what they had set out to do; now, as inadvertent "born-agains," they could get on with the business of living. A few became disenchanted at last with further attempts, regarding themselves as somehow incapable of death, but as still quite capable of becoming maimed—and henceforth of living, if they were careless, a life even worse than the one that had pushed them to the brink originally. The patient who survived the leap from the bridge developed delusions (if delusions they were) of immortality, subsequently abandoning thoughts of suicide altogether. One of those rescued from hanging joined a religious sect emphasizing reincarnation. Another—snatched from death by drug overdose, with only seconds remaining—became an officer of an "Anonymous" organization dedicated to the rehabilitation of addicts; he thus converted his life into something as socially useful as it had been socially destructive before.

A few patients who fully intended to die emerged totally unscathed from their attempts, but still experienced a change of attitude about suicide. One schizophrenic man, for example, despondent over his bleak academic prospects, tried to kill himself with exhaust fumes from the family car; several hours later, he discovered to his bewilderment that he was none the worse for it, because he had mistakenly left on the ventilator. Giving up on inwardly directed aggression after that, he vented his rage upon the house and its belongings for a while. But, as of this writing, he has not been actively suicidal in 20 years.

There is an important lesson in the histories of these suicides *manqués,* over and above the obvious one concerning the limits of revivification. Some of these patients unreservedly and unambivalently sought to die, but did not. Others, though gambling with their lives recklessly, were not hoping to die, but almost did. We ordinarily think, macroscopically and categorically, of life and death, suicide and nonsuicide, as polar opposites—the "on" and "off" positions of some mysterious binary switch. But these patients demonstrate that there is something dicey even about this supposedly two-state system. For some moments at least, these patients existed, like the cat in Schrödinger's thought experiment (Fine, 1986, p. 65), in a thoroughly ambiguous state, resisting any firm definition as to whether they were alive or dead. When the "experiment" was completed (i.e., when the medical team had done its work), there was a certain randomness to the results. Some who had truly wanted to die were saved. Likewise, it *must* be the case that several of the 49 suicides in the PI-500 had entertained a *little* hope of being rescued, yet were not. This would not pertain to the man who blew his brains out with a shotgun the day his therapist transferred off our unit, or to the woman who jumped from her parents' 17th-floor apartment. There were others, however, who took overdoses of a sleeping compound, half expecting a boyfriend (in one instance) or a roommate (in another) to return, and who died because they guessed wrong.

Although it is reassuring to learn that the near-death experiences catalyzed the life forces in several of the almost-suicides—in effect, "curing" them in a way their previous therapy had not yet done—we cannot, of course, rely upon such extreme and unpredictable measures to save other suicidal patients. This is all the more reason, then, to adopt an ultraconservative policy when working with suicidal patients (in some cases, maintaining personal contact via telephone even during vacations; in others, hospitalizing at the first sign of decompensation; etc.). If our efforts succeed, a greater proportion of those who want to die will become more genuinely life-oriented, and fewer of those who secretly wish to go on living need forfeit that wish.

Diekstra (1987), who also cautions us that "suicide threats or gestures and suicide attempts must always be taken seriously" (p. 46), has also advocated assessment of the ratio of expectation of death to expectation of indirectly solving a problem via a suicidal act. Those who begin with *low* lethality–manipulativeness ratios will often progress, if their acts are dismissed or ignored, to *more* lethal attitudes and acts. Would the rate of suicide completion have been higher if the hospital staff entrusted with the care of the PI-500 had been more blasé? Probably. But we can never know precisely, because as clinicians we have neither the moral right nor the stomach to test such a hunch "scientifically."

PARASUICIDE

Suicide gestures that were not truly intended to be fatal are now often collected under the heading "parasuicide" (Kreitman, 1977). Many parasuicidal acts are committed with the intention of manipulating a lover or family member. Others commit these acts in hopes of extricating themselves from an intolerable situation. Here too is "manipulation"—not to get *more* attention from someone, but to get *away* from someone (usually from an abusive intimate). Though many suicide gestures have little actual suicidal *intent* behind them, I continue to use the term "parasuicide" in this section, though Diekstra's (1988) phrase "deliberate self-harm" is more accurate.

Parasuicide is not the exclusive preserve of borderline patients. Clinicians have long felt, however, that nonpsychotic persons who make suicide gestures or who mutilate themselves are "special" and deserve placement in a category that somehow calls attention to this self-injurious propensity. Lately, BPD has become that category. Both the Gunderson and the DSM definitions incorporate manipulative suicide gestures in their diagnostic schemata. Not all BPD patients exhibit this sign; not all nonpsychotic parasuicides are "borderline." But a history of parasuicide makes clinicians feel on surer footing about the diagnosis of BPD than they would in the presence of other signs, such as anger or labile affect. We want, of course, to avoid the triviality of tautology: "Parasuicides are borderline *because* borderline depends in large measure on the presence of parasuicide." Since "borderline" is only a diagnostic construct in the minds of various mental health professionals, and not a pathogen-induced entity like measles, we must at least make sure that as a construct it does not chase its own tail.

What conditional probabilities emerge in the PI-500 with respect to this parasuicide–borderline question? Distinguishing (serious) attempts from (nonserious) gestures is not always easy, even for clinicians on the scene at the time, let alone for those relying upon old records. Besides, the language in the

TABLE 4.4. Patients among the Major Diagnostic Groups Who Made Suicide *Gestures* (but Not Attempts) *before* the Index Admission

Diagnostic group	Total n	Gestures only	
		n	%
Borderlines			
BPD females	145	53	37
BPD males	61	22	36
D females	14	4	29
D males	21	5	24
Other BPO females	22	5	23
Other BPO males	35	4	11
Total	298[a]	93	31
Psychotics			
SZ	99	16	16
SA males	23	1	4
SA females	41	14	34
MDP	39	10	26
SF	36	3	8
Total	238	44	18

[a]This figure does not include the one patient in whom the distinction between BPD and BPO was unclear.

old records was sometimes imprecise. Someone might have spoken of an "attempt" in a case where a patient had ingested 10 aspirins and immediately phoned a relative. Incidents of this sort I amended to "gesture" status. I can only hope that review of the records and my judgment calls kept error within tolerable limits. Table 4.4 shows the results of this review. Among the major diagnostic groups in the PI-500, I could count some 137 patients who, before entering PI, had made only suicide gestures but no attempts. If one called a patient "borderline" (by broad criteria) on the basis of parasuicide alone, one would be right two times out of three (93 of 137, or 68%). This is too wide a margin of error to justify the equation "If parasuicide, then borderline"; yet, for a clinical sign in psychiatry, this degree of correctness is rather impressive. Most parasuicide was concentrated in the BPD population, where over a third (36%) had histories of gestures only. If one relies on DSM criteria, then "gestures only" were concentrated in BPD only to the level of 55% (75 of 137), since 13% of the parasuicidal behavior occurred in dysthymics, anorectics, and patients with other personality disorders who were borderline only by Kernberg criteria.

The predictive power of "parasuicide only" is not very great in the borderlines. Almost all the suicide completers were BPD patients (17 of 19). Of these, 2 of the 10 female completers had made only gestures, as had 4 of the 7 male completers. Of BPD patients who entered PI because of a suicide gesture,

6 of 75 (8%) went on, usually within 4 years, to a completed suicide; however, 11 out of every 12 are still alive at this writing, from 10 to 20 or more years later. Similarly, only two of the nine schizophrenic suicides began their fatal careers with gestures alone; five gave no indication of death wishes at all.

It is worth mentioning here that assessment of parasuicides, suicide attempts, and their relationship to suicide is complicated by the fact that in psychiatry death always looks preventable (certainly in the age range of the PI-500), whereas in oncology—in the case of metastatic melanoma, for example—death always looks inevitable. Yet some melanomas recede spontaneously, and some suicides are, as best one can tell, *not* preventable (though perhaps postponable). Was the weak correlation between parasuicide and real suicide an artifact of the prolonged and excellent care we gave our borderline patients, such that we saved some who would otherwise have died? To a small extent, this may be so. The truth may be unknowable. One could try to compare follow-up results of "matched" patients from different treatment centers with different programs, lengths of stay, and so on. But matched patients are not clones. Dissimilar suicide rates may reflect, not differences in care, but hidden differences in the patients themselves.

At present, we can identify certain high-risk groups (Allebeck, Varla, & Wistedt, 1986; Angst & Clayton, 1986; Michel, 1987), but this does not always provide us with the clues we need to spot individual patients at high risk or to tide them over the vulnerable years when the lethality of their illness is at its height. The deciding factors are not so often diagnoses anyway, but the personality assets and ego strengths of various suicidal patients. Some such patients, when viewed from this perspective, seem clearly salvageable; others do not.

One borderline man, for example, had made a suicide gesture with a few sleeping pills, following a promotion at work for which he felt unqualified and unready. He came to PI against his will and tried to sign out the next day. We confronted him with his suicidality; we pleaded with him; we cajoled him for hours, much as SWAT teams do with "jumpers." Reluctantly, he agreed to stay. This drama repeated itself four or five times during the 26 months he spent on the unit. Throughout this lengthy stay, he spoke of suicide incessantly, and remained anhedonic despite subtoxic doses of antidepressants and a course of electroconvulsive therapy (ECT). He kept aloof from the other patients; for his two therapists, it was "like pulling teeth" to get him to reveal himself. He had no hope for the future, despite his IQ of 137 and his responsible job in engineering. Because of those assets and his caring family, he did not seem hopeless to us at first. But he made no changes at all in 2 years, and we grew pessimistic. When he signed out once again a few months later, our "SWAT team" enthusiasm was gone, and so was he. Three months later, on his 30th birthday, he killed himself—as he always said he would. Fifteen years have now passed since his death, but I still regard this patient as "salvageable," though I do not know what we could have done differently (apart from committing him to the hospital for the rest of his life). His family, his "life situation," did not seem that bad. Perhaps this was the key. There was nothing we could rescue him *from*. Instead, endogenous depressive features were so marked, his social inhibitions so great, as to make life seem an unending torture to him.

The reader may compare this parasuicide/suicide with the story of another borderline patient, whose parasuicide activity also consisted of mild overdoses on three or four occasions before her PI admission. She too spoke of suicide incessantly during the early phases of her 2-year stay, though she became less preoccupied with this theme toward the end. Unlike the man in the preceding vignette, however, she was not anhedonic. Characterologically, she was much more "perky." She was mistrustful and witheringly contemptuous of the hospital personnel for a long time, but made many friends among her fellow-patients. Her family was quite different from the engineer's. She had not become mistrustful without cause. Shortly before her hospitalization, she had been approached incestuously by her father and seduced by an uncle who began by taking advantage of her attractiveness in getting her to pose for "art photos." She had no one to whom she could turn and had resorted to the parasuicidal overdoses alluded to earlier. The message was clear: "Save me from this family!" Many months passed before she could admit *wanting* to be saved, but once this turning point came, she made great strides toward recovery. If we did nothing else, we rescued her from an intolerable environment, and created for her an undisturbed atmosphere within which her various strengths could assert themselves. Fifteen years have elapsed since her discharge, also, except that at follow-up she was very much alive, married, raising a family, and helping to run a successful business. She had made no more suicide gestures since leaving the hospital. Hers is one of dozens of cases in the PI-500 of parasuicide as a cry for help, from someone who had the makings of a gratifying life once the rescue had been accomplished.

Some of our best outcomes had this sort of opening chapter. As a clinical rule, we might "triage" parasuicidal acts in this way: those that reflect genuine hopelessness; those that represent outrageous manipulations of others; and those that signify a cry for help in the face of intolerable life circumstances. Suicide is very likely in the first instance (though many truly hopeless, suicidally inclined patients do not "waste time" with faint gestures; they commit acts of extreme lethality, often with no warning). The manipulative are generally immature and narcissistic. These are the "quintessential" borderlines, who ultimately improve if motivated enough to work on their characterological defects and if disciplined enough to become occupationally self-sufficient. A small percentage of these will ultimately commit suicide, especially if motivation and discipline are of a very low order and if drug or alcohol abuse is also part of the clinical picture. Borderline patients who make suicide gestures within the context of abusive backgrounds are often appealing in personality and quite salvageable (unless the abuse has been overwhelming and protracted). Removal from the traumatizing environment, long-term residential care (especially for adolescents who need only a year or so before college or work), and supportive/ rehabilitative therapy may be sufficient to effect a recovery in such cases, even without much exploration of the deeper conflicts.

Parasuicide, like the more serious attempts, is more worrisome in male than in female patients with BPD: In the PI-500, the BPD males with attempts or parasuicide are now dead of suicide in 20% of cases (5 of 25); the females, in 10% (9 of 88).[3] This warning is especially valid in relation to highly narcissistic young men who measure their worth by impossibly high standards of vocational achievement. The perfectionistic engineer in the example above left himself no other sources of gratification. In the PI-500, several borderline men of average abilities felt humiliated by the high levels of success their fathers had achieved, and have now committed suicide. Our culture makes it easier for a woman than for a man to feel content "just" having built a successful love relationship. As difficult as that is, becoming the head of a large corporation is necessarily a rarer accomplishment (there being fewer such positions). Factors of this sort may account for the "paradox" in which the engineer from the good family is now dead and the woman from the abusive family is now thriving.

Though Kullgren (1988) noted a tendency toward higher completed suicides in a small series of BPD patients with *multiple* as opposed to *single* previous attempts, this correlation did not hold true in the PI-500. Among the latter, 5 of 25 borderlines who had made one serious suicide attempt before the index hospitalization have committed suicide, along with 2 of the 18 who had made multiple previous attempts.

In recounting the two vignettes just above, I am aware that the inevitability of the engineer's suicide may not look so inevitable to the reader. Because the suicide seemed to be an expression of underlying illness—a disease of the brain, if you will—there may be room for doubts: "Perhaps a trial of monoamine oxidase inhibitors . . . perhaps a second course of ECT. . . ." Perhaps. If the reader remains unconvinced, let me offer as a final example a suicide whose inevitability may give the most hardened skeptic pause. This case was set in motion not by illness or by aberration of personality, but by the kind of circumstances that make one a pariah even to oneself.

In one of the earlier cohorts of the PI-500 was a borderline man of 20, admitted because of a suicide gesture with hypnotics. Throughout the year before his hospitalization, his mother, who had been blatantly seductive toward him all his remembered life, had led him into an openly incestuous relationship. A month before he came to our unit, she killed herself with pills he fetched for her from the pharmacy. He carried out his errand already suspecting the purpose to which this prescription would be put. While on the unit he acted the model patient, withheld all mention of his suicidal impulses, and seldom made

---

[3]BPD males with gesture(s) *only* were more apt to commit suicide than BPD females with gesture(s) *only:* 4 of 22 males (18%), compared with 2 of 53 (4%) females. BPD females who had made both gestures and attempts were more likely to commit suicide: 4 of 18, or 22%.

reference to the Sophoclean mold into which his life had been compressed. Actually, the hospital personnel did not know the complete story until after his release. Once he revealed the details some months later, he killed himself with the same medication his mother had used. Unlike his mother, he gave no perceptible warnings beforehand. Naively, one might suppose that a skilled therapist could have helped him "work through" the intolerable guilt, especially because he had, after all, been a victim, not a perpetrator. But his was not a guilt to be worked through. *Tout comprendre, c'est tout pardonner* is not always curative for our patients, any more than it was for Oedipus (who had an even better excuse than our patient; the Theban king had no way of knowing who this Jocasta person was).

As clinicians, we must familiarize ourselves with the statistics: "The risk of suicide, given the suicide of a parent, equals X." I hope that this book will make a contribution to this process. But at the same time as we struggle to rescue every would-be suicide from premature death, we need to be aware that certain circumstances *dictate* suicide, with a compellingness beyond our skills to overturn. Of the 49 suicides in the PI-500, the lives of some half dozen, as best I can judge, had been ruined to this extent. Viewed from another perspective, the majority who committed suicide might have been saved by means already available to psychiatry. As for the remainder, only elimination of the predisposing circumstances would have been curative. We cannot change the past of patients who have already been irremediably traumatized. We can only change the "past" of those yet unborn. And this can be effected only through such measures as reduction of parental abuse and elevation of the general standards of living. These are sociopolitical tasks, not the tasks of individual psychotherapy; their success will reward the next generation, but not the current one. Follow-up studies can play a part in this effort, through their delineation of different *profiles* of persons at high risk for suicide: Which profiles are amenable to pharmacotherapy and psychotherapy? Which are reflective of ills curable only at the societal level?

SELF-MUTILATION

On the continuum of suicidal behavior, self-mutilative acts are ordinarily at the milder extreme. Certain grotesque or extreme examples of self-mutilation include suicidal intent (cutting one's throat); however, the majority of such acts probably express no suicidal intent at all, but rather extreme tension or frustration (Graff & Mallin, 1967; Grunebaum & Klerman, 1967; Menninger, 1935; Pao, 1969b; Pattison & Kahan, 1983; Rosen & Thomas, 1984; Rosenthal, Rinzler, Wallsh, & Klausner, 1972). Often self-mutilation is more dramatic and bloody than, say, a suicide attempt with barbiturates. One of the PI-500 patients burned her initials on her forearm with a cigarette; another criss-crossed the skin of all four extremities with a razor—a flamboyant act,

TABLE 4.5. Self-Mutilation among the Major Diagnostic Groups

Diagnostic group	*n* traced	SMA only	SMA + SG/SA	% with SMA	Completed suicide SMA only	Completed suicide SMA + SG/SA
Borderlines						
BPD females	141	10	20	21.3	0	1
BPD males	52	0	2	3.8	0	0
D females	13	0	0	0	0	0
D males	21	0	0	0	0	0
Other BPO females	21	0	1	4.8	0	1
Other BPO males	27	1	1	7.4	0	0
Totals	273	11	24	12.8	0	2
Psychotics						
SZ	96	1	4	5.3	0	1
SA females	40	2	6	20.0	0	2
SA males	21	0	0	0	0	0
MDP females	15	0	3	20.0	0	0
MDP males	23	0	0	0	0	0
SF	32	2	0	6.3	0	0
Totals	226	5	13	7.9	0	3

Note. SMA, self-mutilative acts; SG, suicide gestures; SA, suicidal acts. Total patients with SMA (borderlines *and* psychotics) = 53 of 499, or 10.6%; total of SMA patients who committed suicide = 5 of 53, or 9.4%.

despite the superficiality of the cuts. It is easy to understand why behavior of this sort stimulates clinicians to make a diagnosis more serious than "neurotic," especially if the patient is past adolescence. Not all self-mutilative behavior leads to hospitalization; a certain proportion of mild cases (very superficial wrist-cutting) are bandaged in emergency rooms and (not always wisely) sent home.

The self-mutilative histories of the 53 PI-500 patients who indulged in these acts may represent some of the more dangerous bands of the self-mutilative spectrum. Borderlines accounted for 54% of the PI-500, but for 66% (35 of 53) of the self-mutilators. Within the (broadly defined) borderline group, 91% of the self-mutilators (32/35) were BPD cases. Almost all were women. These data are spelled out in Table 4.5, and are in line with the observations of Schaffer, Carroll, and Abramowitz (1982) to the effect that nonpsychotic patients who mutilate themselves usually meet the Gunderson or DSM criteria for BPD.

Having divided the self-mutilating patients into two groups—one with a history of suicidal acts prior to the index admission, and one without such a history—I noted that the mutilation-only group contains no patients who have (as yet) gone on to a completed suicide. The sample is admittedly small (*n* = 16), but the result is nonetheless of interest. The finding suggests that the 5 completed suicides among the 37 patients exhibiting both self-mutilation *and* suicidal acts were a function of whatever impelled these patients to the suicidal gestures or attempts (rather than of other factors impelling them to wrist-scratching, etc.). The validity of this correlation needs to be tested in other large-scale follow-up studies.

Similarly in need of further study is the apparent predilection of female patients (especially those with BPD) for self-mutilative behavior. How much do biological factors (e.g., premenstrual shifts in neuroendocrine balance) account for the phenomenon? How much are psychosocial factors responsible (e.g., is such behavior a measure of last resort for a woman entrapped by an abusive man)? Perhaps future follow-up studies of borderline self-mutilators will be able to test the hypothesis emerging from Coid's work (Coid, Allolio, & Rees, 1983): He and his colleagues noted elevations of plasma metenkephalin concentration in a group of habitual self-mutilators. Subjective relief of symptoms after self-mutilation may coincide, as Coid et al. suggest, with a reduction in a neuropeptide that subserves the perception of pain.

TOPICS FOR FUTURE RESEARCH

This chapter on suicide and suicidal behavior should serve to remind the reader both how far we have come in identifying risk factors and how poor is our ability to predict just *which* high-risk patients will actually die by their own hands during some specified interval. Roy (1985) has written an excellent summary of what we do know: For example, about 1% of the general population will eventually die of suicide, and nearly all of the latter will have some diagnosable emotional disorder at the time. Also, the suicide rate in alcoholics is about 75 times that of the general population; 7% of alcoholics commit suicide within 5 years of their latest hospitalization. This is a correlation I "rediscovered" in connection with the PI-500. Roy's comment that 10% of schizophrenics die by suicide is a confirmation of the impressions generated by the present study (where, thus far, almost 10% of the schizophrenics have now committed suicide). All such estimates need to be interpreted in the light of cultural factors; presumably, the figures would be higher for comparable diagnostic groups in "high-risk" populations or countries (Hungary, Sweden), and lower in low-risk populations (Italy, American blacks).

Pokorny (1983) has made it plain that mere identification of high-risk populations affords us little predictive ability vis-à-vis individual patients: In his large-*n* sample, only half the eventual suicides belonged to his "high-risk" subgroup, and only 1 patient in 20 among the "high-risk" patients actually died. Even adding certain unusual factors to our computers enhances our predictive powers only slightly. Hankoff (1980) drew attention, for example, to the heightened occurrence of suicide in psychiatric units undergoing rotation of therapists or abrupt changes in treatment ideology or morale. We saw this in connection with the last cohort of the PI-500. All this still accounts for only a small percentage of the variance.

We should remember that the data we do have stem largely from persons with *less* than the most severe forms of suicidality. Gardner and Cowdry (1985, p. 391), in their excellent article on suicidal behavior in BPD, divided self-destructive tendencies into four broad categories: those associated with melancholia, impulsive/retributive rage, communicative parasuicidal gestures, and self-mutilation to relieve dysphoria. But the most determined among, say, the melancholic kill themselves after careful planning and on their first try. Although we can identify some of the gross risk factors in such persons (e.g., age, sex, employment, marital status), we can learn very little about the true nature of their immediate or past psychological environments. What if almost all such suicides were linked with intense maternal rejection or with withering humiliation at work or at home? Would the offending parties be likely to come forward with such information? As it is, the worst-risk patients are known only to the police and to the coroners, except in cases of miraculous survival (see "Almost-Suicides," above).

The PI-500 study points to hostility and aggression as strong predictors in those who are already suicide-prone. Klerman, Lavori, and Rice (1985), for example, showed that the incidence of depression varies considerably according to year of birth; that onset of depression is occurring earlier than in the past; and that the calendar years associated with increased rates of depression correlate with the years associated with higher-than-expected suicide rates. My impression is that, in recent years, young people (i.e., adolescents and young adults) susceptible to depression/hopelessness are for some reason also more likely to convert their despair into lethal action, the more so if fueled by rage and fury. Wetzel, Reich, Murphy, Province, and Miller (1987), in their meticulous study of suicide rates in white and nonwhite men and women during the half century beginning in 1933, examined the effects of age, of birth cohort, and of the period of time within which suicides were occurring. They drew attention not only to the increasing risk for suicide in the third decade of life (especially in white males), but also to the decreasing risk in middle-aged and older people. Their findings suggested that certain social changes in America were intervening so as to reduce risk during the second half of life, while other social changes were heightening the risk for those under 40.

The most important social change operating to undermine one's ability to resist the temptation of suicide is, in the opinion of many (Brent et al., 1988; Murphy, 1988; Rich, Fowler, Fogarty, & Young, 1988), substance abuse. Since the mid-1960s, abuse of illicit drugs has been a persistent and pervasive factor affecting those who are just entering young adult life (as the patients of the PI-500 were), more than those who are just exiting this phase. Alcohol abuse has become more prevalent also, and has begun to affect certain social groups in the United States where the alcoholism rate has traditionally been low. If serious depressive disorders are occurring at earlier ages (for whatever still-to-be-elucidated reasons), and if persons in the age range 15–30 are now more likely to abuse alcohol and other disinhibiting drugs, the suicide rate may indeed increase appreciably just for this one reason. (For further discussion of issues pertaining to substance abuse, see Chapter Nine.)

Doubtless the situation is more complex, with other factors also accounting for some of the variance. One possibility is that a higher divorce rate may be leading to a higher proportion of children with poor support systems and of girls reared with and sexually abused by stepfathers, leading in turn to heightened risk for BPD and suicidal acts. Diekstra and Moritz (1987), in their excellent overview of suicide among adolescents, cite the divorce factor as important for other reasons, applicable probably to a higher proportion of potential suicide completers: Not only has the increasing divorce rate in developing countries over the past two decades exposed a large number of young persons to a weakened support systems, but it has made them vulnerable to rejection by one or another parent. Diekstra and Moritz also mention the diminishing rates of church affiliation as another factor weakening ties to one's social group. It is noteworthy that within the PI-500 (and by no means confined to this small segment of our population) many turned eventually to one or another major religion, unconventional religion, or commune, as an antidote to the anomie to which Diekstra and Moritz allude (see also "Religious Cults," Appendix B). Holinger, Offer, and Zola (1988) have speculated that increasing proportions of adolescents in the population as a whole during recent times may have heightened competition for jobs, and thus may have heightened the suicide risk among persons with depression or low self-esteem. Violence in the home may also contribute in an analogous way. It remains unclear whether the families in our country are actually becoming more violent, or whether we have merely begun to unearth secrets whose frequency has perhaps not changed much from one era to another.

There is, at all events, reason to hope that in a generation new factors will have emerged—ones that relate more to the particular psychological past of high-risk persons—so that our predictive powers will be fairly respectable even on behalf of individual patients.

Parental Morbidity, Subsequent Morbidity, and Striking "Borderline" Characteristics in the Borderline Patients

PSYCHIATRIC ILLNESS IN THE PARENTS OF BORDERLINE PATIENTS

A number of investigators have studied the incidence of psychiatric illness in the close relatives of borderline patients (Akiskal, 1981; Andrulonis, Glueck, Stroebel, & Vogel, 1982; Links, Steiner, & Huxley, 1988; Stone, Kahn, & Flye, 1981). Many have noted a heightened incidence of affective illness in the families of borderlines, compared with the families of schizophrenic (SZ) patients. This difference has not always held when patients with DSM-defined borderline personality disorder (BPD) were compared with those manifesting other personality disorders (Barasch, Frances, Hurt, Clarkin, & Cohen, 1985). The proportion of close relatives with alcoholism has been particularly striking (Links et al., 1988).[1] The significance of this correlation is not always clear. The symptomatology and abnormal personality development that characterize BPD could come about as expressions of the genetic liability associated with some types of alcoholism. Or the instability, abusiveness, and sexual molestation that often accompany the alcoholic family might be themselves engender the clinical picture of BPD. SZ, in contrast, is rare in the families of BPD patients.

For the PI-500, I have better information about their parents than about

---

[1]In the Andrulonis et al. (1982) series, the first-degree relatives of borderline patients were often alcoholics (35%), though the proportion of alcoholic first-degree relatives of the schizophrenics in this series was equally high (36%).

TABLE 5.1. Psychiatric Illness in the Parents of Borderline and Schizophrenic Patients

Diagnostic group	n, all biological parents[a]	Parental illness					n, parents with these conditions
		Alcoholism	MAD	BPD	SD	Probable SZ	
BPD males	48	7	4	2	0	0	12[b]
BPD females	78	15	3	3	0	0	20
BPD × MAD males	66	6	4	3	0	0	11[c]
BPD × MAD females	203	22	21	2	2	0	45[d]
Total BPD	395	50	32	10	2	0	88
D	72	1	13	0	1	2	17
Other BPO	107	8	9	1	3	1	21[e]
SZ	198	8	13	1	4	4	25[f]

[a]Adoptive parents excluded.
[b]12 = 13 minus 1 (MAD × alcoholism).
[c]11 = 13 minus 1 (MAD × alcoholism) minus 1 (BPD × MAD).
[d]45 = 47 minus 1 (SZ × alcoholism) minus 1 (BPD × MAD).
[e]21 = 22 minus 1 (MAD × BPD).
[f]25 = 26 minus 1 (MAD × alcoholism).

their siblings. If we put to one side "probable" and "spectrum" cases of the functional psychoses, or those cases where a parent had been "psychotic" without a reliable diagnosis, then the major differences between groups show up in relation to alcoholism. Table 5.1 presents the data concerning the ill parents of the SZ patients and of the various borderline subgroups. Patients with BPD were more likely to have alcoholic parents than were the dysthymic (D) and other borderline personality organization (BPO) patients, $\chi^2 = 7.8$, $df = 1$, $p < .01$. Parental alcoholism was also greater among the BPD than among the SZ patients, $\chi^2 = 11.1$, $p < .001$.

Significant differences did not emerge when I focused on "certain" as opposed to "probable" SZ in the parents. If one includes "probable" SZ, there did appear to be more schizophrenic parents among the SZ than among the BPD patients ($p < .01$). In addition, the SZ patients were more apt to have parents who were "paranoid," "delusionally jealous," or "schizotypal" (13 of 198) than were the BPD patients (9 of 395). Major affective disorder (MAD) was more common in the parents of the dysthymic than of the BPD patients ($p < .01$), but the difference between the BPD and SZ groups in this regard was not significant.

The next section of this chapter discusses in more detail the occurrence of manic–depressive psychosis (MDP) among parents of borderline patients, as well as the number of patients initially diagnosed as borderline who went on to develop MDP.

PARENTAL AND SUBSEQUENT
MANIC–DEPRESSIVE PSYCHOSIS
AMONG THE BORDERLINES

I began the follow-up of the PI-500 hoping not only to sketch the natural history of borderline and related conditions, but also to shed light on the relationship between borderline and affective disorders. In my earlier papers (Stone, 1977; Stone et al., 1981), my colleagues and I put forward the hypothesis that a large proportion of borderline conditions, perhaps 60%, arose out of genetic predisposition to MDP. Placed in evidence to support this contention was our observation that many borderlines had one or more first-degree relatives with unipolar or bipolar forms of MDP. A number of authors subsequently submitted similar findings (Akiskal, 1981; Andrulonis et al., 1982), and also spoke of a causative relationship in a subgroup of borderline patients. This seemed plausible whether one began with "borderlines" defined by broad or by restrictive criteria. A number of other authors challenged these conclusions (Kroll, 1988; Kroll, Carey, & Sines, 1985; Loranger, Oldham, & Tulis, 1982; Pope, Jonas, & Hudson, 1983; Rutter, 1987; Torgersen, 1984). Torgersen (1984) drew attention to the fact that many borderlines had no such affective pedigrees; what we were claiming as "causation" was merely correlation or overlap of essentially different entities. Barasch et al. (1985) showed that depressive illness, in particular, was indeed common in the families of patients with DSM-defined BPD, but was also (and about equally) common in the close relatives of patients with other types of personality disorders. These data cast doubt upon any claims of *specificity* regarding the power of "risk genes" for MDP to engender *borderline,* as opposed to other, personality disorders.

Now that the lives of the 299 borderlines in the PI-500 have unfolded over a span of 10 to 25 years since their discharge from the hospital, I am in a position to re-examine these issues from a vantage point not available when my colleagues and I published our initial hunches. The sample size is also considerably larger than that of our earlier (or indeed of any subsequent) studies, even when the sample is shorn of those patients not meeting DSM criteria for BPD.

In this section, I direct attention to just those patients ($n = 26$) who, having been diagnosed as borderline upon admission, went on to develop some type of MDP during the years between discharge and follow-up. The ratio of this diagnostic conversion (or *addition,* in those cases where the borderline features were still very much in evidence) was the same, whether I began with the broad-criteria borderlines (26 of 299, or 8.7%) or with the BPD patients only (17 of 205, or 8.3%).

It will be a useful mental exercise to suppress for the moment our usual tendency as diagnosticians to speak in absolute terms. The most treacherous words here are "is" and "are." Once we claim that such-and-such patient "is" borderline, we begin to convince ourselves that we have stumbled upon something as real, as susceptible to external validation, as finding tubercle bacilli in a coughing person. In psychiatry, we are rarely offered anything so neat. Instead, we must deal with conditions that evolve over time (prodigious stretches of time, in many instances), and that we are compelled by clinical urgency to diagnose from just one brief temporal segment—rather as though we were obliged to guess the contents of a hero sandwich from a random slice. The younger the patient, the more difficult the task, for here we are again given merely the butt end of the "sandwich" from which to make our section, with the longer remaining portion to be supplied to us slowly over the next 10 or so years. Patients whom psychiatrists label "borderline" are usually young; in the PI-500, a quarter of the patients were adolescents under 18. Initially, even looking at the cross-sectional view revealed to us not a clearly recognizable picture (equivalent to the tubercle bacilli in the example above), but rather a patchwork quilt of signs and symptoms, of whose individual pieces we had then to create (if we could) some meaningful pattern.

Borderlines Who Became Unipolar

The nine patients diagnosed as borderline at PI who went on to manifest a picture of unipolar recurrent depression in the years to come were an older group when first seen; their average age was 26 (range = 19–35). One of the patients was already the subject of controversy, inasmuch as his clinical signs were also compatible with a mild agitated depression. Self-mutilation and suicide gestures were noted in all but three cases.

In retrospect, the crisis that led to initial hospitalization could be understood as the first, and therefore not as yet "recurrent," major depressive episode in the life of a unipolar patient. One of these patients, 19 years old on admission, grew convinced that his condition would hold him back all his life; he committed suicide 5 years later. His therapist at PI had found him "vague, inaccessible, and eerie" and had been unable to establish rapport with him. The remaining eight had an average Global Assessment Scale (GAS) score at follow-up of 62 (range = 35–75), indicating good overall functioning but with continuing mild symptoms. One was a successful executive, married with three children. His score would have been much higher, were it not for occasional waves of depression that passed over him at unpredictable times and for which he took antidepressants.

In their 1985 paper, Barasch et al. reported that 6 of 10 patients diagnosed as having BPD in 1979 were still so diagnosed 3 years later; the original impression thus had a predictive sensitivity of 60%. But this was a small sample and a brief interval. At intervals of 15 to over 20 years, this predictive power may fizzle out: Of the eight still-alive PI borderlines who went on to become "unipolar," only two continued at follow-up to exhibit the angry, impulsive, and self-injurious features of BPD. The other six, five of whom I interviewed personally at follow-up, would no longer qualify as Kernberg borderlines either. These were now well-functioning persons, indistinguishable (with one exception) from their neighbors. They were affected by transitory periods of pessimism and gloom, which they were able to conceal from those around them. The exception was a woman with a rather saturnine (depressed/irritable) disposition, whom her coworkers experienced as cranky and joyless. Only three of the eight were ever rehospitalized (one who remained and two who no longer remained "borderlines" at follow-up).

With respect to family background, these nine borderline-turned-unipolar patients had six parents with unipolar depression and one with nonrecurrent major depression. Of the 18 parents, that is, 39% were unipolar or had a severe depression; one had committed suicide. Five of the families contained at least one such parent.

One might advance the hypothesis that, in these five families at least, risk genes were transmitted that substantially heightened the likelihood of a subsequent affective disorder. The latter manifested itself first as a "borderline condition," usually in late adolescence, and then went on years later to take on the clinical coloration of unipolar depression—the same condition diagnosed in the parent(s) a generation earlier.

Borderlines Who Developed Atypical or Bipolar Affective Disorders

The 17 PI-500 borderlines who went on to develop bipolar illness, atypical depression, or bipolar II illness (episodes of hypomania plus severe depression) were more numerous and somewhat younger than their unipolar-to-be counterparts. The average age for these patients was 22.8 (range = 15–39); four were 17 or younger on admission. Some already showed some signs of atypical depression (making them examples of BPD × atypical depression comorbidity) during their hospitalization. This is in line with Soloff, George, Nathan, and Schulz's (1987) observation that such comorbidity is common (41% in their series) in a BPD population.

Although in most series the incidence of severe affective illness in the families of bipolars is as great as in the families of unipolars, the parents of these 17 borderlines showed full-blown forms of MDP in only 2 instances of 34 (5.9%)—the father of one patient, the mother of another. Both were bipolar. Major but nonpsychotic depressions were noted in another four parents. Altogether, six parents (17.6%) showed some form of serious affective illness. SZ was mentioned in the history of one of the mothers and in one sibling. Two other siblings were bipolar. About a third of the families (6 of 17, or 35%) had at least one affectively ill first-degree relative.

The mean GAS score at follow-up in this subgroup was 60.4 (i.e., essentially the same as for the unipolar-to-be patients). The range was broader (10–85). There have been no suicides, though four made serious attempts before coming to PI and one patient became strongly suicidal in the time immediately preceding follow-up, after the loss of a love relationship.

The same argument made on behalf of the borderlines with unipolar parents and a unipolar evolution seems plausible for several of those with bipolars among their close relatives and a bipolar evolution. Actually, the lines need not be so clearly drawn, since unipolar patients sometimes have bipolar relatives and vice versa. The bipolar relatives of the PI-500 patients who were diagnosed as MDP on re-examination of their admission records were to be found more often in the families of the *bipolar* patients; only rarely were they found in the families of the *unipolar* patients. Among the latter, one had a father with "manic temperament" (a *forme fruste* of bipolar MDP). She became alcoholic, was wildly impulsive, and eventually committed suicide.

Some of the bipolar and bipolar II patients (on admission) would have been diagnosed as having BPD by DSM criteria, were it not for the overshadowing psychotic affective features. Bipolar II patients in general often show the impulsivity, aggressivity, flamboyance, and lability that are characteristic of DSM or Gunderson borderlines. It is not surprising that some of the PI-500 borderlines evolved into bipolar and bipolar II patients over the years. It is a little surprising that more ended up unipolar than bipolar II, given the similarity of the clinical picture of the latter to BPD. Possibly this discrepancy is a reflection of a heightened likelihood that unipolar and "unipolar-to-be" suicidally inclined patients will be hospitalized at some point, in comparison to bipolar-to-be borderlines. The latter are often outgoing, recover from loss more readily, and come to the attention of clinics and private practitioners more often than that of hospitals for long-term care.

Several of the patients who became bipolar responded particularly well to lithium and had been well for many years by the time of follow-up. One future bipolar II patient who was given to "speaking in tongues" (see "Religious Cults," Appendix B) while at PI had been asymptomatic for 15 years, was married, and was raising three children. Another eventual bipolar patient abused marijuana and was in and out of psychosis after leaving PI; however, once he stopped using the drug, he became well, worked, and raised a family. Still another, a gifted artist, had been well while on lithium for 17 years.

Some of the borderlines-turned-manic, however, were still quite symptomatic at follow-up; some, with very active forms of bipolar illness, were in the midst of a manic episode and were hospitalized at the time I traced them. Others had severe personality disorders that appeared to lower their ceiling of potential. These disorders were compatible with one of the Kraepelinian temperaments associated with MDP (most often, manic/irritable or cyclothymic). At least five of the bipolar-to-be borderlines raised the complaint so often voiced by bipolar manic–depressives—namely, that projects once begun were often interrupted or abandoned because of a resurgence of the illness. This was especially true of the "rapid cyclers" and in women with premenstrual aggravation of their mood disorder. Some had, reluctantly, to shift from a desired career to jobs that could be taken up or dropped in accordance with their mood of the moment. These former patients have gone into free-lance editing, driving cabs, home-based computer work, crafts, and other similar pursuits not wedded to rigid 9–5 schedules.

The fate of the affectively ill borderlines, many of whom, as I have tried to demonstrate, may best be regarded as attenuated cases of MDP, seems inextricably bound up with the attribute of *aggressivity*. The quintessential borderline—that is, the bipolar II, impulsive, histrionic, labile, suicide-gesture-prone, rageful patient—shows aggressivity in all its forms. Angst and Clayton (1986), in their discussion of the premorbid personalities of depressive and bipolar patients, mention that "the whole concept of aggression is confusing. . . . One must differentiate between irritability, anger, hostility and aggression; between aggressive thoughts alone, or with aggressive actions" (p. 527). Affectively ill borderlines, especially of the bipolar II type, often demonstrate this entire gamut, though not always in the same proportions. Those who commit suicide or are suicide-prone have usually exhibited a long-standing style of angry, impulsive decision-making (Crumley, 1981). Angst and Clayton also noted heightened nervousness, aggressivity, and depressiveness in unipolars when compared with a control group—in other words, greater instability in bipolars. Their findings would probably be applicable to our bipolar II patients and to many patients my colleagues and I are currently calling "borderline."

The implications of aggressivity for suicide potential are of critical importance. As noted elsewhere (see Chapter Four), completed suicide in the large borderline population of the PI-500 was limited almost entirely to those meeting the DSM criteria for BPD, which specifically include anger. In the relatively nonhostile, nonaggressive dysthymic borderlines who failed to meet DSM criteria, there have been no suicides.

In any given patient, it is not always clear what constitutes the major source of the aggressivity. In some borderlines, such as the ones referred to in this section, genetic predisposition appears to play a major role. This predisposition may interact in an unfortunate synergism with hostile responses from the parents. But even the latter do not always stem purely from pre-existing characterological problems in the parents. Some borderlines, as children, were remarkably colicky, tantrumy, provocative, and unruly when compared to their siblings. They drove their otherwise fairly reasonable parents to the edge. The "angry" parents, as they remember them years later, were in large measure creatures of their (the patients') own making. In other cases, of course, one or both parents were chronically hostile and were experienced as such by every other member of the family. As I mention elsewhere (see Chapter Seven), there are all too many cases in which the aggressivity in a borderline is most likely a reflexive trait, formed in imitation of an in defense against outrageous treatment by the parents. Some of the PI-500 patients, for example, were abused by a manic father. Here, nature and nurture intermixed in such a way as to give a double dose of aggressivity: innate plus induced.

Kernberg's (1975) useful concept of innate aggression, or Bergeret's (1984) concept of a *violence fondamentale,* would appear to overlap considerably with the concept of aggressivity (presumably biologically based), as alluded to here and in the paper of Angst and Clayton (1986). Certain patients (adolescents, especially) with "minimal brain damage," hyperkinetic syndromes, and temporal lobe epilepsy with partial complex seizures also show what might be viewed as a surplus of innate aggression. Perhaps in MDP there is a "true" surplus (unipolar < bipolar), whereas in "minimal brain damage" there may be an ordinary complement of aggressivity, insufficiently modulated because of the brain dysfunction. Someday we may be able to pinpoint specific central nervous system (CNS) pathways, mediated by dopaminergic or other neurotransmitters, that subserve the phenomena of aggressivity (see Pickar, 1986).

Another trait found with some frequency in affectively ill borderlines of the (more common) depressed type is anhedonia. The hypomanic, bipolar II types of affective disorder are less often associated with this diminished capacity for pleasure in borderlines. This may play a role in determining which borderlines will ever require hospitalization, especially over the long term, and which will have a good or a bad prognosis. Each subtype has advantages and disadvantages. In the bipolar II type, one often sees lability and impulsivity against a backdrop of histrionic, extraverted, and narcissistic characteristics. This is the kind of patient for whom Klein and Davis (1969) created the category "hysteroid dysphoria." Manipulative suicide gestures are more common than frank suicide attempts. Hospitalizations may be necessary at times, but are often brief. These patients will appear as the sickest of one's outpatient roster or as the healthiest of one's inpatients. Their pleasure sense is usually well developed; many such patients are indeed sensation-seeking and tend to collapse when sources of intense pleasure momentarily dry up. A broken romance may thus trigger an acute episode.

The unipolar-like borderlines, in contrast, often exhibit anhedonia. They are experienced by others as dour, pessimistic, perpetually anxious, and overly sensitive to criticism. Though less impulsive than the bipolar II borderlines, their suicidal behavior is apt to be more serious. When hurt they "stay down" longer, because they lack the keen pleasure sense that allows, say, a lovelorn bipolar II borderline to snap out of a depression at the prospect of a new lover. Klein and Davis (1969) have drawn attention to the relative ease with which "hysteroid dysphoric" patients can be flattered, humored, or otherwise "jollied" out of their depression. The anhedonic patient is not only more vulnerable to rejection, but, having learned the dreadful consequences of rejection (suicidal depression), will often learn to avoid intimate relationships altogether. Several of the PI-500 borderlines who (1) managed not to make a completed suicide attempt and (2) went on to become unipolar became inclined over the years toward the solitary life. At follow-up, they were "workaholics," perpetually gloomy individuals—but alive.

Comments

Although 8% is an impressive figure for the risk of BPD evolving into one or
another form of MDP, it cannot by itself silence the critics who do not accept
as likely the hypothesis that BPD and MDP may be at times interrelated (with
"risk genes" for MDP sometimes expressing themselves phenotypically as
BPD). Neither do the aforementioned articles in this section prove the null
hypothesis. The criticism has for the most part been derived from studies
containing very few subjects, or else from chart review. The present study, by
the same token, did not rely upon a standardized questionnaire and interview of
the nearly 1,100 biological parents. Our social service staff did, however, have
prolonged contact with almost all the parents. The numbers I cite regarding
parents who were hospitalized for affective illness, who committed suicide, and
so forth are trustworthy—the more so as I have had a chance to verify certain
questionable allusions in the old records or to discover, as part of the follow-up
process, instances of family mental illness occurring after the index patient left
the hospital.

I think we are now in a position to make a more convincing statement than
was hitherto possible—one that may settle, or at least quiet, the controversy
about BPD and affective illness. The statement hinges primarily on the matter of
etiological heterogeneity, and secondarily on that of sample variation. The
borderline syndrome, whether defined broadly, more narrowly (as in DSM), or
more precisely still (as by Gunderson), is simply not etiologically unitary. One
should think of it more as one does of "dropsy" (the 18th-century appellation
for congestive heart failure). The more physicians explored dropsy, the more
causes they found, until they eventually recognized it as a "final common
pathway" resulting from a multiplicity of sources. If 20, or 10, or (worse yet)
only 5 borderlines in 100 have families with pedigrees loaded heavily for MDP,
the statistician can easily enough "prove" that the relationship is merely a
"chance" one. Yet several of those pedigrees may contain close relatives with
very nearly the same clinical picture when they were the same age as the patient,
along with other close relatives with classic unipolar or bipolar conditions. We
know enough now about certain factors that place children at high risk for
MDP, but that may be decisive for BPD. Extreme irritability, moodiness,
impulsivity, tantrumy outbursts, and the like are especially common in these
situations. I have outlined a number of the relevant characteristics in Table 5.2.
If a young person goes on to develop in 8, 10, or 15 years a classical form of
MDP (as some of our PI-500 borderlines did), it seems to me that we could cut
through a lot of criticism with Occam's razor—and claim that in *this* patient, at
any rate, the BPD and MDP were different sides of the same coin, which turned
up at different phases during the course of that person's life.

Furthermore, I am willing to claim that some particular series of borderline
patients may be especially rich in just such pedigrees. The investigator stationed

TABLE 5.2. Traits, Symptoms, and Attributes Noted with Above-Expected Frequency in Children of Manic–Depressive Parents

A. Relevant taxonomic axes

1. Extraverted (related to manic temperament)
   Outgoing, exhibitionistic, clowning, expressive, creative, immature

2. Inhibited (related to depressive temperament)
   Unsociable, perfectionistic, shy, pessimistic, tense conscientious

3. Impulsive (related to irritable temperament)
   Poor impulse control, fidgety, distractible, aggressive, "conduct disorders," alienation of potential friends

B. Various characteristics and associated conditions

1. Attention deficit disorder	10. Moodiness
2. Brighter than average	11. Neurological soft signs
3. Creativity	12. Self-regulatory difficulties with attempts
4. Early reading ability	at "self-cure" through abuse of alcohol
5. Excitability	and drugs
6. Exuberance	13. Separation anxiety
7. Hyperactivity	14. Tantrums
8. Imaginativeness	15. Verbal > Performance scores on IQ tests
9. Modulation difficulties	16. Work capacity impaired

Note. Adapted from Kron et al. (1982, pp. 280–281) and from Kraepelin (1921).

at a treatment center where those are indeed these local conditions must inevitably conclude that in such-and-such percentage of cases, BPD is a phenotype of MDP risk. One might encounter these "local conditions," for example, in a largely urban patient population whose families were comparatively less inclined to abuse their children physically, sexually, or emotionally. I regard the PI-500 as an illustrative sample.

My experience as I write these tendentious remarks is now a quarter-century greater than it was during my residency at PI. I have done clinical research involving extensive interviewing of borderline patients for various periods of time—in rural America, in American cities far from New York, and in many foreign countries (Sweden, France, Switzerland, Thailand, Australia, Israel, Hungary, etc.). I now recognize that there are many samples of borderline patients in which very different conditions obtain. In Brisbane, Australia, for example, the two dozen borderlines I either interviewed or learned about through case presentations had almost no affectively ill relatives. Many had alcoholic parents. But the rates of incest and physical abuse were strikingly high (incest alone, over 50%; one *or* the other form of abuse, about 90%). The same was true in samples with which I became familiar at treatment facilities in rural New Hampshire, in Seattle, and in Topeka. Had I taken my training at one of those centers, my theoretical stance would have overlapped with that of Rutter or Pope—until I encountered samples of a quite different kind in New York City, or Hartford, or Paris, or Lyons, or wherever. In Scandinavia, young people tend to be more reserved than is customary in America; their "border lines" appear more schizotypal on average than ours do. Some make suicide gestures, but impulsivity and inordinate display of anger are less common. Their ill relatives are more often schizoid or depressed, and less often bipolar, compared with, say, those of the PI-500.

In Table 5.3, I have described the BPD → MDP subgroup of patients and have included data concerning psychiatric disorders in their parents. (These patients are indicated by plus signs in the "DSM-III BPD?" column.)

In conclusion, rather than to assert simplistically that BPD "is" or "is not" a manifestation of MDP, it would henceforth seem more prudent to report that in one's borderline series X% of the patients appear to have developed the BPD syndrome on the basis of strong loading for MDP; Y%, on the basis of severe abuse in early life; and Z%, because of an interaction (as best one can tell) of unfavorable factors from both sources. There will be a remainder, of varying size, of cases that evolved out of constitutional factors unrelated to MDP (cf. Andrulonis et al.'s [1981] series of "episodic dyscontrol" cases in adolescents). For still other borderlines, a question mark will hang over their cases, perhaps for many years, and we will be unable to compartmentalize the etiological factors with any certainty.

PARENTAL AND SUBSEQUENT MORBIDITY AMONG THE DYSTHYMIC BORDERLINES

The D borderlines had the best average outcomes of any major diagnostic group within the PI-500. Their median GAS score at follow-up was 70. Fifty percent showed clinical recovery (GAS > 70); 73.5% were "well" (GAS > 60); and none of the 34 traced patients (out of 36 total) has committed suicide thus far. They were the most likely to marry and have children. Some of the reasons for this encouraging picture lay concealed not too far beneath the surface—in the layer of initial diagnostic criteria. These were the patients who exhibited BPO but showed fewer than five items when assessed by DSM criteria, though they *did* meet criteria for MAD. With respect to DSM, the D patients usually did *not* show impulsivity or inordinate anger. Fewer of them, in other words, manifested the kind of hostility that ruins close personal relationships; nor were they chaotic, given to scenes, recklessness, hysterical outbursts, or the like. One would find these patients, in the older typology of Grinker, nearer the neurotic end of the spectrum, as Type IV "anaclitically depressed" patients.

Nine of the D patients went on to develop more fully recognizable affective disorders—bipolar or bipolar II in six instances, unipolar in three. Two of the bipolar patients had had hypomanic episodes along with the depressive episodes before coming to the unit. Their personalities were cyclothymic. Table 5.3 shows the follow-up and family data on these nine patients (they are indicated by minus signs in the "DSM-III BPD?" column).

TABLE 5.3. Borderline Patients Who Developed MDP

Patient no.	Sex	Follow-up GAS score	DSM-III BPD?[a]	Still had BPD at follow-up?	Parents' illness	
					Father	Mother
Borderline → unipolar depression						
1	F	64	+	−	−	MDE
2	F	35	+	+	−	−
3	M	Su	+	N/A	−	−
4	F	69	+	−	U	Su
5	F	67	+	−	U	−
6	M	75	−	N/A	U	PDE
7	M	73	−	N/A	U	−
8	F	51	+	+	−	−
9	F	64	−	N/A	−	−
Borderline → bipolar II illness						
1	M	50	−	N/A[b]	B	MDE
2	F	55	+	+	SZ	−
3	F	52	+	+	−	−
4	F	85	+	−	−	−
5	F	31	+	+	Ti	−
Borderline → atypical depression						
1	F	40	+	+	−	−
Borderline → bipolar I illness						
1	F	70	+	−	−	−
2	M	73	−	N/A	Td	B
3	F	80	+	−	Tm	−
4	F	63	+	−	−	−
5	M	81	−	N/A	−	−
6	M	58	−	N/A	−	−
7	F	73	+	−	−	−
8	F	70	−	N/A	−	−
9	M	10	−	N/A	−	−
10	F	60	+	−	−	MDE
11	M	78	+	−	−	−

Note. B, bipolar; MDE, major depressive episode(s), not hospitalized; N/A, not applicable; PDE, psychotic depressive episode(s); Su, committed suicide; SZ, schizophrenia; Td, depressed temperament; Ti, irritable temperament; Tm, manic temperament; U, unipolar depression.

[a]The nine BSD-negative patients constitute the D group (see "Parental and Subsequent Morbidity among the Dysthymic Borderlines").

[b]Became alcoholic.

A family history of MDP was common among the D patients. Eleven of the patients had one or both parents who were unipolar (seven instances), bipolar (three instances), or psychotically depressed (two instances). One might view the D patients as attenuated variants of the BPD × MAD group. Many authors have attested to the frequent association of BPD or BPD traits with affective disorder, including, most recently, Manos, Vasilopoulous, and Sotiriou (1987). Not surprisingly, one commonly finds affective illness in the families of both BPD × MAD and D patients.

Both incest and parental abuse were rare in the backgrounds of the D patients. This may have contributed to their not emerging as BPD cases to begin with as they entered adult life, and also to their more favorable life trajectories. In contrast to the BPD group, where extremely adverse environmental factors were often added to whatever constitutional disadvantages may have existed beforehand, the D patients had as a rule only minor environmental disadvantages to cope with. The one incest case, though transgenerational, involved an uncle instead of a father. This patient was doing reasonably at follow-up (GAS score = 69). The patient at greatest initial disadvantage had been living in a series of foster homes after the suicide of his mother. She killed herself shortly after the father, an abusive man who threatened her with her life, obtained his release from a mental hospital. The patient is one of the two members of the D group I have been unable to trace.

The patients who went on to develop MDP had the same median GAS score as the D group in general. One of the patients required hospitalization at about the time of my follow-up contact and had been in and out of hospitals, working only sporadically at low-level jobs, since leaving our unit. Another, whose father had been taking lithium for bipolar illness, was functioning marginally. He had an irritable temperament, was mildly alcoholic, and had few friends and only an irregular (though high-level) work history. The least symptomatic of these patients (GAS score = 81) was enjoying a lucrative success in the art world at follow-up, though before his hospitalization at PI he had gotten into skirmishes with the law over passing bad checks. He was the only D patient with a history of even mildly antisocial traits. The most successful D → MDP case at follow-up (though with a lower GAS score), who had become unipolar, had a strong family history of depressive disorders; despite his occasional bouts of depression, he was managing a large business, was a devoted family man, and was also active in the community.

Because of their comparative stability, the D patients were more often good candidates for expressive psychotherapy than were the BPD patients. Two have themselves become clinical psychologists with successful practices.

Those who did least well tended to have either fairly marked MAD comorbidity or else a prognostically unfavorable personality subtype (e.g., schizoid or passive–dependent).

BORDERLINE PATIENTS AND THE SCHIZOPHRENIA SPECTRUM

Patients with Schizotypal Personality as a Subset of the Borderline Group

A generation ago, diagnosticians confronted with patients who would currently be diagnosed as having "schizotypal personality" (STP) called them "borderline schizophrenics" (Stone, 1985c). Psychogeneticists had limned the characteristics of these patients in descriptive language in that era, having been at pains to discern attenuated forms of schizophrenic endowment among relatives of those exhibiting the full-blown form of the illness (Kety, Rosenthal, Wender, & Schulsinger, 1968). Later, the DSM incorporated those clinical features with the best discriminating power (vis-à-vis neighboring diagnostic entities) into the description of STP. The concepts are not identical, since Kety et al.'s "borderline schizophrenia" implies genetic kinship to SZ, a point not stressed in DSM.

Up through the 1960s, "borderline" often meant "borderline schizophrenia." The "schizophrenia" in this instance referred to the broad, Bleulerian concept, not to the tighter and clinically more ominous definition to be found in DSM-III and in Feighner et al.'s (1972) criteria. The conflation of items— some borrowed from Kernberg (1967), some from Gunderson and Singer (1975)—that now makes up the DSM category of BPD was implicit in the older usage. Formerly, that is, the term "borderline" stood for a range of disorders characterized by *the strong presence of either or both sets of (BPD or STP) items*.

These prefatory remarks are necessary if readers are to understand why I have chosen to discuss STP under the "borderline" heading, even though the DSM uses the terms disjunctively. In clinical practice, BPD and STP are, in effect, variants of an overarching concept "borderline between neurosis and psychosis," the individual items of both often showing up in the same patient. To take but one example, most BPD patients exhibit "identity disturbance" (see below). But so do the majority of patients with STP, whose definition nonetheless does not include that item. Still, there are patients whose clinical profile includes only (or almost only) the STP items, or else those of BPD. We may consider these the "pure types." As I have mentioned elsewhere (Stone, 1985c), we do not often see schizotypal patients in the hospital, because they seldom make the flagrant suicide gestures or outright attempts on their life that DSM-defined BPD patients are apt to do. Schizotypal patients present themselves instead in the clinic or in one's private office—introverted, marginal, but getting by. I have seen more schizotypal patients from among my private patients than I could find within the PI-500 (Stone, 1985d). In that article, I mentioned the fact that I encountered frank (and hospitalized) cases of SZ in the parents and siblings of my schizotypal patients much more often than would have been expected in the general population. This was noted, also, to a more

TABLE 5.4. Patients with STP or STP Traits

Patient no.	Sex	BPD?	MAD?	Psychiatric illness in parents		Follow-up GAS score
				Father	Mother	
STP, "pure types"						
1	M	–	–	–	–	65
2	M	–	–	–	–	50
3	M	–	–	–	SZ	53
4	M	–	–	MD	–	71
5	M	–	–	Alc	–	84
6	F	–	–[a]	–	–	Su
STP, "mixed types"						
7	M	+	+	–	–	N/T
8	F	+	+	SZ	–	55
9	F	–	+	Alc	P	83
10	F	+	+	–	P	51
Prominent STP traits short of DSM-defined STP						
11	M	+	+	Alc	P	76
12	M	+	–	–	–	52
13	M	–	+	SZ	Su	N/T
14	M	+	+	P	STP	72
15	M	–	–	–	–	60
16	M	+	–	–	–	40

Note. Alc, alcoholism; MD, major depression; N/T, not traced; P, paranoia; Su, committed suicide; SZ, schizophrenia.

modest degree in the families of the 16 patients with STP ($n = 10$) or STP traits ($n = 6$) in the PI-500 sample of *broad-definition* borderlines. These 16 patients comprise just over 5% of the latter group of 299; only 2.5%, if we exclude those with concomitant MAD ($n = 8$).

Table 5.4 shows the interrelationships among the schizotypal patients with respect to BPD and MAD.

In the combined group—those showing DSM-defined STP, plus those with prominent STP traits but falling short of DSM criteria—the male preponderance was about 2:1. Only 2% of the broadly defined borderline group were "pure types" (STP without concomitant BPD). The average outcome GAS score for all 16 schizotypal patients was only slightly lower than for all borderlines (62.4 as opposed to 66.4); the range was relatively narrow (40–84), apart from the one suicide. For the traced, still-alive schizotypals without concomitant MAD ($n =$

9), the average GAS score was the same (62). Those without BPD (the "pure types"; $n = 6$) had an average score of 63.8. The "mixed" group (STP × BPD; $n = 3$ traced) had an average score of 63.5. Essentially, therefore, there were no differences among the various subgroups.

Perhaps a more accurate picture emerges if we reflect that, of the 14 traced patients in this STP/STP-trait group, 6 were clinically well at follow-up (GAS scores > 60). Hazardous as it is to make pronouncements based upon such a small series, one might speculate that these patients (including those with STP × BPD) were less likely to *recover* (i.e., to have GAS scores > 70) than are borderlines without STP features, about two-thirds of whom are now well.

The one schizotypal patient with MAD but no BPD is now doing well. This patient, a woman who at follow-up was happily married and raising two small children, had a few difficult years just after leaving PI; she remained briefly within an ungratifying marriage, from which she extricated herself with the help of some additional office psychotherapy. Moderately depressed while at PI, she had been asymptomatic for years by follow-up, and was no longer as shy as she was on our unit. She kept in close touch with her parents every week. One would no longer diagnose her as having "STP." In general warmth and effectiveness, she leads a life indistinguishable from that of her neighbors.

The other particularly successful schizotypal patient (follow-up GAS score = 84) represents an unexpectedly positive outcome (see also Chapter Fifteen). He began as an extremely shy adolescent, spiritually but also physically self-lacerating, who at the time of his admission was nearly immobilized with compulsive rituals. After his discharge from the hospital, he eventually completed graduate school, got an advanced degree, married, and had two children.

Of the two schizotypals with the worst outcomes (apart from the suicide), one was the abused child who lived for a while as a vagrant (see "Parental Brutality," Chapter Seven; "Missing Persons, Vagrants, and the Homeless," Appendix B). The other was a suspicious and hostile man who never worked steadily and who once killed someone in a dispute.

A Borderline Patient Who Became Schizophrenic

Whereas some 26 of the PI-500 borderlines went on during the follow-up interval to develop MDP, only one developed SZ. Originally, his clinical picture was that of combined STP, BPD, and MAD (depression). The STP features overshadowed the others in this "mixed borderline" condition. His thinking was paranoid, as he was preoccupied with fantasies of violence. These were directed sometimes against others and sometimes against himself, but were never acted out. Nineteen years later, the patient—supported by disability insurance and living alone in a small room—reported to me, "I'm still hopeful about the future; I still think a lot about violence; I still get anxious if I try to work." He added, "I don't like the kind of work I can do, like being a messenger, because my potential is higher, so it's humiliating . . . doesn't seem manly." It was unclear whether he had ever worked; he told me he had, intermittently, some years ago, but his parents and therapist related to me that he had not. He had been rehospitalized for short stays on many occasions, usually because of paranoid ideation and anxiety.

A number of investigators (Akiskal et al., 1985; Rutter, 1987) have commented on the rarity of a schizophrenic evolution in cases of DSM-defined BPD. This seems generally true, particularly in our culture. In Scandinavia, the frequency of STP features is greater in the "borderline" population, though it remains unclear whether this evolution is encountered more often.

A Borderline Patient Who Developed Schizoaffective Psychosis

The evolution of BPD into schizoaffective psychosis (SA) also occurred just once in the PI-500. This patient, a woman in her early 20s when admitted, showed mostly depressive symptoms at first, along with impulsivity and irascibility. Over the years, the irascibility progressed under stress to the level of combativeness, even with family members. Separations from those close to her and from therapists provoked delusory ideation, often erotomanic in nature, necessitating brief hospitalizations on many occasions. During calmer intervals she was able to work, often for almost up to a year at a stretch. She maintained close friendships. Her love relationships were stormy; she often picked over-controlling and abusive men. Her medication regimen usually consisted of a phenothiazine plus an antidepressant, although the latter seemed at times to engender manic episodes. Erotomanic and eccentric religious/philosophic preoccupations persisted even at times when she was euthymic. The variability and complexity of her clinical picture led to related shifts in diagnostic labeling over the course of her illness: "mixed borderline" (i.e., with MAD and STP features), "SA," and "SA, functioning at the borderline level." "Occasion variance" of this sort is common in schizoaffectives followed over long periods of time (Stone, 1980a).

STRIKING "BORDERLINE" CHARACTERISTICS EXHIBITED BY THE BORDERLINE PATIENTS

In this section, I discuss two characteristics included in the major definitions of "borderline" that some PI-500 borderlines exhibited in striking or extreme ways: identity disturbance and chaotic impulsivity.

Identity Disturbance

Kernberg (1967) singled out "identity disturbance" as a key item in his definition of BPO; he relied here upon Erikson's (1956; cf. also Stone, 1985b) description of "identity diffusion." As Erikson mentioned, there comes a time "when the young individual finds himself exposed to a combination of experiences which demand his simultaneous commitment to *physical intimacy* . . . , to decisive *occupational choice,* to energetic *competition,* and to *psychosocial self-definition*" (cited in Stone, 1985b, p. 239; italics in original). It is the gross failure to negotiate this maturational step that constitutes identity diffusion. This deficit is often announced quite openly, as when someone habitually expresses pain and bewilderment about not knowing "who I really am." In others, the trouble is more subtle, manifesting itself as simultaneous, paradoxical assertions of quite opposite attitudes and convictions about matters important to one's sense of identity. Not all persons making these contrary assertions are aware (until someone points out the discrepancy) of their "double-think" and general lack of integration.

When the prevailing notions of what constituted a "borderline" case were abstracted from the original definitions (chiefly those of Kernberg, 1967, and Gunderson & Singer, 1975), and woven into the DSM definition (Spitzer, Endicott, & Gibbon, 1979), identity disturbance was included—no longer as a necessary item (as in the Kernberg system), but as one of eight items in the DSM checklist. In the latter system, polythetic in nature (because only five of the eight items are required for the diagnosis), identity disturbance will not always figure in the diagnosis of "borderline." As Clarkin, Widiger, Frances, Hurt, and Gilmore (1983) have shown in a clinic population of BPD patients, "identity disturbance" was present only in three-quarters of the cases. One will also encounter patients who exhibit a quieter form of identity disturbance (such as the albino girl born of black parents, mentioned by Akiskal, 1981), unaccompanied by the fanfare of (DSM-specified) borderline storminess and aggressivity. These patients would be accounted "borderline" by the Kernberg criteria but not by those of DSM.

To do justice to both the psychoanalytic and the phenomenological conceptions of "borderline," I have presented data in many sections of this follow-up study according to both schemata. Naturally, I feel on surer ground in the presence of cases exemplifying the Kernberg, Gunderson and Singer, and DSM definitions all at once; here, I can offer my data and my impressions without parenthetical remarks or footnotes. These cases usually are embodiments of still another diagnostic concept, "hysteroid dysphoria," as adumbrated in the writings of D. Klein (Klein, 1977; Klein & Davis, 1969). The utility and validity of this concept have subsequently been challenged by Spitzer and Williams (1982); nonetheless, the "hysteroid dysphoria" patient is usually the quintessential borderline, satisfying all criteria in all the diagnostic systems.

The most striking example of borderline "identity disturbance"—not because it was the most severe or most pervasive, but because its presence was the most eloquently expressed—was that of a woman in her late 20s. She was of markedly histrionic personality and had made a "stagey" suicide gesture after a romantic breakup. She complained of intense loneliness and feelings of isolation. After the breakup, she abused alcohol and ate chocolates compulsively. In the hospital, her mood, labile under the best of circumstances, was dysphoric, characterized by feelings of hopelessness, inadequacy, and sadness. Her life had been hectic—a succession of minor triumphs and major failures, stormy love affairs, and strained relations with her family. The paradoxical quality of her object relations came through in her comments about her father, alternately depicted as a "vicious, cruel bastard" and "my romantic hero whom I madly love." With respect to her identity, she told her therapist, with a despair that did not intrude too heavily upon her wit and dramatic flair, "I have no idea whether I'm beautiful or ugly, talented or pedestrian, a bitch or a saint, crazy or a genius! How do people gauge such things? You're the doctor; you tell *me!*"

Chaotic Impulsivity

Though impulsivity is, arguably, the key item of BPD (Livesley, Reiffer, Sheldon, & West, 1987), some borderline patients exhibited this trait in the extreme. One might designate these extreme examples as "chaotic": patients whose preadmission lives were characterized by drug abuse, wildness, promiscuity, frequent rage outbursts, tumultuous relationships (whether at home or with intimates), run-ins with the law, running away from home—in other words, patients who were maximally irresponsible, unpredictable, and tempestuous. Not surprisingly, chaotic patients were grossly overrepresented among the borderlines with the worst outcomes. Almost invariably, borderline-level patients who were chaotic also fulfilled BPD criteria.

Of the 19 BPD patients whose impulsivity reached the chaotic level, only 1 ended up among the best-outcome group. She had been a "wild" adolescent: promiscuous, drug-abusing, unable to stay with one person or see one task through to completion. After eloping from our unit, she disappeared for almost 10 years; finally, she was rescued by a man who insisted she join Alcoholics Anonymous (AA). Her life took an abrupt upturn, and she remained well (completed professional training, worked steadily, married, and raised a child) thereafter. Another alcoholic (but non-BPD) borderline patient also made a dramatic recovery after AA. He was chaotic before and for 8 years after his stay on our unit. During the latter period, he behaved as though his actions were determined by an internal "bad-luck" magnet. The disasters of which his life at that time was an unbroken chain included the following: He took a job at a pharmacy and the next day banged into a cabinet, spilling hundreds of bottles and thousands of pills (along with the shards of the broken bottles) onto the floor. Fired from that job, he then became a traveling salesman; his travels took him no further than the tree into which he "racked" the company car a few days after he started work. His next stop would have been jail had not his family grudgingly reimbursed the company. And so on, until he joined AA; as with the preceding patient, this was the turning point. In the 7 years prior to follow-up he worked steadily, and at the time of follow-up was supporting his wife and their first child, born the week after I first spoke with him.

As for those with worst outcomes, half the BPD patients were also chaotic. These included a woman, once arraigned for child molestation, who had been jailed for shoplifting; an arsonist (both suicides); an imposter (see Appendix A); a man who shot three people to death (see "Gradations of Antisociality," Chapter Six); and a woman enjoined because of her abuse from visiting her own child. All the chaotic borderlines except two abused alcohol, marijuana, or LSD before (and usually after) the index hospitalization.

Personality Subtypes among the Borderline Patients

An unavoidable hazard of *long-term* follow-up studies is the inevitable discovery, given an interval of 15 or 20 years, of factors one would consider important at follow-up that were customarily ignored at the time the baseline data were first accumulated. We failed to assess or else to record impressions about many personality factors that hindsight now tells us were important. In regard to the PI-500, we were dimly aware during the initial evaluations that generally likeable patients—regardless of diagnosis—would probably do better in the long run than patients the staff found irksome or difficult. For a year and a half (1969–1970), we actually rated newly admitted patients on a rudimentary scale of "likeableness" by circling a number from −10 to +10. For most of the PI-500, however, even this assessment is not available.

We may have ignored this factor in part because psychiatric and especially psychoanalytic training in prior generations discouraged us from making value judgments. We could legitimately view our patients as the victims of this or that combination of early circumstances, parental influences, or the like, but we could not legitimately view them as "nice" or "good" versus "unpleasant" or "bad." We were no more blind than were laypeople to the fact that compassionate people usually ended up as more successful, interpersonally and occupationally, than did those who treated others shabbily. But, unlike laypeople, mental health professionals were expected not to say this out loud.

The delineation of the personality disorders in DSM-III (Axis II), along with the current interest in developing sophisticated instruments for personality assessments (see Loranger, Susman, Oldham, & Russakoff, 1987), has enhanced our awareness of the personality dimension in our diagnostic evaluation. But Axis I and Axis II diagnoses account for only a portion of the variance in *outcome*.

Not all patients with antisocial personality (ASP), for example, are unlikeable or unsalvageable. Some of the PI-500 borderlines with ASP were charming and appealing. Though irresponsible and disrespectful of convention at the time they were hospitalized, they were free of malice and never committed acts of violence. Many of these patients, as they matured into their 30s and 40s, mellowed without further treatment into trustworthy, respectable members of their community.

The investigator can readily drown in the ocean of personality variables that look promising as predictors of outcome. We could discuss outcome from the vantage point of the personality disorders enumerated in DSM-III-R. Many borderline patients exhibit enough abnormal traits to warrant a secondary diagnosis from among the dozen or so types in Axis II. Clinicians have begun to speak of this situation as one of "comorbidity." This phraseology can be misleading, I believe, because a patient with borderline personality disorder (BPD) and simultaneous narcissistic personality disorder (NPD) does not have two separate conditions in the same sense as does the patient who presents with glaucoma and an ulcer. Rather, the patient has a particular and quite unified personality—various aspects of which we regroup for heuristic purposes under two headings. When we come to make generalizations, we confront this dilemma: Should we include "BPD × NPD" patients in our discussion of borderlines, or of narcissistic patients, or both? Or should we exclude such patients from a discussion of BPD by itself or of NPD by itself, on the grounds that they are not "pure types"? How large a series must we have before we can find enough BPD patients without "comorbidity" to permit statistical analysis? If the pure types are rare (and they are!), perhaps we should simply regard the descriptions in the manual as archetypes—Platonic ideals, in effect—and confine our efforts to real patients, each of whom is a bewildering *Gemisch* of abnormal traits belonging to half a dozen "disorders" and of normal traits not even to be found in the manual. Where these latter strengths largely override the personality weaknesses, the outcome may be much more favorable than we would have forecast on the basis of the personality disorder diagnosis alone. Lamentably, the reverse is also true, as we have noted: Some of the talented, attractive, and personable abuse victims in this series nevertheless killed themselves.

The way to proceed through these complexities is, I suspect, to begin with the examination of one or two variables in large groups, knowing that the results will be simplistic and superficial, and then to examine the necessarily smaller subgroups that share a larger number of variables in common. This approach is analogous to shifting from a coarse to a medium lens in the inspection of a histological specimen.

CLASSIFICATION OF THE BORDERLINES INTO PERSONALITY SUBTYPE GROUPS

With respect to the PI-500, I found it easier to reconstruct, through the old records and through memory, the personality subtypes of the borderline-level patients. In the patients with a psychosis, the latter often submerged personality factors in such a way as to obscure what they had been like before they became ill. (Later in this chapter, I discuss this point at greater length.)

I find it useful to analyze personality along *dimensional* as well as along categorical lines. We may regard any Axis II category, for example, as a dimension, in regard to which each patient may show no traits, a few traits, or enough to qualify for the disorder in question. A patient with BPD may thus have schizotypal personality (STP) as well ("BPD × STP"), and show pronounced narcissistic and less pronounced paranoid traits. The resultant *profile* will be comparable in many ways to the Minnesota Multiphasic Personality Inventory (MMPI) profile of the same patient. Borderline patients frequently show characteristics not easily captured by the standard manual, yet rather well delineated in other compilations. Kernberg's (1967) description of the "infantile" personality, for example, contains elements of the histrionic personality, along with childlike poutiness and demandingness (reminiscent of NPD) and the sort of ragefulness or crankiness ("unreasonableness") alluded to in Kraepelin's (1921) description of the "irritable temperament."

In Table 6.1, I have compartmentalized the 206 patients with BPD into some 20 subgroups (the number assigned to each reflects the code number I used in the computer). These reflect the Axis II personality disorder subtypes, along with several others borrowed from the psychoanalytic literature ("infantile," "depressive") and the temperament literature ("cyclothymic," "hypomanic," "irritable/explosive," etc.) (see Kröber, 1988). Avoidant patients with classic phobias (of elevators, bridges, etc.) I called "phobic." I classified these borderline patients in accordance with their next most prominent set of abnormal personality characteristics. Usually these were marked enough to warrant a "comorbidity" diagnosis in DSM; sometimes the traits fell short of the standard criteria.

Because the resultant groups were relatively small, I recorded only three levels of outcome: Global Assessment Scale (GAS) scores > 60 ("well"), GAS scores = 1–60, and suicide. Generalizations are hazardous even in groups of 10, but I felt it justifiable to construct a graph (Figure 6.1) showing the percentages of traced patients currently well (GAS scores > 60) for personality subtypes with at least this number. As Figure 6.1 shows, the BPD subgroups did not perform much differently from the whole-group average (63% of the BPDs were well at follow-up), except for the irritable/explosive and the antisocial patients, both of whom did less well than average, and for the obsessive–compulsive patients, who did better than average. Arguably, the BPD × obsessive–compulsive patients who did not commit suicide did better than the group average: Their average follow-up GAS score was 76 (*SD* = 9), more than a decile better than that of the remaining 160 nonsuicide BPD patients (63.8), *t* (two-tailed) = 2.87, *p* < .001.

Taken one subgroup at a time, BPD patients whose predominant traits were in the DSM "eccentric" cluster ("Cluster A"; paranoid/schizoid/schizotypal) were too few to permit generalization. When all borderline-level patients were included (not just those with BPD), their collective number rose to 18 traced. These included 8 who were well at follow-up (45%) and 2 suicides.

TABLE 6.1. Outcome in Traced BPD Patients According to Predominant Personality Pattern

Code	Predominant personality pattern	n	n untraced	Follow-up GAS scores >60	1–60	Suicide	% traced patients now well (GAS scores > 60)
1	BPD × ASP	15	2	1	9	3	7.7
2	BPD × avoidant	4	0	0	4	0	0.0
3	BPD × depressive	15	1	10	2	2	71.4
3.1	BPD × depressive–masochistic	25	0	17	7	1	68.0
4	BPD × histrionic	21	0	15	4	2	71.4
5	BPD × hypomanic	0	–	–	–	–	–
6	BPD × irritable/explosive	20	1	9	9	1	47.4
7	BPD × NPD or prominent NPD traits	19	1	14	3	1	77.8
8	BPD × obsessive–compulsive	19	2	15	1	1	88.2
9	BPD × paranoid	3	0	1	2	0	33.3
10	BPD × phobic (with discrete phobias)	5	1	3	1	0	75.0
11	BPD × passive–aggressive	11	0	8	2	1	72.7
12	BPD × passive–dependent	12	2	8	2	0	80.0
13	BPD × schizoid	2	0	1	0	1	50.0
13.1	BPD × STP	3	1	0	2	0	0.0
14	BPD × infantile	28	2	18	6	2	69.2
15	BPD × abrasive	1	0	0	0	1	0.0
16	BPD × inadequate	0	–	–	–	–	–
17	BPD × cyclothymic	2	0	2	0	0	100.0
18	BPD × sadistic	1	0	0	0	1	0.0
	Totals	206	13	122 (63.2%)	54 (28%)	17 (8.8%)	63.2 (average)

[a]*n* traced = 193, or 93.7%. These figures reflect a more recent tabulation (compared with Chapter Three), reflecting a larger number of traced patients.

Prominent "comorbidity" with traits in this cluster may, in other words, have had a negative effect upon long-term outcome. This would not be surprising, given the handicaps that paranoid/schizoid traits impose upon socialization.[1]

[1]One should keep in mind, with respect to schizotypal patients, that clinicians cannot distinguish very clearly between *actual* schizotypal and *actual* BPD patients. *Prototypical* cases are rare. Instead, varying degrees of "admixture" are often present, given the existence (on DSM-category-based criteria) of either one (Serban, Conte, & Plutchik, 1987). See also "Borderline Patients and the Schizophrenia Spectrum" in Chapter Five.

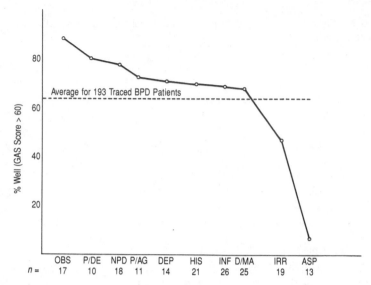

FIGURE 6.1. Percentage well (GAS scores > 60) at follow-up: BPD patients in personality subtypes with at least 10 traced patients. OBS, obsessive–compulsive; P/DE, passive–dependent; NPD, narcissistic; P/AG, passive–aggressive; DEP, depressive; HIS, histrionic; INF, infantile; D/MA, depressive–masochistic; IRR, irritable/explosive; ASP, antisocial.

Suicides were not especially frequent in any of the personality subtypes, with the exception of BPD × ASP (3 of 13 traced, or 23%; this figure did not quite reach statistical significance).

OUTCOMES FOR THE LARGER PERSONALITY SUBTYPE GROUPS

One can better appreciate the impact of certain personality subtypes upon outcome by inspecting the distributions of follow-up GAS scores. Given the wide differences in outcomes within each group, the *median* score provides a more trustworthy index of typical function than does the mean. Figure 6.2 shows the median scores for patients in the larger subgroups vis-à-vis comorbidity.

Patients with Antisocial Personality

Among the borderline patients with ASP, to look at one subgroup on a case-by-case basis (Figure 6.3), those who met BPD criteria were, with one exception, always *below* the median; those without BPD were at or above this

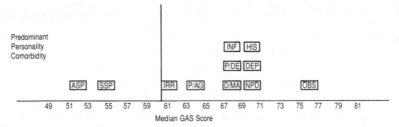

FIGURE 6.2. Borderlines of various predominant personality comorbidity (subtypes with at least 10 members): Median GAS scores at follow-up. SSP, schizoid/STP/paranoid (DSM "Cluster A"); other abbreviations as in Figure 6.1.

level. This suggests that the impulsive, hostile, rageful, and self-injurious traits of the BPD × ASP patients rendered them even more vulnerable to a bad outcome than was true when ASP was unaccompanied by these attributes. The three suicides were also BPD × ASP.

The Worst, Median, and Best Cases

Since the outliers as well as the typical patients within any one personality type are of special interest, I sketch briefly the nature of the worst, median, and best cases among the ASP patients still living, before turning to a more detailed discussion of gradations of antisociality. I have described the suicides in the separate chapter on that subject (see Chapter Four).

The worst ASP patient was an adolescent reared in a chaotic and violent home where a genetic factor for combativeness seemed to be operating in both parental lines. This man murdered three persons and is still incarcerated; he is discussed further below. The median patient was a man who had eloped from PI and then lived a vagrant's life, moving from one community and one odd job to

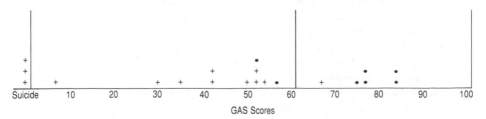

FIGURE 6.3. Distribution of GAS scores at follow-up in antisocial borderlines. Plus signs indicate BPD patients; dots indicate other borderlines.

another. He married, sired two children, and quickly divorced, leaving the children in the care of their mother. He abused drugs and alcohol until shortly before follow-up, and was jailed briefly on a sex charge. A church group rescued him, helped him get off drugs, and rehabilitated him; at follow-up, he was living alone near a family member and supporting himself through steadier employment. His irascibility, once a serious problem, was now under better control. The best ASP patient had run away from home as an adolescent because of his abusive, alcoholic mother. He spent several months at PI, but left without any recognizable improvement. Never belligerent or abusive like the first two patients, he got by for a few years at various menial jobs, drinking excessively and "conning" family members into supporting him. Finally, he joined Alcoholics Anonymous (AA); at follow-up, he was working effectively in the alcohol rehabilitation field, was married, and had recently become a father. All three men had IQs of 125 when tested at the hospital.

Gradations of Antisociality

Antisocial Personality with Crimes of Violence. The status of ASP within the taxonomy of psychiatric disorders is complex and controversial. Cleckley (1976) has reviewed the subject in his monograph on the psychopath. More recently, Blackburn (1988) challenged Cleckley's notion of the "psychopath," also taking psychiatry to task for confusing acts of law-breaking (now incorporated into the DSM definition of ASP) with personality traits, strictly defined. Some psychopaths are charming, nonviolent, irresponsible, and so on, and remain just this side of the law. Some mass murderers are not irresponsible, glib, or the like, but commit heinous crimes. If one defined "psychopaths" (or whatever label one used instead) *purely* via personality traits, the list might include "unempathic," "cold," "hostile," "aggressive," "self-centered," "exploitative," and "irresponsible." Many, *but not all,* such persons habitually commit antisocial or delinquent or criminal acts. However we choose to define this abnormality of personality, we must also deal with the *continuum* (dimensional) aspects, since individuals exhibiting these qualities will vary from mild to extreme. Even the spectrum of murderers has many subtle bands of demarcation.

In Table 6.2 I offer a spectrum of antisociality, compartmentalized into a "worst" region, containing those who murder with malice and after torture of their victims; a "mildest" region, containing persons guilty of no worse than truancy or petty thievery; and an arbitrary number of intermediate zones. Together with the abstract descriptions of the successive bands of this spectrum, I have provided examples from the biographies of notorious antisocial persons and from the ranks of the PI-500 borderlines who were "comorbid" for ASP.

I believe there are practical consequences to the placement of antisocial persons along such a spectrum. There may be predictive value, regarding treatability and long-term outcome, in whether someone in adolescence or early

TABLE 6.2. Gradations of Antisociality

Spectrum of antisociality: mildest to worst forms	Examples from the literature	Examples from the PI-500 borderlines
Mildest: impulsive, irresponsible, dishonest (but nonviolent) in petty ways		Borderline male, alcoholic for several years, irresponsible and in minor trouble with the law, until enrolled in AA
Impulsive, irresponsible, dishonest (but nonviolent) in major ways		Borderline male, alcoholic and destructive of property through carelessness, until enrolled in AA
Lifelong antisociality, "white-collar crimes" (e.g., embezzlement)		BPD male, imposter
Career criminal, nonviolent, or threatening but not actually harming (larceny, robbery)		Borderline male, arrested for theft on several occasions after PI, but not traced recently
Violent, but only upon extreme provocation, in self-defense	Ricky Kyle (Finstad, 1987); Wayne Dresbach (Mewshaw, 1980); both patricides	Borderline male, matricide
Sadistic, but without premeditation to hurt		Two BPD males, one of whom eventually committed suicide; both were verbally abusive to women
Habitual violence (including lethal) upon small provocation	Murderer Marlene Olive (Levine, 1982); murderer Gary Gilmore (Mailer, 1979)	BPD male (a Marine) who killed three people in a bar
Malice with intent to hurt or endanger, but not to kill	Rapist Fred Coe (Olsen, 1972); torturer Cameron Hooker (McGuire & Norton, 1988)	
Malice with intent to kill; no torture	Murderer Chester Gillette (Brandon, 1986); murderers James Giesick and Sam Corey (Dillmann, 1986)	BPD male, arsonist, responsible for three deaths
Worst: Malice with torture of victims	Serial killers: Gerald Gallego (Biondi & Hecox, 1987); John Wayne Gacy (Cahill, 1986); Dennis Nilsen (Masters, 1985)	

adult life manifests extreme or only mild degrees of antisocial behavior or of unempathic personality. Because of the many variables of personality, however, no simply constructed, linear spectrum can do full justice to all the examples in a whole society. Some who commit vicious acts do so as members of organized crime, but are good family members outside "business hours." There are many puzzling cases that do not fit neatly within the spectrum; the PI-500 contained several examples of its own.

Where, for instance, are we to place one of the PI adolescents who, in seeking to kill one boy (he believed that the boy had "wronged" him), ended up killing (via arson) not the boy himself but three others in his family? This patient had come from an intact, nonviolent, and reasonably nurturing home, and was a "genius" according to his IQ tests. He had never had friends, however (and has not to this day, 18 years later), and remained an irritable and dour "loner." I learned of his bungled vengeance murders personally, when he was caught trying to harm one of his fellow-patients in the hospital. An adolescent when these acts occurred, he was at first unsuspected, and when suspected went unprosecuted. In recent years he has lived as a schizoid "loner" (cf. Gallwey, 1985). He was never in trouble with the authorities.

Less "inhuman" (and more able to evoke sympathy) is the story of another borderline adolescent admitted to PI because of incorrigible behavior and proneness to violence. His hyperkinetic nervous system may have owed more to constitution than to rearing, but the direction of his impulses was certainly influenced by his chaotic home. Both parents were hyperexcitable, irascible, and physically abusive, their violence spending itself either on each other or on their son. The municipal social services agencies had identified them, in a characteristic euphemism, as a "multiple-problem family"—one that remained impervious to whatever ameliorative measures the social workers tried to institute.

The patient eloped after about 5 months on our unit, still in his 14th year. Nothing was heard of him until 3 years later, when we learned (from the newspapers) that he had lied about his age and joined the Marines; a few weeks later, he had sauntered into a bar on a Saturday night and shot three patrons to death with his M-1. He was incarcerated soon after and remains in jail to this day. This young man was hostile and without friends, but, unlike the patient just mentioned, could also be viewed as the victim of uncommonly abusive parenting. Perhaps he represents the coalescence of nature and nurture at their extreme worst: This man had two violent grandfathers in addition to his violent parents, plus a violent uncle and any number of violent cousins, all of whom showed hairtrigger violence upon trifling provocations and all of whom exhibited the same congenital skin anomaly (cf. Norris, 1988).

Antisocial Personality without Crimes of Violence.   Nine percent of the PI-500 exhibited ASP, either fully enough to meet DSM-III criteria (6%) or nearly so (3%). Of these 49 patients, 39 were borderline by broad criteria, and 26 exhibited BPD by DSM criteria. The remainder consisted of one with schizophrenia (SZ), three with manic–depressive psychosis (MDP), and six with a schizophreniform psychosis (SF) precipitated by hallucinogens. This means that those with a psychosis were rarely antisocial, whereas the borderlines were so in about one of eight cases (39 of 299, or 13%). The low trace rate of 72.3 in the 33 patients with ASP by DSM criteria is a reflection of the difficulties in locating individuals many years later (fathers who have abandoned their families), patients who have been fleeing from the law, etc.). Since, during our preadmission screening, we rarely accepted patients with known histories of violence, the PI antisocial patients are not representative of antisociality (or "psychopathy") in the general population. Females accounted for 29% ($n =$ 14) of the group: half the milder (ASP trait) cases, but only 5 of the 33 cases with ASP comorbidity. They were more often unruly than violent, having been referred because of drug abuse, truancy, or shoplifting.

Aggressivity was more common in the males, as would be expected. There were several who set fires, brandished guns (one eventually killed someone), or stole on a larger scale. One was the imposter (whose case is described in Appendix A). While there were at least eight confirmed alcoholics (including four females), almost all the antisocial patients abused substances—often the whole anthology of currently available "street" drugs.

As a rule, the home environment in these 49 patients was significantly more disruptive than what was reported by the other patients, including the non-ASP borderlines. Using a broad definition of "early loss" (desertion by a parent, death of a parent before age 16, divorce before age 16, suicide of a parent, adoption), I found that the borderlines with ASP were more than twice as likely as the non-ASP borderlines to have experienced a severe childhood loss (27 of 39 vs. 87 of 260), $\chi^2 = 18, p < .001$. Often the home was not so much "broken" as *disintegrated,* with caretakers and their children scattering in all directions and retaining ties with no one. (The patients who sustained an early loss of some sort are described in more detail in Chapter Seven.)

Half the adoptees in the PI-500 were antisocial: In the whole series, 1 patient in 40 was adopted, as against 1 in 7 among the ASPs. One patient was told that she was adopted, though in actuality she was the natural child of her father by a mistress about whom she was never told; she was raised by the father with his wife, a violent schizophrenic who brutalized the patient until, at 14, she ran away into a life of drug abuse, promiscuity, and petty thievery. When admitted to PI, she aroused great sympathy from the treating staff, was a model of deportment on the unit, and was depressed upon release rather than impulsive. She became agoraphobic and still abused drugs, but was no longer antisocial. After a few years of a tortured existence, feeling unable to work or fashion any kind of meaningful life, she committed suicide.

At least eight of the ASP patients had one alcoholic parent; one had two such parents who were continuously quarrelsome and abusive, eventually divorcing when their daughter was 12. She spent over a year at PI and seemed headed for social recovery, but killed herself a few months after her release.

Family discord, including high "expressed emotion" (see Leff & Vaughn, 1980), was the rule even in the 11 families that stayed together. This factor appeared to contribute as greatly to the development of ASP as did divorce, death, and desertion. Forty percent of the homes of these patients were, or became, fatherless. This is nearly double the rate noted in the PI-500 as a whole.

The presence of ASP augurs poorly for intensive psychotherapy; dyadic therapies of any sort are usually insufficient in this situation, because of the need for stringent limit-setting over and above whatever might be said in the one-to-one sessions. The PI therapists usually felt frustrated when working with ASP patients, saw little results for their efforts, saw how often these patients eloped or signed out against advice, and in general came to assume a dismal prognosis. Rarely were any of them considered "improved" at the time of discharge. The one borderline with ASP who *was* considered "improved" failed to return home the evening he was discharged, called his family once from another part of the country, and has never been heard from since (see "Missing Persons, Vagrants, and the Homeless," Appendix B).

But those who predicted disaster were often wrong, too. About one of the borderline × ASP males, a staff member said, "There has been no major breakthrough in therapy, and the likelihood is so minimal that there is nothing to be gained from continued hospitalization." He was returned to his argumentative and chaotic home. At follow-up 18 years later, he was an executive in a large chemical corporation, was married, and was abstaining completely from the alcohol and other substances he abused as an adolescent.

The realm of nonviolent ASP patients is as rich in subdivisions as that of violent ASPs (see Table 6.2). There are, for example, the reckless but not violent, the violent, the impulsive but not violent, the slick, the "Jean Valjean" types (who steal food to keep alive), and the outcasts. Some outcasts were rejected by disturbed and outrageously unfair parents; others became outcasts because of a kind of innate disruptiveness of the sort that would exhaust the patience of the calmest parent. At the hospital, of course, we saw very few of the polished, sociopathic charmer types (of the sort portrayed in the "high-society jewel thief" movies of the 1930s), since a well-functioning con-man would not end up in a psychiatric hospital.

Among the traced borderline × ASP patients, the females tended to have higher follow-up GAS scores (by 10 points) than the males. This is in accord with common clinical impressions. The female ASP patients were seldom aggressive or delinquent. Many were adolescent girls of fundamentally good constitution and obedient disposition, turned away from home by a rejecting mother or else seduced by an alcoholic/sociopathic father until they ran away to what they hoped was a better environment. They became street gamines, taking up with strangers (who also misused them), stealing trifles here and there to keep alive. Several were "persons in need of supervision" (PINS) cases, remanded to our unit by the municipal social agencies in lieu of placement in a reformatory. At follow-up, one of these girls was the deputy mayor of a town in the West; another was a leader of her local PTA; a third helped run an agency for wayward minors such as she herself had once been.

The borderline × ASP males were more often headstrong, arrogant, insubordinate, and wild as adolescents. Some were glib and superficially appealing; others were sullen, irritable, and contentious. The male ASPs with the three best outcomes at follow-up had become a manufacturer, a successful businessman, and an alcohol rehabilitation counselor, respectively. All were married with children. The hospital personnel would never have forecast such improvement when these patients had left the hospital; one, in particular, the staff found quite repugnant because of his menacing and coarse behavior.

Whereas the manufacturer felt that the hospital had saved his life, the connection between treatment and eventual recovery in those ASP patients who did well was seldom perceptible. Usually they had not gotten along well with the hospital staff, or vice versa. At best, the hospital seemed to serve as an interruption in what had been a downward spiral, allowing some of these patients to "spin out" of their dive. Their ultimate salvation often enough came in the form of an "Anonymous" group or of a religious sect—in other words, some powerful and supportive system external to their own psyches.

In future follow-up studies of ASP patients, certain "soft signs" may turn out to be important for their predictive value. Likeableness is one such measure (Woollcott, 1985). Though we unfortunately did not record our impressions about this attribute in any consistent manner, I have the impression that most of the ASP patients whom the staff found likeable eventually did well; those regarded as hostile only seldom recovered. As always, there are exceptions. The most destructive homes can crush anyone: For instance, the appealing woman who ran away from home after having been beaten by her adoptive mother later committed suicide. But the coarse and menacing man, as mentioned, mellowed over the years and became a successful store proprietor.

Patients with Irritable Personality

Though DSM-III-R does not recognize irritable personality, it does acknowledge something similar (and similar also to "episodic dyscontrol"; see Appendix A) under the heading "intermittent explosive disorder" (312.34). The patients I have called "irritable personalities" show the features of Kraepelin's (1921) "irritable temperament"—a constitutionally based disorder of temperament noted in certain patients with MDP and their relatives (see also Rutter, 1987). These persons are habitually impulsive and aggressive, not merely *episodically* assaultive or destructive, as in the case of intermittent explosive disorder.

As a group, the irritable borderlines' median GAS score at follow-up was just at the edge between well and not well (61), though their outcomes were not as poor as those of either the "Cluster A" patients (paranoid/schizoid/schizotypal) patients or the ASP patients. Furthermore, some of the patients with predominant ASP were markedly irritable; I could easily have classified them under this rubric, had they not been even more strikingly antisocial. Two murderers and an arsonist were among these BPD × ASP × irritable patients. Although the best of the irritable borderlines have mellowed considerably (the pathologically jealous man (see Appendix A) became a well-functioning professional; a man formerly violent toward his provocative parents became an extraordinarily successful and no longer irascible businessman), the worst retained this disadvantageous trait. The man who killed his mother and then attempted suicide was an irritable borderline when hospitalized 25 years ago. His mother was chronically abusive and far more irritable than he; this was a case of murder provoked.

I have described one of the typical BPD × irritable personality patients elsewhere in this book under "Episodic Dyscontrol" (see Appendix A). Another typical case was a man (whose GAS score at follow-up was also 61) who was irascible, argumentative, and occasionally assaultive, and was once jailed for a few days on account of a theft. He continued the same way after he left PI until a few years later, when a consultant, noticing some hypomanic traits as well, suggested a trial of lithium. Apart from a few relapses when he discontinued the medication, he became considerably calmer and less argumentative, and had been so for years at follow-up. He was working at a craft and supporting himself, but remained leery of close involvements, lest the inevitable tensions in an intimate relationship reawaken his irascibility. This patient represents one of the instances of borderline conditions evolving into one or another variety (here, bipolar) of MDP (see Chapter Five).

An alcoholic woman whom the courts enjoined from seeing her child because of her abusiveness was one of the poorer-functioning irritable BPD patients (GAS score at follow-up = 21). Her case serves as an excellent demonstration of the true impact of personality. On the unit at the same time as this woman was another, hospitalized because of chronic schizophrenic psychosis. She was a "flower child" of the 1960s: soft-spoken, fée, unconventional, but liked by everyone because of her charm and her accomplished flute-playing. Twenty years later, she emerged as one of the best-functioning schizophrenic patients, still eccentric in her ideas and ill at ease in crowds, but pursuing her musical talents with the encouragement of her admiring and protective husband. By virtue of a more pleasing personality, this "psychotic" patient had a follow-up GAS score more than 40 points higher than that of the irritable borderline patient.

Though this irritable temperament group (within *all* borderlines) contains only one suicide (with 24 of 27 traced), the *risk* for suicide among such patients may be, in general, rather marked—if not in the PI-500, then perhaps in larger and more heterogeneous series of such patients. Graves (1988), working on the large epidemiological study of long-term outcome in medical students inaugurated in the 1940s by Caroline Thomas at Johns Hopkins, offered data to the effect that irritability was the strongest predictor of future suicide among the 25 items of the questionnaire given the 1,337 students at the outset. The four other predictors to emerge from this study were (in the order of their efficacy) the urge to be alone, urinary frequency, diminished appetite, and sleep difficulties. In similar fashion, Mogul (1988) noted marked increases in suicide attempters (vs. nonattempters) of uncontrolled anger, as well as of anxiety, drug abuse, and premenstrual syndrome (PMS). All of these observations are in line with the point made here and elsewhere (Weissman, Fox, & Klerman, 1973), that suicide risk is not so great in the merely depressed as in the angry, hostile, irritable, *and* depressed patient. That is, The BPD patient with anger and impulsivity will be at higher risk than will the BPD patient lacking those two items.

Patients with Narcissistic Personality

I have already described narcissistic borderlines in considerable detail elsewhere (Stone, 1989b). As I mentioned there, BPD patients with mild to moderate narcissistic features were distributed, as to gender, in the same proportions as BPD patients in general. But the 14 meeting DSM-III criteria for NPD (which are stricter than the DSM-III-R criteria) showed a male preponderance (71% male, as opposed to 29% male in the BPD group as a whole). Ronningstam and Gunderson (1989) noted a similar male preponderance in their series. This disparity may be a reflection of the specific items chosen for the DSM diagnosis, some of which (lack of empathy, preoccupation with power and success) may be more common among males than females in our culture. Perhaps minor manifestations of narcissism (vanity, primping) are more common in women, whereas men are more apt to show the more serious traits, such as ruthlessness, extreme arrogance, and so on. BPD patients exhibiting the dual "comorbidity" NPD × ASP were almost all male in the PI-500: 12 of 13, or 92%. Kernberg (1987) gathers these patients under the apt heading "malignant narcissism." This combination usually predicted an abysmal outcome (11 traced; average GAS score = 46; suicide rate = 18%); only one such patient was doing well at follow-up. The other narcissistic patients, in contrast, are doing about the same as the BPD patients in general. Regarding theories on the development of NPD, the reader should consult Russell (1985).

The GAS scores do not, of course, tell the whole story. We cannot easily gather systematic data in a retrospective follow-up study about the intimate daily life of the traced patients. Were some of the narcissistic borderlines, for example, though successful at work and in the grosser measures of social functioning, more critical of their partners, less tolerant of foibles, and so on, than the depressive or dependent patients? To garner reliable material on such questions, we would need to know not only the former patients, but also their friends, family members, spouses, and coworkers long enough to get the "real" story. This would be a lifetime's work, even assuming that one could gain entrée to the patients' circles of intimates to such a broad extent. Instead, I can offer only a few anecdotal impressions.

Five borderline-level women with NPD (three with BPD) achieved follow-up GAS scores of 84. During their hospital stays, they had been haughty, aloof, disdainful, preoccupied with success, envious, and in some cases exploitative. One had made a serious suicide attempt as her marriage deteriorated; she seemed emotionally unreachable while on the unit, imperious, proud, and hypercritical.

Toward the end of her lengthy stay, she softened considerably. Her depression was more visible; she also became more open with her therapist and less sarcastic toward the staff. Continuing to work with this therapist for several years after her discharge, she eventually divorced, resumed graduate school work, remarried, had two children, and at follow-up was a professional woman successful both in career and in marriage. One would not now classify her as narcissistic, or, indeed, as borderline. Another of these women was married at follow-up, without children, highly successful in a business she launched several years earlier. The BPD traits were gone or in abeyance; she was still rather aloof and self-centered. People would still characterize her as "narcissistic," though she no longer showed enough items to elicit a DSM-III-R diagnosis of NPD. I suspect (but do not know) that she was more brittle and less forgiving than the first-mentioned women, although both were functioning in the superior range on the relatively coarse measures of the GAS.

The worst-functioning patient in this subgroup was a woman (follow-up GAS score = 31) whose background was much more traumatic (physical and sexual abuse) than that of the two women described above; she also had more serious affective symptoms. She held a responsible job for many years, but after a long love relationship failed, she rapidly deteriorated, becoming dysfunctional at work and actively suicidal. Rehospitalized briefly and maintained on antidepressants, she was leading a precarious life at follow-up, perched on the edge of self-destruction. Vanity and hostility were as discernible in her personality now as they were at the hospital 20 years ago.

Patients with Obsessive–Compulsive Personality

One of the more surprising findings concerning personality subtypes was the generally good outcome among the borderlines with obsessive–compulsive "comorbidity." Seven out of eight are now well. In the path toward normal psychosexual development enunciated by the psychoanalytic pioneers, "obsessives" were fixated at the anal stage—a notch below the "hysterics," who were situated nearer to the genital level. This theory created a bias inclining its adherents to regard the obsessives as "sicker." Yet one encountered hysteric patients who were clearly more disturbed than the average run of obsessives. To preserve the model, the former became known as "hysteroid" (Easser & Lesser, 1965). Kernberg (1967) preferred the term "infantile" (hysteric traits combined with poutiness, anger, demandingness, etc.).

Elsewhere (Stone, 1980b), I have suggested that men and women with histrionic or with obsessive–compulsive personalities are, in any large population, about equally advantaged and disadvantaged, though the advantages may be distributed disproportionately in relation to certain life stresses. Histrionic traits, characterized by overemotionality, may have a utility in problematic intimate partnerships, where the crucial step in settling differences is often to "get out the feelings." Obsessive traits, of which underemotionality, perfectionism, excessive neatness, and restraint are typical examples, create obvious problems in intimate contexts; however, they may solve equally knotty problems in the occupational sphere and in the matter of tolerating being alone. Since the patients of the PI-500 were, as they left the hospital, more concerned with issues of survival (how to support themselves, how to get through a weekend alone) than with the fine points of intimate relationships, perhaps the obsessives (provided they were not overwhelmed with repetitive thoughts) had an easier time adjusting than did the patients with predominantly histrionic or depressive traits. Certainly their work record is impressive. Included among the 27 borderline obsessives at follow-up were a manufacturer, two physicians, an accountant, a psychologist, three lawyers, a real estate developer, an editor, an engineer, a philanthropist, an electronics technician, and an artist of international reputation. Even the one suicide was an engineer.

Patients with Histrionic Personality

Among the 25 borderlines with histrionic features (all female, all traced), outcome differences seemed related more to life events than to the remainder of their accompanying personality traits. Of the two suicides, for example, one had been an incest victim (father and brothers); the other had had a markedly seductive father. The most disabled of those still alive at follow-up was another incest victim (father) who remained self-destructive and unable to work consistently or to sustain relationships. Another, from a poor and chaotic home, became a prostitute; still another, from a wealthy but emotionally arid home, became a drug addict (GAS score for both = 52). Three of the four with best outcomes (GAS scores = 87, 88, 91, 92) were also incest victims, but their fathers were in general more kindly disposed toward their daughters; their acts of molestation were rare and of a less serious nature. One of the four was a recovered alcoholic at follow-up.

Patients with Infantile Personality

Among the borderlines with infantile personality (32 traced out of 35, all female), the presence or absence of affective comorbidity seemed determinative in several cases. One of the patients showed a schizoaffective (SA) evolution. She had been unable to work steadily during the 5 years prior to follow-up, and was wildly impulsive and chaotic in her relationships with men, alternating between desperate clinging and outbursts of rage. She had been rehospitalized repeatedly for suicide gestures. The worst-functioning of those still alive (GAS score = 30)

points up the arbitrariness of placing chaotic patients in this or that compartment of personality types. Described by her family at the time of follow-up as
moody, irritable, self-destructive, spiteful, and episodically abusive, she showed
depressive, irritable, passive–aggressive, and antisocial traits, in varying proportions at various times. She was in a psychiatric hospital because of suicide
gestures when I contacted the family.

The best-functioning of these patients had grown up in a loving but
turbulent family with overintrusive parents, in reaction to whom she became a
moody and hostile adolescent. A talented musician, she spent only a few months
on our unit before she left to resume her studies. She subsequently married, had
a child, and pursued her career with good success for many years (follow-up GAS
score = 87). Another patient who did quite well (GAS score = 74) was the
more remarkable for having been raised in a much worse environment. Her
father had molested her sexually when she was 5 years of age. As an adolescent,
she became a runaway and an addict. She had many difficult years after leaving
the unit (a failed marriage, a continuing drug problem), but eventually returned
to school, conquered her drug habit, entered a sustained and stable relationship,
and began working (with excellent commendations) in one of the helping
professions.

Patients with Depressive or Depressive–Masochistic Features

Many of the borderline patients I have categorized as "depressive" or
"depressive–masochistic" were also dysthymic by DSM criteria, especially the
former, and did not show enough angry and irritable traits to exemplify BPD.
In a few, one could see a mixture of narcissistic or avoidant or obsessional traits,
but paranoid and irritable traits were rare. Only 1 of these 53 patients (of whom
I traced 52) had features of ASP, and those only during her late adolescence,
after her abusive mother provoked her into running away. She became
promiscuous and alcoholic for several years; after leaving the unit, she became
agoraphobic; some 5 years later she committed suicide. About a third of these
patients (8 of 25 depressives; 11 of 26 depressive–masochistics) had at least one
first-degree relative with affective disorder (bipolar in 4 cases); another 3 had an
alcoholic parent. These figures do not exceed those for the borderline patients
in general.

The worst-functioning of the depressive patients, apart from the two
suicides, was a man with concomitant avoidant traits who had worked steadily
since leaving the unit, but who at follow-up was leading a constricted life with
no sexual partners and with almost no social contacts. The most successful was
a woman who made a suicide gesture following the death of her mother. She
spent the better part of a year on the unit, working with a therapist whom she

felt (correctly, as it happened) was ineffective and insensitive to her needs. She finally eloped from the unit, amidst gloomy prognosticians by the staff; enrolled in graduate school; married; and became a community leader of such prominence as to preclude further description. She never sought and apparently did not need therapy in any form during the intervening 20 years.

One of the depressive borderlines with a course and outcome more typical of this subgroup was a woman who became alcoholic after leaving the hospital, eventually brought herself under control via AA, and at follow-up was working full-time in an administrative capacity. There were few keen pleasures in her life; her marriage was ungratifying, and she was not very happy. But by all external criteria she was functioning smoothly; as her family mentioned, no one would know she had ever been ill.

In contrast to the masochistic patients, who appeared to contribute actively to their own suffering, the depressive borderlines more often seemed ill-fated, as though born under an unlucky star. With the exception of the woman who let herself be seduced by one of the staff and who then killed herself, these patients did not go out of their way to make themselves miserable. Some were the "high-risk" offspring of parents who had MDP, but were otherwise adequate and nurturing. A few came from abysmal families where both parents were alcoholic and abusive.

One of the "high-risk" patients (two first-degree relatives with unipolar depression) illustrates an important point concerning the measure of outcome—namely, that even as useful a scale as the GAS cannot convey the total picture, especially where not all the important segments of life are on the same level. This man was one of the most successful of all the patients in the PI-500, not only in his work (at follow-up, he was running a large business) but in his marriage and civic involvement. Yet he remained susceptible to episodes of depression that came over him unexpectedly "like a black cloud descending," as he phrased it; for these, he periodically took antidepressants or an occasional "refresher course" of psychotherapy. Because he was still moderately symptomatic, his follow-up GAS was 73, even though in every other respect his life resembled that of the patients in the 90s decile.

Unlike the passive–aggressive, infantile, narcissistic, or irritable borderlines, whose hostility was more intense and nearer the surface, the depressive (including masochistic) patients were as a group less hostile, more apt to blame themselves (whether or not they had been blameworthy), and more vulnerable to the special set of painful emotions engendered by unrequited love—pining, *Sehnsucht*, or what Milan Kundera (1980) attempted to define by the indefinable *litost*: a state of "torment caused by a sudden insight into one's own miserable self" (p. 122). This intropunitiveness, coupled with introspectiveness and a tendency to form strong bonds of attachment (prominent features in this group), did not always guarantee these patients a good outcome, but did make many of them good candidates for intensive psychotherapy. Again, those who did *not* do well were usually burdened with serious forms of affective illness or else with severe early traumata. A masochistic (× BPD) woman with a follow-up GAS score of 45 was a victim of father–daughter incest, which exerted more damaging effects upon object relations than her charm and attractiveness could overcome. The best-functioning patient described her long period of "rough sledding" after leaving the unit: She continued to feel depressed and inadequate, and made several suicide gestures, until she managed to complete graduate school about 5 years later. At follow-up, she was married, working at a high professional level involving community work, and raising three children (GAS score = 91). Whereas she had been rather morose and uncommunicative on the unit, she was now cheerful, optimistic, and outgoing; in effect, she was "no longer the same person." This former patient was one of several who complained that the hospital kept her too long and held her back from advancing with her studies.

Patients with Passive–Aggressive Features

Because their personalities are characterized more by inhibition than by action, more by fearfulness than aggression, the depressive and masochistic patients might also be grouped with DSM's "Cluster C"—a point to consider for DSM-IV. (The DSM clusters are discussed further below.) The remaining borderlines with secondary pathology in this cluster—the (passive–)dependent and passive–aggressive patients—ultimately did reasonably well, with median GAS scores in the mid-60s. This was the case despite the general unresponsiveness of the passive–aggressive patients to psychotherapy: Their sulkiness, lack of cooperation, and wariness of authority undermined the efforts of therapists and ancillary staff alike.

Of the passive–aggressive borderlines still alive (15, all traced), the highest- and lowest-functioning were as similar as fraternal twins and were admitted within the same year. The most handicapped was a chaotically impulsive woman, talented but rebellious as an adolescent, who lived in and out of counterculture communes and residential treatment centers after eloping from our unit when she was 17. She was promiscuous, put a baby up for adoption, was raped, and was never able to work. Her story is puzzling in many ways. Her family was nurturing and remained intact; she had an IQ of 131; her early years were free of loss or trauma. Nevertheless, at menarche she was abusing marijuana, amphetamines, and on rare occasions LSD. Her drug abuse accounted for much of the deterioration in her late adolescence, but probably cannot explain her continuing rebelliousness and impulsivity over 20 years later.

The best-functioning of the passive–aggressive patients did not meet the BPD criteria, but also began abusing marijuana and amphetamines after puberty. He grew up in an intact and nurturing family as well, and had an IQ of 133, similar to that of the impulsive woman. Spending over a year on the unit, also when he was 17, he seemed more committed to treatment and less rebellious. After discharge, he entered graduate school; at follow-up, he had been supporting himself for 19 years in an occupation that gave him considerable satisfaction (GAS score = 90). One might think that something would leap out of the pages—if not of their lengthy admissions notes, then at least from the notes of their subsequent course—that would explain the 50-point difference in these patients' follow-up GAS scores. So far, this something has eluded me.

Interestingly, the "median" passive–aggressive patient (who *did* meet the BPD criteria) was admitted in the same year and at nearly the same age (16) as the two described above. She came from a middle-class Jewish family like the other two, but her parents had divorced when she was young. She began abusing marijuana and mescaline after menarche, and changed from a shy young girl into an unruly adolescent with a "chip on my shoulder." Following a lengthy stay on the unit, she became part of the counterculture for several years, supporting herself through her skills in theatrical stage design. She tried a number of different therapies (some conventional, some faddish), and maintained a number of long-lasting relationships with men. The passive–aggressive traits apparent during her hospitalization may have been mobilized, or intensified, by the drug abuse. In the years immediately prior to follow-up, she gave up these drugs and manifested once again the shy, avoidant traits that had characterized her childhood years.

Patients with Passive–Dependent Features

The passive–dependent borderlines (whom DSM would now call simply "dependent personalities") were another group whose typical outcome was in the average range. One might have anticipated that they would do worse, because they had less ambition, less drive, and less resilience than many of the obsessive–compulsive or narcissistic borderlines. But "gumption" is not the only ingredient of successful life: Some of the dependent patients had jobs at follow-up that were less remunerative or exciting than those of, say, their obsessive–compulsive counterparts, yet a number had distinguished themselves for their community-mindedness and personal appeal. One such dependent patient, whose harmony and "inner" success are surely the equal of the more showy success of some of the obsessive executives, was a woman with BPD who devoted her life to the poor within a large religious commune in a foreign country. Her follow-up score of 68 does not capture the selflessness and high purpose that animated her life after she left the hospital.

The highest-functioning of the patients with dependent personality was a man, also with BPD initially, who at follow-up was neither borderline nor dependent. When hospitalized 20 years ago, he had suffered a brief psychotic episode under the influence of hallucinogenic drugs and alcohol. Every member of his family, with the exception of one sibling, was alcoholic. His course after he left our unit went steadily uphill. He gave up alcohol, somehow managing to do so without the help of AA, and graduated first in a large class of business students. At follow-up, he was running an important corporation, was a leader in his community, was married, and had three children. He was one of the two patients in the PI-500 with a follow-up GAS score of 95. Alcoholism, incidentally, was a common problem among the dependent patients; 8 of the 21 were alcoholic. All of these patients gave up drinking with the exception of one man who, partly for this reason, was the worst-functioning of the 19 traced patients. He had been heavily involved in a variety of illicit drugs, including cocaine years before its popularity; he rarely worked and was on disability at follow-up. He had little motivation for anything, and was unable to complete scholastic or other tasks. Probably his heavy and continuing use of marijuana contributed significantly to this listlessness.

Avoidant and Phobic Patients

Borderline patients with avoidant comorbidity were too few to support generalizations unless I combined them with those who had a classic phobia—usually, agoraphobia. (Agoraphobia is discussed at greater length in Chapter Ten.) Only 8 of the 13 I traced in this combined group had BPD; of these, 4 were incest victims. The median GAS score among the 13 (65) belies the fact that this group as a whole functioned poorly, both socially and occupationally. Most were leading constricted lives at follow-up, as one might expect from their lack of ease in most human encounters. One remained agoraphobic for 24 years, despite several rehospitalizations and several courses of supportive and behavioral therapy. Another was married briefly, divorced, and returned to her parents' home, where she had remained housebound for 12 years at follow-up. Three of the four incest victims (all three were daughters molested by fathers) appear to have been permanently crippled by their experiences. One took refuge in a religious cult; another lived a hermetic life after a few unhappy love affairs at about the time of her hospitalization. Both made several suicide gestures before admission to our unit, as did the third young woman, who avoided relationships with men for the 15 years between her departure from our unit and follow-up.

The best-functioning of the BPD × phobic patients was a woman whose father was also severely agoraphobic. He grew quite possessive of her when he and her mother divorced early in the patient's adolescence. She remained nearly immobilized by her symptoms for 7 years, 2 of which were spent on our unit. Behavior therapy for agoraphobics was new and poorly understood at the time (the 1960s). Fortunately, she responded to a psychotherapy that focused sometimes on the here-and-now, sometimes on the relationships with her father. Upon leaving the unit she acquired a "transitional object" in the form of a pet dog, in whose presence she could do her errands free of anxiety. I have followed her yearly for the past 25 years, during which time she married, raised two children, and worked effectively both in community affairs and at her place of employment (GAS score at most recent follow-up = 78).

The best-functioning of the 13 patients in the combined avoidant–phobic group was a man without the BPD characteristics, who recovered rapidly upon leaving the unit without any further therapy. He overcame his shyness and the generally inhibited personality he brought with him to our unit, to the point of becoming the chief executive officer of a large manufacturing concern. A few weeks before I spoke with him, he and his wife had their first child. This vignette may serve to illustrate a clinical hunch about "avoidant" characteristics— namely, that if one develops shyness from having been abused, molested, or humiliated, the shyness is difficult to overcome. One remains an "avoidant personality." In the absence of such traumata, one may in time become much more self-confident, so that one can shed one's shyness and leave it behind.

THE MOST "NEGATIVE" PATIENTS

Despite the fairly wide range of personality types in the PI-500, ours was not a random sample of the population, or even of the psychiatrically ill population. Because we were able to screen most of our prospective patients, we excluded as many as we accepted. Having felt instinctively that markedly paranoid, aggressive, or antisocial patients would be poor candidates for intensive psychotherapy, we were hesitant about admitting them. Symptomatically, our patients were for the most part very ill—delusional, destructive, drug-abusing, and so on—yet the majority had favorable personality traits, likeable qualities, and other counterbalancing assets.

This leaves me in a position to comment only briefly on the most "negative" kinds of patients: We had few to begin with, and they proved to be the most difficult to trace. For example, I would very much like to know what became of the haughty and venomously spiteful borderline man, brutalized by his father and turned out onto the streets, who elicited from Harold Searles the remark (after the patient had "stonewalled" him for 40 minutes), "I want you to know this is *not* the worst interview I have ever done!" I am equally curious about the borderline adolescent whom we were persuaded to accept on our unit after he and his father, the latter a "higher-up" in a notorious organized-crime family, chased their valet with a rifle for (allegedly) carrying on an affair with the patient's mother. Though hospitalized ostensibly for "depression," both these men were antisocial; the second was also bellicose. I have found neither of them. One of the most aggressive antisocial patients whom I did locate had been administratively discharged because of chronic flouting of the dormitory regulations and because of his cruel treatment of several young women on the unit.

He abused drugs before and for many years after the index hospitalization. After his discharge, he worked sporadically, married briefly, was rehospitalized once, and at follow-up was still manipulative and dependent upon his family (GAS score = 49).

SUBTYPE CLUSTERS AND PERSONALITY DIMENSIONS AMONG THE BORDERLINES

Subtype Clusters

Comparing the obsessive–compulsive patients with the "Cluster A"[2] (paranoid/schizoid/schizotypal) patients, we see that they appear distinguishable not only phenomenologically but prognostically. Median GAS scores at follow-up were higher in the obsessives by two deciles. The obsessives also outperformed the other patients in "Cluster C"—the passive–dependent and passive–aggressive. The same is true if we merge the avoidant and phobic borderlines into one group with 13 traced patients: Their median GAS score (65) was also about a decile lower. I agree with the impression of Hyler and Lyons (1988) that the obsessive–compulsives probably belong in their own separate category, whereas the avoidant, passive–dependent, and passive–aggressive can meaningfully be grouped as the "anxious" cluster, and the paranoid/schizoid/schizotypal as the "eccentric" or "asocial" cluster. Creating an "unstable" cluster from the histrionic, NPD, BPD, and ASP patients likewise seems tenable, although many narcissistic patients in office practice are not particularly unstable. These clusters, incidentally, are not dissimilar to the three personality dimensions delineated in the other Scandinavian literature: the "substable," the "subvalid," and the "subsolid" (Bech, Allerup, & Rosenberg, 1978).

For the sake of simplicity, we might coalesce certain subgroups within the borderline domain of the PI-500: Those with infantile personality were similar to the histrionics, though more irritable and less well integrated; the depressives and the depressive–masochistics were similar, as were the avoidant patients and the classic "phobics." This would yield the distribution indicated in Figure 6.4. The preponderance of the histrionic/infantile and depressive/depressive–masochistic subtypes is related to their frequency within the population of female borderlines, who in turn comprised two-thirds of the borderline domain.

---

[2]For didactic purposes, DSM-III-R has compartmentalized the personality disorders into an "eccentric" cluster ("A"), consisting of the paranoid, schizoid, and the schizotypal; a "dramatic" cluster ("B"), consisting of the antisocial, borderline, histrionic, and narcissistic; and an "anxious" cluster ("C"), containing the avoidant, passive–dependent, obsessive–compulsive, and passive–aggressive.

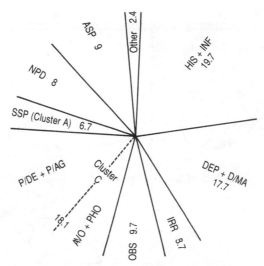

FIGURE 6.4. Subtype clusters within the PI-500 borderlines (traced and untraced). AVO, avoidant; PHO, phobic; other abbreviations as in Figures 6.1 and 6.2.

Personality Dimensions

We may also regroup the patients within a field reflecting certain important *dimensions* of personality that lie at a higher level of abstraction from the subtypes themselves. Because of the difficulties of illustrating more than three dimensions at once, I chose for Figure 6.5 "active" versus "passive," "extraverted" versus "introverted," and "more ill" versus "less ill." This figure may make clearer than the preceding diagrams that I included in my analysis of personality both the types outlined in Axis II and the Kraepelinian temperaments associated with MDP (depressive, manic, irritable, cyclothymic). Though the latter resemble some of the entities described in Axis I (depressive neuroses, cyclothymia), I felt that the DSM does not adequately capture this area of psychopathology. Admittedly, some persons develop "irritable" or "depressive" personalities more because of early traumata than because of risk genes for MDP, so these two subtypes are less reliable indices of MDP than are the (hypo) manic or cyclothymic.

Even this complicated diagram cannot do justice to the interrelationships among the various categories of personality, especially when we inspect the extreme regions of these necessarily arbitrary compartments. Extremely histrionic patients, for example, are apt to show strong narcissistic traits. Extremely narcissistic persons (especially males) are apt to be antisocial (or, more accurately, "psychopathic," according to Cleckley's [1976] description). Infantile personality is an overlap region between histrionic and irritable. Some extremely histrionic patients are unusually outgoing and "charged up"; they are also

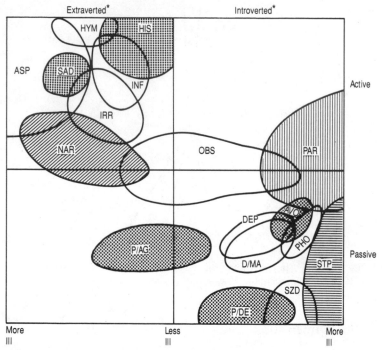

FIGURE 6.5. Personality subtypes of borderline patients on the dimensions of "active" versus "passive," "extraverted" versus "introverted," and "more ill" versus "less ill." HYM, hypomanic; PAR, paranoid; SAD, sadistic; SZD, schizoid; other abbreviations as in preceding figures. (*cf. Jung, 1921.)

hypomanic (especially certain borderline females with bipolar II affective disorder). Many antisocial, sadistic, and irritable persons have strong paranoid traits (not properly reflected in the diagram). What we are dealing with is a complex set of conditional probabilities: Given a predominant personality of Type X, what are the likelihoods of coexisting traits belonging to Types A, B, C, D . . . ? Few types are mutually exclusive. I do not think that one finds schizoid patients who are at the same time hypomanic. Most other combinations are possible, and many of the resulting profiles appear to have important prognostic consequences. The more common patterns will often resemble the typical MMPI profile of BPD patients (Resnick et al., 1988). Unusual patterns may be associated with an atypical course.

The *least* successful of the still-alive obsessive–compulsive patients, for example, was a man with marked avoidant and paranoid traits, as well as BPD. His father had ridiculed him mercilessly during his adolescence, shattering his self-esteem. At follow-up 17 years later, the patient was still leading a meager life, mostly isolated, working sporadically at odd jobs well below the level for which his postgraduate training had prepared him (GAS score = 52). The most successful obsessive, in contrast, was a borderline-level woman with mild infantile and narcissistic traits. She completed graduate school with honors after leaving the hospital; at follow-up, she had a wide circle of friends and a number of absorbing hobbies (GAS score = 90). Unlike the first patient, she did not have a traumatic history. These factors can often be quite difficult to tease apart, since parental humiliation may contribute importantly to development along paranoid and avoidant lines (Frosch, 1981); later, the clinician may view either the personality factor or the traumatic factor as the chief culprit, depending on the factors' relative weights or upon the clinician's theoretical bias.

The reader interested in other abstract systems of personality will find Cloninger's (1986) article on biosocial theory most valuable. He focused on three dimensions of personality: novelty-seeking, harm avoidance, and reward dependence. Each may be high or low ("N, n"; "H, h"; "R, r") in any given person. Cloninger characterized a number of the personality types I have been discussing, in accordance with their specific pattern. For example, in Cloninger's schema, histrionic = N h R; antisocial = N h r; passive–aggressive = N H R; explosive/schizoid = N II r; passive–dependent = n H R; obsessional = n H r; cyclothymic = n h R; and the "imperturbable schizoid" = n h r. Most patients with BPD exhibit the N h R pattern (especially the females) or the N h r pattern (especially the males), since impulsive novelty-seeking is a defining characteristic. But, as I have noted, most of the patterns Cloninger outlined may have existed within the PI-500 BPD patients and certainly within the broadly defined borderline group, with the exception of the "imperturbable schizoid."

A WORD ON PERSONALITY SUBTYPES AMONG SCHIZOPHRENIC PATIENTS

The schizophrenic patients in the PI-500, as noted earlier, showed much less diversity of underlying personality traits than did the borderlines. During the acute phase of their illness, their florid symptoms often masked these traits, rendering diagnosis of the personality component futile. One had to rely instead on anamnestic material or on the surfacing of various personality attributes, once the psychosis subsided. I could not always discern which traits were predominant, since in several instances the admixture of schizoid and paranoid traits, or of schizoid and obsessive–compulsive traits, was rather evenly balanced. Here I used as my guide the majority opinion as expressed in the old records. Arieti (1977) once estimated that a quarter of schizophrenics were schizoid in their premorbid personality. In the present series, 22 of the 99 schizophrenics were distinctly schizoid, yielding a ratio similar to Arieti's. However, half the obsessive–compulsive and nearly all the paranoid patients had schizoid traits as well; the latter were merely overshadowed by traits belonging to these first two categories. The median follow-up GAS scores in both the paranoid and schizoid groups were nearly the same (30 and 36), as were the suicide rates (14.7% and 13.6%, respectively).

In contrast, the schizophrenics with a predominantly obsessive–compulsive personality, though a small group, appeared to do significantly better. Their median GAS score (56) was over two deciles higher than that of the paranoid group ($SD = 16.5$ in both), $t = 4.2$, p (two-tailed) $< .01$. This seemingly robust finding is not so easy to interpret, however, if we take into consideration that two of the nine obsessives met DSM criteria for SZ initially, but did not evolve along the lines customary for "true" schizophrenics, nor would their clinical picture at follow-up support a diagnosis of SZ. One had a break into SZ (by all appearances), lasting 9 months, during her last year of college. Her delusions, hallucinations, and peculiarities of speech gradually cleared while she was on the unit. She then eloped from the unit, returned to school, completed a professional course, and obtained a high administrative position. During the 24-year follow-up interval, she never had another breakdown and never required or sought psychiatric care. It is unclear whether she would be appropriately grouped among the schizophrenics, as simply a recovered case, or whether she should have been placed among the "schizophreniform" patients, had we used follow-up rather than initial diagnosis as our distinguishing criterion.

Another of the obsessive schizophrenics who was functioning well at follow-up retained an area of eccentric religious thinking that surfaced when he was under stress. Whereas he used to lose perspective and become psychotically engulfed in this mode of thought years ago, now he was able to recognize it as it began to happen, and to re-establish contact with his therapist. He and the preceding patient (current GAS scores $= 81$ and 80, respectively) represent the best outcomes in the SZ group.

The woman who underwent lobotomy (see Appendix B) was another well-functioning obsessive–compulsive "schizophrenic." I have used quotation marks here, because, like the first patient, she was schizophrenic by DSM-III criteria when initially evaluated, but after her operation was free of the signs and symptoms that would trigger this diagnosis.

Whereas the recovered schizophrenics with obsessive–compulsive personality had pleasant and conventional social façades pre- and postmorbidly, the poorer-functioning patients in this category were handicapped by certain peculiarities of behavior. One man was awkward in gait and had numerous facial tics and mannerisms that alienated him from others. His therapist was innovative enough (I speak of 20 years ago) to use videotape playback of his behavior to educate him about his eccentricities, but the latter never really disappeared. Another similar patient could not bring herself to sit down during her sessions or throughout much of her day on the unit. This was not phenothiazine-induced akathisia (she was not on medications at the time), but rather a behavioral aftereffect of her preoccupation with catching germs from other people who had sat down before her.

The schizophrenic patients with paranoid personality alienated others more because of their hostility and mistrustfulness than because of their mannerisms. Several were violent, including one man who committed murder, another who was killed while committing a crime, a third who was assaultive, and a fourth who burned down part of his parents' house. One disappeared for several years, living as a homeless person (see Appendix B). Only 1 of the 34 traced patients was socially well adjusted at follow-up. Only one ever married, and she was divorced at follow-up—a woman living in a commune and no longer involved with her children.

Those whose predominant traits were schizoid included a woman who had been friendless and a "loner" throughout her life and defiant as an adolescent. She began abusing drugs at about the time of her menarche, became promiscuous, and was raped twice before her hospitalization. In the 18 years of follow-up her behavior grew less chaotic, though she never worked and continued to depend upon support from her family. Paranoid tendencies continued as well, mainly in her avoidance of her (in reality benevolent) family, lest they "harm" her. The best-functioning schizoid SZs were two men, each of whom went through 7 or 8 difficult years after leaving our unit, requiring several rehospitalizations along the way. Both were then able, without further treatment, to work steadily and marry. One completed graduate school and was self-employed at follow-up; the other became a civil engineer. Neither had children. The engineer derived a sense of structure and of community from a religious foundation. Unlike most of the schizophrenics, whose work records were spotty or nonexistent, this man was a "workaholic." Neither man came from an abusive background, though both had suffered the loss of a parent during their growing up. The median-scoring schizoid patient (GAS score = 35) remained quite disabled at follow-up—living at home, not working, and still exhibiting paranoid ideation as well. He continued to imagine himself a great inventor, periodically sending off never-to-be-answered letters to the patent office. Another, whose follow-up GAS score was 32, had been incapacitated since leaving our unit, having made several serious suicide attempts in the 17-year follow-up interval. These led to lengthy rehospitalizations. His course has been consistent with that of a schizoaffective patient. At the time of the index hospitalization he showed considerable artistic talent, but he was never able to pursue this remuneratively or consistently. Sometimes he did portraits of the other patients in the hospital where he resided at follow-up, though on one occasion he flew into a rage and smashed his easel.

GENERAL COMMENTS

In the preceding pages, I have tried to show some of the ways in which personality influences outcome. I am painfully aware that I have been able to mine only the shallowest layers; so many of the factors have remained either hidden in layers below our powers of penetration or else merged with the more recognizable skeins in such a way as to elude detection. Among the schizophrenics, most personality differences were swallowed up in the severity of the underlying illness, much as though one had mixed a teaspoon of orange juice in a bottle of ink. Although the obsessive–compulsive schizophrenics fared better than the average, the other subgroups either showed mean GAS scores that were indistinguishable or were numerically too small to permit meaningful analysis. Among the borderlines, personality factors were far more impressive as determinants of different life courses, but even here the gross distinctions I could assess (Axis II "comorbidity," etc.) accounted for less of the variance than might rightfully belong to personality as a whole. For example, the fate of borderline patients who were free of any obvious constitutional predisposition and whose families were not abusive seems *mostly* a function of personality differences—the ones we can measure easily plus the subtle ones, such as responsibility, perseverance, and the other assets Kolb (1982) enumerated. These positive attributes cut across the archetypes outlined in DSM, as do a large number of other negative qualities seldom mentioned in discussions of person-ality: tactlessness, rigidity, scrupulosity, and pettiness. Any of these, in the extreme, can exert major effects on the life course.

Interactions among the various dimensions create even greater complexity and probably account for a sizeable fraction of variance. An avoidant, overly sensitive obsessive–compulsive borderline may shy away from certain job opportunities, give up on dating after the first polite refusal, and so forth, whereas a more assertive and less easily bruised counterpart may get both the job and the date. After a long interval (10 or 20 years), the originally subtle differences get magnified, like two beams of light a millimeter apart near their origin but miles apart by the time they reach the moon. Because of this "sensitive dependence on initial conditions" (Gleick, 1987), the one patient is found leading a gratifying life at follow-up while the other is still languishing on the sidelines.

As a result of my preliminary assessments, I am tempted to make the generalization that a borderline patient with a pleasing personality, whose "Axis II" traits belong mostly to the favorable subtypes (obsessive–compulsive, histrionic, depressive, etc.) will probably be well (GAS score > 60, among other measures) 10 or 15 years after initial evaluation. This clinical improvement will itself be more sensitively dependent upon life's conditions than would be so with someone who was never emotionally ill to begin with. Thus, divorce, death of a loved one, job loss, or the like may "throw" the recovered borderline patient, bringing about a recrudescence of symptoms. McGlashan (1986a) noted this kind of evolution in some of the Chestnut Lodge borderlines as they crossed into their 40s and faced dissolution of a marriage and a weakened support system. In some instances personality was again a key variable, as in the case of the tenuously organized borderline woman in the PI-500 who killed herself in her 40s shortly after her divorce. She had alienated her husband with her abrasiveness and petulance. But a fragile patient with a much more agreeable personality may succumb just because of rotten luck (e.g., a spouse may unexpectedly drop dead, and the death may then precipitate severe depression and suicide).

By the same token, a borderline patient with the above-mentioned positive traits who has a markedly negative life course will often turn out, upon re-examination of the old records, to have been traumatized as a child, or to have come from a family laden with emotionally disturbed members, or both.

The Impact of Life Events: Early Loss, Incest, and Parental Brutality

This chapter concerns certain life events occurring during childhood and adolescence, and the impact they appear to have exerted upon the lives of some of the patients in the PI-500.

The literature on life events is large and ever-expanding. One can find articles pertaining to many different psychodiagnostic categories as well as to various forms of physical illness. Cross and Hirschfeld (1986), for example, report on correlations between certain stressful events and later suicide. Paykel, Rao, and Taylor (1984) comment on life stress in relation to milder forms of depression; Hudgens, Morrison, and Barchha (1967), Benjaminsen (1985), and Faravelli (1986), upon the severer forms of affective disorder; and Seivewright (1987), on the connection between life events and personality disorders. Canton and Fraccon (1985) concentrate on schizophrenia (SZ). Gyllenhammer and Wistedt (1987) note an inverse relationship between the "endogenous"-ness of a psychiatric disorder and the likelihood of life events as precipitants. Morrison, Hudgens, and Barchha (1968), reporting on a larger-scale study, discuss psychiatric illnesses in general. Murphy and Brown (1980) mention the high psychiatric morbidity in physically ill patients and outline the often complicated links between life events and organic illness, where psychiatric disturbance may be an intervening variable.

Because I had to rely chiefly upon the old records, and secondarily upon my memory and the collective memories of my colleagues, I have better information on certain gross traumatic events (such as parental death or abandonment, physical brutality, or sexual molestation) than I do of verbal abuse, shaming of children, crushing of children's spirits by smashing toys in a fit of anger, and the like—all potentially pathogenic life events, but ones that the therapists did not always set down in writing during the intake interviews years ago. For these reasons, I confine this chapter to early loss and to familial abuse, both sexual and physical.

EARLY LOSS

Early loss of a parent or other primary caretaker, whether through death, separation, or some other cause, may contribute to the development of emotional illness—sometimes as a primary "agent"; more often, as a negative factor that exposes pre-existing fragility in a young person already vulnerable because of adverse constitution or environment. Premature loss occasionally acts as a "proximate cause" of illness, as when an adolescent runs away from home within days of a parent's abandoning the family or makes a suicide attempt the week after the death of a parent. More often, however, the time intervals between loss and the psychiatric disorder (as clinicians come to recognize) are rather long, and causal connections are more tenuous. Hostile divorce, for example, may lead to custody battles, to a daughter's ending up with an alcoholic and seductive father or stepfather, to fosterage, or to a host of other deleterious situations that gradually undermine emotional well-being. These stresses may actualize a potential case of SZ, making it recognizable several years "ahead of schedule," or may, through a series of interrelated adverse events, convert a potentially normal adolescent into a case of borderline personality disorder (BPD).

In my review of the PI-500 records, I divided early losses into a number of categories, to facilitate the assessment of their impact upon the lives of the traced patients. These categories are as follows:

1. Death of a parent before age 16.
2. Death of a parent within 2 years of the patient's hospitalization.
3. Divorce of the parents before age 16.
4. Abandonment by a parent.
5. Death of a primary caretaker other than a parent within 2 years of hospitalization.
6. Suicide of a parent.
7. Adoption.
8. Critical illness of a parent (death imminent) at the time the patient was hospitalized.
9. Placement in foster care or in an orphanage.
10. Death of a sibling who had been alive during more than 5 years of the patient's life.
11. Separation(s) of more than 6 months (at a time) from a primary caretaker.
12. Birth out of wedlock (patient never knew the father).
13. Death of a stepparent before age 16.

Cross and Hirschfeld (1986), in their review of psychosocial factors and suicidal behavior, mention the connection between early loss of parents or other important caretakers and eventual suicide or attempted suicide ("parasuicide").

TABLE 7.1. The Incidence of Early Loss in the Major Diagnostic Groups

Diagnostic group	n	Any loss		No loss	
		n	%	n	%
All borderlines	297[a]	113	38	184	62
Borderline × ASP	44	26	59	18	41[b]
Borderline, no ASP	253	87	34	166	66
Borderline suicides	19	11	58	8	42
SZ	99	39	39	60	61
SA	64	20	31	44	69
SA female suicides	9	3	33	6	67
MDP	39	19	49	20	51
SF	36	24	67	12	33[c]
Total	535	213	40	322	60

[a]Does not include 2 not classifiable as BPD or not BPD.
[b]Compared with borderline, no ASP: $\chi^2 = 9.70$, $df = 1$, $p < .01$.
[c]Compared with borderline, no ASP: $\chi^2 = 13.9$, $df = 1$, $p < .001$.

Suicide attempters come from broken homes two or three times as often as persons of similar age in the general population; Dorpat, Jackson, and Ripley (1965) give a figure of 69%. Others emphasize the frequency of divorce and desertion as opposed to death of a parent (Crook & Raskin, 1975; Morgan, Burns-Cox, Pocock, & Pottles, 1975), commenting that suicide attempters often describe their parents as quarrelsome, unsympathetic, or cruel. In one study, family life was twice as likely to be "chaotic" among attempters as among controls (Adam, Bouckoms, & Streiner, 1982).

Because there was no control group for the PI-500, epidemiologically speaking, I have had to make do with estimates of early loss based on studies conducted in the United States during the same span of years (1963–1976) and with persons similar in age to the patient cohorts. These reports generally present figures in the 20% range for some significant early loss in the normal young adult population (Seligman, Gleser, Rauh, & Harris, 1974; Wahl, 1954). The incidence of combined early losses in the lives of the PI-500 is about double this average. Table 7.1 shows the percentages for the major diagnostic groups, singly and in the aggregate. This table also highlights the patterns of early loss in a few special subgroups (viz., borderlines with antisocial personality [ASP] and borderline suicide completers).

Three subgroups showed a reversal of the 40% loss/60% no loss pattern noted in most of the groups: The borderlines dead from suicide, the borderlines with ASP, and the schizophreniform (SF) patients all showed a pattern of 60% loss/40% no loss. Given that patients with drug psychosis made up the bulk of the SF group, these averages suggest that early loss contributes to the development of antisocial traits, especially in adolescent males, and also to the risk of *completed* suicide. For schizophreniform patients, early loss may weaken support systems, force adolescents to rely more on a peer group than on the remaining parent or caretaker, and incline them in the direction of deviant and drug-abusing peers rather than conventional peers. Constitutionally, the schizophreniform patients did not appear more at risk for a psychosis than patients in other categories: 28% of their parents were psychiatrically ill (including seven with severe depression, two with SZ, and four with substance abuse)—a similar proportion to that noted in the families of the borderlines. But in early losses, the schizophreniform patients exceeded the borderline suicides and the antisocial borderlines: Two out of three had suffered the death or separation of a parent—the highest such ratio in any diagnostic group of the PI-500. Parental death or desertion was more common than divorce: 22% of the schizophreniform patients had experienced divorce, as compared with 34% of the antisocial borderlines. Five of the schizophreniform patients were also antisocial, including one who became drug-addicted during a stormy adolescence following the death of his mother (this patient subsequently recovered) and another whose mother died when he was 1, whose father was hospitalized for years for SZ, and who was raised partly in orphanages and partly by an uncle. This man, who almost killed a girlfriend, was, at follow-up, in an institution for the rehabilitation of addicts.

In many instances, premature loss was a factor contributing to subsequent mental illness—in a subtle manner not easily charted and not readily captured in statistical tables of "life events." But in other instances, the red thread linking the early loss to later damage, though winding in its path and tangled with other threads along the way, remained well within view. Here, however, the charts and tables fail us and we must rely upon anecdote. The following vignette is illustrative.

A schizoaffective (SA) woman of 18 entered our hospital because of a suicide attempt with sleeping pills. Her mother had died the year before after a protracted bout with cancer. Several weeks after the mother's death, the patient took a potentially fatal overdose of hypnotics and was accidentally discovered by a next-door neighbor who had a key to the house. The patient was hospitalized elsewhere, revived, and released. The same scenario repeated itself 5 months later; this time her sister discovered her. Hospitalized once again, she quickly formed an erotic transference to the psychiatrist. He informed her as tactfully as he knew how that hers were feelings to be talked out rather than acted out, whereupon she made yet another suicide attempt. This led to her hospitalization at PI. Throughout her 19-month stay, she was guarded, evasive, and seductive. She did reveal that, after her mother became ill, her father took to fondling her breasts, lying next to her, and so forth, as though she were her mother's replacement. Toward the latter part of her stay on our unit, and unbeknownst to her therapist, she became enmeshed in a sexual affair with one of the male nurses. Shortly after her release, she made demands upon the nurse's time that he declined to meet. A day later she hanged herself.

In this case, the death of the mother stimulated the father's incestuous activities, leaving the patient to deal with two overwhelming stresses instead of one. A dependent girl throughout adolescence, she sought relief via the formation of a tight bond that at the same time re-enacted the familial boundary violation. The therapist at the second hospital did not cross the boundary; this left her lonely but not guilt-ridden. The male nurse, meeting her more than halfway but later rejecting her, left her both lonely *and* guilty. Either feeling may have prompted the suicidal behavior. Loss, in this instance, unleashed a tragic sequence of events, through its effects upon the patient and her equally bereaved father—a sequence that might never have unfolded but for the premature death of the mother. In the section on schizoaffectives in Chapter Twelve, incidentally, I relate an almost identical scenario where the outcome was unexpectedly good.

INCEST

Background

In the past decade, reticence about incest has been decreasing. Women are far more likely to have been incest victims than men, and are coming forward much more often than was once the case to share with mental health professionals what happened to them during their earlier years. The taboo is so great that many people still cannot believe that the incidence of incestuous experiences is as high as recent reports suggest—as though what we are now hearing about stems from fantasy and "retrospective falsification" on the part of women with unresolved Oedipal strivings. The psychoanalytic pioneers, albeit trailblazers with respect to the discovery of childhood sexuality, did not quite discover the lost continent of actual incest, though they brushed past it many times.

I owe my own awareness of this reality to the psychologist Barbara Brooks, my colleague at the New York Hospital in Westchester during the late 1970s. Having devoted her PhD dissertation to the topic, she was more attuned to the possibility of a valid incest history than were the rest of the treatment staff; she spotted a particularly horrendous example in a patient under her care on my unit (a young woman impregnated by her father, who then left her to hitchhike the 100 miles back from the abortion clinic). We began to inquire more carefully about various forms of sexual abuse and molestation in all our patients, from which it developed that about half the borderline females had an incest history. This history was less apt to be present in the borderline males or in the other diagnostic groups (cf. Zanarini, Gundersen, Marino, Schwartz, & Frankenburg, 1989). There was a wide range of severity, with forced intercourse with a father at one extreme to unforced petting with a sibling at the other.

Recent estimates placed the incidence of an incest history (broadly defined) at about 5% for women in the United States (Finkelhor, 1984). In a methodical epidemiological study by Diana Russell and her colleagues in San Francisco (Russell, 1986), the incidence of incest in some form was found to be even higher: 16%. Surveys in the latter study were carried out, wherever possible, by women of the same ethnic background as the potential respondents; this may have enhanced cooperation with the research team. All authors who have devoted themselves to the topic agree that the incidence of sexual molestation in all forms (i.e., by parents, relatives, acquaintances, and strangers) is much higher than that of incest alone: A third to a half of women report such experiences. (The figures vary in accordance with the cutoff point in age used by the questionnaires; use of age 18 raises the percentages over those obtained when age 15 is used). Among the findings in Russell's study were the following: a greater incidence of incest in higher- than in lower-income families; about double the incidence in Latino families (20%) compared to Asian families (8%); and a greater incidence in Catholic and Protestant families (17% and 18%, respectively) than in Jewish families (10%). Other characteristics of the family background of incest victims (the frequency of paternal alcoholism or violence, maternal illness, etc.) are provided in Herman's (1981) monograph and in the book by Blair and Rita Justice (1979). Forward and Buck (1979) offer a number of clinical vignettes demonstrating the serious effects of incest. A useful questionnaire for obtaining information on sexual history (including possible incest history) is appended to the book by Kempe and Kempe (1984). Goodwin (1982) and Goodwin, Cheeves, and Connell (1988) have shown the effects of *extreme* incestuous abuse.

My estimate of the incest histories in the PI-500 has been affected by biases in opposite directions. In many instances I have had to rely upon the old records. Although these were detailed and reasonably complete concerning most relevant issues, allusions to incest were often soft-pedaled or suppressed altogether in cases where such a history had been detected. In the era of the PI-500, we were scarcely more prepared to believe in the possibility of incest than were Freud and the pioneer generation of analysts. We seldom inquired about such matters minutely and were therefore dependent upon the (occasional) candor or (customary) reticence of the patients and their families. All this would tend to lower my estimate of the frequency. Counterbalancing the inadequacy of the original charts were my own memory and the recollections of my colleagues—the former therapists, who often knew a good deal more than had been recorded in the charts. A number of relatives also came forward and volunteered to me information concerning incest that had never been revealed to the therapists or found its way into the old charts. In one instance, eager to set the record straight, an aunt told me of how her niece (our former patient) had been sexually molested by her brother (the father of that patient).

Tables 7.2, 7.3, and 7.4 represent my best reconstruction of this material, using as my guideline the three-tiered definition of incest (most to least severe)

TABLE 7.2. Incest Histories in Female Patients

| Diagnostic group | n | Patients with incest history | |
		n	%
Borderline (broad criteria)	181	35	19.3[a]
BPD	145	28	19.3
SZ	39	2	5.2[a]
SA	41	11	26.8
MDP	15	2	13.3
SF	9	0	0

[a]Borderline > SZ: $\chi^2 = 4.6$, $df = 1$, $p < .05$.

adumbrated in Russell's book (1986, p. 99). Because my information was not always detailed or reliable enough to tabulate according to the 18 gradations Russell outlines ("1. Rape: forcible genital intercourse" to "18. Nonforcible sexual kissing, intentional sexual touching of buttocks, thigh, leg or clothed breasts or genitals"), I have used only the three broad categories. In three instances there had been molestation by more than one relative (father, two brothers; mother, brother, and stepfather; father and stepfather). Some form of father–daughter incest had occurred in 25 of the 35 borderline female incest victims; in another 9, brother–sister incest had occurred. The rarest forms were mother–daughter (two) and uncle–niece (one).

Borderline and Other Female Incest Victims

The mean Global Assessment Scale (GAS) scores for the borderline female incest victims, two of whom were untraced (all borderline, 65.7; BPD, 63.3), and their suicide rate (3 of 35, or 8.6%) do not differ from the corresponding figures for the borderline females as a group. This should not be interpreted as signifying that the incest was without harmful effects. There was a tendency for the incest victims to remain more impaired at follow-up (10–23 years later): 37% had GAS scores < 60, whereas only a fourth of those who were not incest victims had scores in this range. But, more importantly, the incest and its psychological sequelae appeared to play a definitive role in the pathogenesis of the borderline condition that brought the patients to our attention in the first place (cf. Barnard & Hirsch, 1985). Given the multiplicity of variables that interact in the shaping of psychiatric conditions, this may strike the reader as conjectural.

To drive the point home about the pathogenicity of experienced incest would require a discussion too lengthy for a book focused on outcome; I have discussed the issue elsewhere in some detail (Stone, 1985a, 1990). Suffice it to say here that incest, particularly when initiated by a relative of the generation

TABLE 7.3. Female Incest Victims within the Borderline Domain

Patient no.	Severity level/offender[a]	Follow-up GAS score	Psychiatric illness in parents[b]		Comments
			Father	Mother	
BPD patients					
1	U-F	75		PsyD	
2	U-F	55			
3	1-F	37	V		Father attempted rape
4	1-F	74	ASP		Molestation at age 5; father then expelled
5	1-B; 2-SF; 3-M	85			
6	3-F	69	Bip II		Father petted, attempted intercourse
7	2-F	62			
8	1-B	55	V		
9	1-SF	30			Intercourse with stepfather
10	1-B	70			
11	U-F	55	Alc	PsyD	
12	1-F; M	53	MDP		
13	3-F	80	Alc, V		Patient witnessed father's violence toward mother
14	1-B	68	PerD	Alc	
15	2-F	54		UD	
16	1-F	88	PerD	Alc	
17	U-F	Su	D		
18	1-SB; 3-SF	71			
19	3-F	64	Alc, Su	Alc, Su	
20	1-B	31	V		Brother hostile; family rejected patient
21	2-F	82	UD	BPD	
22	1-F	58	PerD	Alc	
23	1-B; 1-F	Su	ASP, NPD, Alc		Father drove several siblings to suicide
24	1-F	45			
25	2-F	63	Alc		
26	1-B	Su	Alc	Alc	
27	1-B	74		Alc	
28	2-F	84	Alc		
D patients					
1	1-M	70			Mother, on one occasion
2	U-F	71	PerD, V		Father petted her in shower
3	1-Un	69			
Other BPO patients					
1	2-M	81			
2	2-F	42		MAD	
3	U-F	70			
4	3-F	68	Alc		

[a]Severity levels: 1, most severe; 2, severe; 3, least severe; U, uncertain. Offenders: F, father; B, brother; SF, stepfather; SB, stepbrother, M, mother; Un, uncle

[b]Psychiatric illness: Alc, alcoholism; Bip II, bipolar II MDP; PerD, (unspecified) personality disorder; PsyD, psychotic depression; Su, suicide; UD, unipolar depression; V, violent. Other abbreviations are as used throughout text.

TABLE 7.4. Other Patients with an Incest History

Patient no.	Severity level/offender[a]	Follow-up GAS score	Psychiatric illness in parents[b]		Comments
			Father	Mother	
Borderline males					
1 (BPD)	1-SF	90			
2 (BPD)	1-B	72	PerD	BPD	
3 (BPD)	2-S	75			
4 (BPD)	1-B	85			
5 (other BPO)	1-S	51			
6 (other BPO)	3-M	86			Mother very seductive, some sexual touching
7 (BPD)	1-M	Su		UD, Su	Mother seduced, had intercourse
8 (BPD)	1-M	Su	(adoptee)		Mother seduced, had intercourse
SZ patients					
1 (F)	2-F	50	PerD		
2 (M)	1-SB	45		SA, Su	Seduced by stepbrother
3 (M)	1-Un	80	PerD		
4 (F)	1-F	42	Alc		Father attempted intercourse
5 (M)	1-M	Su			Tried to rape mother
SA patients					
1 (F)	2-F	62	PerD, V		
2 (F)	2-F	62		SZ	
3 (F)	2-F	55		SZ	
4 (F)	1-F	Su	PerD		
5 (F)	3-F	38			
6 (F)	2-F	Su	Alc		
7 (F)	3-F	73	PerD, Alc	PsyD, Alc	
8 (F)	2-F	52		BPD	Father masturbated her
9 (F)	1-F	Untraced	V, PerD		Father had intercourse
10 (M)	1-M	71	V, PerD	SA	
11 (F)	U-F	67	PerD		
12 (F)	3-SF	37	Alc	Alc	
MDP patients					
1 (M)	1-M	45		SZ	
2 (F)	2-Un	47			
3 (F)	3-F	50		MDP	
SF patients					
1 (M)	1-B	36	SZ		
2 (M)	2-M	70		SZ	

[a]Severity levels: See Table 7.3. Offenders: S, sister; others as in Table 7.3.
[b]See Table 7.3.

124

older than the victim, constitutes a betrayal of both the trust and the love that characterize the attitude of the younger person toward that relative; in other words, there is a gross misappropriation of the emotional funds invested in one's supposed protector. Brutality, of course, represents a similar betrayal. Forced or sadistic forms of incest, where aggression and sexuality are intertwined, have, *a fortiori*, even worse effects than unforced incest. Since the patterns relating to intimacy, learned in childhood, act as the template for intimate partnerships in adult life, the incest victim · comes into adult life severely handicapped. Overstimulated, exploited, loving and hating the incestuous sexual partner at the same time, the incest victim tends to mistrust, adore, and hate by turns; to exploit byways of symbolic revenge; and otherwise to disrupt potentially harmonious relations with love partners. The object-relational attitudes that evolve out of the incest experience and the chaotic behavior these attitudes foster constitute the very features, in many instances, by which we define a borderline condition among our adult patients. Some incest victims, in other words, manifest the identity confusion, ambivalence, self-destructiveness, and impulsivity that make up some of the DSM, Kernberg, and Gunderson, criteria for borderline conditions. Along with these qualities, they often are intolerant of being alone, and they show an affect hunger and sensation-seeking tendencies that disrupt any efforts to perfect a skill or master a trade.

Among the female borderlines of the PI-500, one became so "turned off" to men because of forced genital contact with an older brother as to opt for a homosexual life. In addition, she was self-mutilative and self-destructive for many years prior to follow-up, missing suicide by a hair on several occasions. Another left her husband precipitously when her daughter reached the age (13) when she, as an adolescent, had been "gang-raped" by her father and four brothers; she was convinced that her husband (who was not at all of that type) was going to misuse her daughter in the same way. Several had sexual relations with their therapists before coming to PI. I have noted that women who become victimized in boundary violations of this kind very often have an incest history. Another—feeling herself to be a pariah, doomed to a tortured exist-ence—killed herself shortly after her wedding.

Because of the secrecy in which the topic of incest is ordinarily enveloped, the therapists and supporting staff were often misled as to the patients' real history and as a result would sometimes defend a therapeutic approach that was, in the light of what later emerged, contraindicated. A case in point concerns the mother of one of the PI-500 borderlines who told the patient that her father was "dead," whereas he was in fact alive and trying to locate her. This seemed monstrous to us—to have denied her daughter contact with her own father for over 10 years. But "contact" is the key word here: It came out later that the father had engaged in sex with his daughter when she was a young child. The mother forced him to leave the home, divorced, moved away, and chose (in a quite pardonable deception) to tell the daughter her father had "died." Before we realized what had happened, we urged the mother to permit "normal relations" with the father to resume—which the mother stubbornly, and wisely, refused to do. This patient has done well over the years (GAS score at follow-up = 74); I suspect that her good outcome is in part a function of the mother's decisive action, which prevented further damage and helped compensate for that damage by affording her more years of a healthier environment.

Incestuous experiences tended to be most pathogenic when they (1) were transgenerational (father, uncle); (2) involved force; (3) were chronic; and (4) occurred well within the span of the victim's memory. When most or all of these conditions were present, the resulting deformation of the personality often showed the following characteristics: compulsive sexuality; impulsivity; a propensity toward relationships involving boundary violations; sadomasochism; extreme jealousy; abuse of alcohol or drugs; and the pervasive sense of being a pariah. One could add an intense *cynicism,* inasmuch as the incest victim knew about "what adults do" long before ordinary children did, and also saw through the hypocrisy of the offending male (often enough, a father regarded with respect by the community) and the naîveté of the other betrayed party (usually the mother).

Apropos of compulsive sexuality, Yates (1987) has outlined a number of characteristics relative to sexually molested girls and boys, under the heading of "eroticized children." These include (1) exclusive emphasis on sex as a tension-relieving mechanism; (2) overly intense, personalized relationships; (3) exaggerated orientation toward libidinal experience ("seeking, expecting, yearning for further sexual experience"); and (4) difficulty in differentiating sexual from nonsexual touching (p. 258). In a similar vein, Edelberg and Tange (1987) mention the frequent feelings of anxiety and guilt in incest victims, along with boundary problems and loyalty problems within the family (p. 137). Elsewhere (Stone, 1990), I have presented an extensive catalog of symptoms, personality traits, and syndromes associated with incest. Some of the more severe effects of incest and early overstimulation are visible in the harrowing story of the sociopathic Diane Downs, the events of whose life progressed from father–daughter incest to marriage, divorce, and her eventually shooting to death her three children when she found them "getting in the way" of a new romance (Rule, 1987).

The borderline woman mentioned above who killed herself after her wedding exemplified many of these qualities. She had come from a wealthy family prominent for several generations in the Midwest. Sexual abuse (by her father and brothers) began when she was 8 and continued throughout her adolescence. She developed a whole host of psychiatric problems, beginning at menarche. There were several hospitalizations before and after the one at PI. A woman of no meager talent or charm, she had a wide circle of admirers, drawn to her in part because of her "spontaneity." The latter was more in the nature of a reckless impulsivity, manifesting itself as promiscuity, drug abuse, and wild partying. This image of spontaneity derived in part from her willingness to break social conventions. Those who knew her could see behind the glamorous façade—the depression, loneliness, self-hatred, and sense of impermanence about identity.

Women of this sort, if they identify with anything, identify with men's devaluation and exploitation of them. People become what they are called; these women saw themselves as "things" (more specifically, as playthings), to be used and discarded. In their estimation, at least, their lives were of no value—something to throw away, either in frank suicide (as in the preceding case) or in a kind of suicidal risk-taking and disregard of self. The best-known example in the Western world of this phenomenon is Marilyn Monroe. The details of her life have been set forth in the excellent biography by Summers (1985). In Monroe's life, childhood sexual molestation by boarders took the place of incest; she did not know her real father. In the end, she threw her life away in a setting of increasing drug abuse and in a series of acts that had the same *meaning* as suicide, even if (as several of her biographers contend) she did not intend *literally* to die on the particular night in August 1962 when her life ended. Women *made* into self-destructive borderlines through incest or sexual molestation of a particularly exploitative kind may be said to exemplify the "Marilyn Monroe syndrome." There were at least four such in the PI-500, including another suicide and two others whose lives have been tormented and joyless throughout the posthospital years.

In incest cases where accompanying sadism is extreme, the end result may be an induced psychosis, mimicking the prototypical psychoses (especially SZ), yet without any suggestion of hereditary abnormality. One may find hallucinations, persecutory delusions, nightmares of being attacked by men, and depersonalization—that is, a posttraumatic stress disorder (PTSD) of psychotic proporstions (see Breslau & Davis, 1987). (For a fuller discussion of PTSD, see Chapter Ten.)

At least three of the incest victims diagnosed as SA in the PI-500 were sexually brutalized by their fathers. One was delusional, unable to speak a coherent sentence while at PI, and markedly evasive and secretive (as are most such patients). She eloped after 4 months on the unit. Fortunately, she ran back to her mother (and to a nonabusive environment) rather than to her (divorced) father. Her psychosis lifted, and over the next 12 years she improved markedly. At follow-up, she was employed full-time and had recently become engaged. But the other two committed suicide. One had been raped by her father and, after leaving PI, drowned herself. The other became sexually involved with a recreational therapist at the hospital and hanged herself when the affair was discovered.

Another kind of induced psychosis common among victims of sadistic incest is multiple personality (see Appendix A).

What can be said concerning mitigating circumstances? Seven of the borderline incest victims had follow-up GAS scores of 80 or greater. A "most severe" form of incest (on Russell's scale) was present only in one. This case involved a father, but the sexual contacts were not tinged with physical cruelty. Even so, the patient, having eloped from PI, was "missing" for many years. She became alcoholic, was rescued by Alcoholics Anonymous (AA), and was doing unusually well at follow-up (working at a responsible job, married, raising a family). In the other six cases, there were milder forms of father–daughter incest (petting, cuddling, no nudity on the father's part) in four, brother–sister sex in one, and mother–daughter sexual *frottage* in another. All seven were in stable marriages at follow-up, whereas only 3 of the 11 with GAS scores < 60 had married (including two who committed suicide).

Whether the female incest victims of the current generation will fare better than those of the 1960s and 1970s is a question for future follow-up studies to answer. There was no group therapy in the era of the PI-500 devoted specifically to incest victims, as there is today. One of the positive effects of the women's liberation movement has been to reduce the shame that once was attached to having an incestuous "secret." This may account for the candor in some of the former patients with whom I spoke in the course of the follow-up. Perhaps this new openness will mean that sexually abused women (the less traumatized ones, at least) will be more accessible patients, with a better prognosis, than their counterparts of the generation before. Greater reliance on female therapists, especially in the initial stages of treatment, may help reduce the likelihood of boundary violations and of certain forms of "acting out" (e.g., sexual affairs with a male patient of the same therapist—as occurred with several incest victims in the PI-500).

It would take us rather far afield to discuss in detail the ethological implications of father–daughter (and other older male–younger female) incest; yet these considerations have great relevance to (1) the recurrence of the phenomenon generation after generation and (2) the female preponderance in most samples of borderline patients. Briefly, there are strong sociocultural reasons for young women to seek the protection of older males and for males to enforce via incest the loyalty and companionship of younger female relatives. These sociocultural, perhaps ultimately species-biological, forces operate much less strongly between mothers and sons. Oedipus aside, there are not many reasons for mothers to seek the protection of or to cohabit with their sons. The Oedipus "complex" may be universal in Western culture, but actual mother–son (aunt–nephew, etc.) incest is rare, whereas father–daughter incest forms part of the background of 5% or more of women in our country (Finkelhor, 1984; Russell, 1986). Psychopathologically, many of these women become "borderline"—enough (in my opinion) to account for much of the variance in the observed female–male ratio in this condition. Ethologically, many of these women pursue the "fast" (promiscuous, impulsive) as opposed to the "coy" coping strategy. Both unconscious behavior programs tend to have a certain survival value that perpetuates their respective personality types within a culture. One can speak here of a "balanced polymorphism" that maintains these types in rather fixed ratios down through the years. A most rewarding discussion of this polymorphism and of its evolutionary stability is to be found in the work of Dawkins (1976, pp. 151–178).

The most impressive piece of evidence within the follow-up study for the specific borderline pathogenicity of older male–younger female incest is the marked difference in its frequency between the borderlines and the prototypical schizophrenics (see Table 7.2). One might have to enlarge the diagnostic shutter to include the schizoaffectives (many of whom resembled the borderlines in symptomatology but were more seriously ill). Family chaos was certainly common among the schizophrenics, yet in the PI sample the schizophrenics were rarely incest victims.

Alcoholism in the parents played a significant role in the early lives of the borderline (and to a lesser extent of the schizoaffective) female incest victims. The borderline incest victims were more apt to have an alcoholic parent than were other female borderlines (13 of 56 in the incest victims; 9 of 147 in the remainder), $\chi^2 = 12.3$, $df = 1$, $p < .001$.

Males with an Incest History

An incest history was less common among the males of the PI-500 (female–male ratio = 4:1). I was able to pinpoint 15 (see Table 7.4): 8 borderlines, 3 with SZ, 1 with SA, 1 with manic–depressive psychosis (MDP), and 2 with SF. I would characterize only a few as *victims,* since this phase implies being overpowered and humiliated. A male sodomized by his father, for example, would be an incest victim. The closest approximation among the PI-500 consisted of a borderline male seduced by his stepfather. In this case the ill effects cannot have been very lasting (though the incest contributed to the anxieties that led to the hospitalization): At follow-up, this man was extremely successful both in his marriage and in his business, and had become a prominent citizen in his community.

Though mother–son incest is believed to be quite rare, there were five instances among the males in which the mother was the initiator, another where the mother stopped short of genital contact, and a last instance in which the patient attempted to rape his mother. Four of the five mothers in the serious cases where chronically psychotic (two schizophrenic, one schizoaffective, one unipolar depressive who committed suicide) and hospitalized on various occasions. The fifth, the adoptive mother of a borderline patient, had bipolar illness but had not been hospitalized; her son, after years of drug abuse and chaotic living, killed himself.

In the remaining cases of males with incest histories, the sexual involvement was with a sister, cousin, or younger brother. The relative absence of lasting psychological damage in this latter group probably stems from the absence of force. The young men in this group felt varying degrees of *guilt,* but did not feel particularly cheapened or humiliated.

PARENTAL BRUTALITY

In their excellent contribution to the study of physical and sexual abuse in the histories of psychiatric patients, A. Jacobson, Koehler, and Jones-Brown (1987) noted that only 9% of the abuse histories elicited during research interviews (of 100 patients) were mentioned in the original records. The reader should bear this observation in mind as I describe the parental brutality factor vis-à-vis the PI-500. I have had to rely chiefly on the old records, since I was able to interview only a small proportion of the former patients directly. Considering that just about 9–10% of an iceberg is exposed to view, the findings of Jacobson et al. can well be likened to the proverbial tip of that glacial structure.

It is well known that abuse begets abuse. Children who have been the victims of parental brutality (and not merely a rare spanking for something even the child understood was wrong) tend later on to behave abusively toward their own spouses and children (see Brassard, Germain, & Hart, 1987; Knutson & Mehm, 1988; Oliver, 1988; Van Hasselt, Morrison, Bellack, & Hersen, 1988); however, as Widom (1989) notes, the majority of abused children do not become delinquent or violent.

Effects of Brutality on Borderline Patients

Since "inappropriate anger" is now one of the important ingredients of the borderline syndrome, it should not be surprising to find in the background of borderline patients factors conducive to inordinate anger and aggressiveness. Elsewhere (see Chapter Five), I have examined possible constitutional abnormalities in borderlines, including organic brain damage and predisposition to bipolar illness. Here, I shift the spotlight to the most important environmental factor: namely, brutality on the part of the primary caretakers during childhood—in effect, the inordinate anger of the parents.

The parents (and their surrogates) of the PI-500 turn out to have been, on average, a remarkably temperate lot, exploding into physical violence toward their children in barely 8% of the cases. Of interest is the finding that the distribution of this phenomenon across diagnostic groups was uneven: Parental physical brutality was rare among the psychotic patients (14 of 243, or 5.8%), but more common among the borderlines (32 of 299, or 10.7%), $\chi^2 = 4.21$, $p < .05$. Table 7.5 shows the distribution across the major diagnostic groups.

There are many samples of borderline patients, both elsewhere in this country and around the world, where the figures are distressingly higher (Stone, Unwin, Beacham, & Swenson, 1988). At the Beth Israel Hospital in New York City, where I was consultant during 1984–1985, nearly all the borderline patients (hospitalized or in clinic) had traumatic childhoods. Some of the stories beggar description. One violent and antisocial borderline man, for example, had been suspended upside down by his feet outside his family's 12th-story apartment, as his alcoholic father yelled at him, "If you don't shut up, I'm gonna let go!"

The 46 identified victims (there may have been others) of parental brutality in the PI-500 were seldom exposed to the most grotesque forms of abuse, such

TABLE 7.5. History of Parental Brutality within the Major Diagnostic Groups

Diagnostic group	n	Patients with parental brutality	
		n	%
BPD	206	23	11.2
D	36	1	2.7
Other BPO	57	8	14.0
SZ	99	5	5.1
SA	64	3	4.7
MDP	39	2	5.1
SF	36	4	11.1

as the one sketched above. One came close, having experienced a kind of "soul murder" at the hands of his irascible father. When the patient was 17, he timorously asked his father to tell him about the "birds and the bees." His father's outrage at the "impertinence" of this question went well beyond even the level of parental reaction prevalent in the still prudish '60s: He took his son's photograph from the mantelpiece, smashed it to smithereens on the floor, and stomped on it, screaming, "Sex education you want! *I'll* educate *you!*" This young man then made a suicide gesture; he spent a year and a half on our unit, but killed himself shortly thereafter. We rarely saw, however, the kind of psychogenic madness (often showing up as multiple personality or SF) that is sometimes induced by chronic and intense brutalization.

It is noteworthy that the median GAS score of the BPD brutality victims (suicides apart) was a decile lower than the median score for the incest victims (55 as against 68), suggesting that parental violence was more noxious than sexual molestation. This possibility is fortified by the observation that the two groups overlapped only slightly: Just five of the BPD incest victims were also victims of parental brutality.

The deviation from the typical follow-up GAS is even more striking in the BPD patients than in the borderline group (i.e., all those with borderline personality organization [BPO]) as a whole. Figure 7.1 shows how the poorer outcomes were concentrated in the BPD subgroup. Table 7.6 provides additional details concerning gender, severity of abuse, and offending relatives. From Table 7.6, one can reconstruct the median outcome for the BPD abuse victims (*including* suicides): That score is 53, or lower still than the median score in the borderline group in general.

The series is too small and must rely too much on retrospective evaluation for us to assess whether the level of parental abuse was (1) greater in the BPD victims than in the other borderlines, or (2) if so, therefore a valid causative factor in their developing certain of the BPD traits (inordinate anger, self-damaging acts, impulsivity). We would, in effect, be studying whether some BPD patients could also be understood as examples of PTSD. I feel that this is

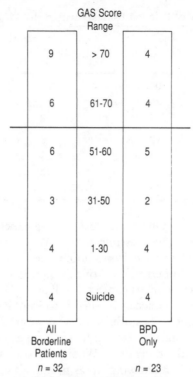

GAS Score
Range

9	> 70	4
6	61-70	4
6	51-60	5
3	31-50	2
4	1-30	4
4	Suicide	4

All
Borderline
Patients

n = 32

BPD
Only

n = 23

FIGURE 7.1. Outcome in traced borderlines with history of parental brutality.

probably the case, but the subject deserves more systematic study and follow-up before the question can be answered definitively (cf. Kolb, 1987).

The median GAS score alone, in any case, does not give a full picture of the effects of parental brutality. If one lumps together suicide and murder as two species of violence (opposite in valence but equal in degree), then the rate of extreme violence in the 32 borderline victims approaches 20%: There were four suicides and two murderers. Since all six had BPD, the rate of extreme violence within the BPD group was even higher: 6 of 23, or 26%. One of the latter was provoked by his chronically abusive and mercilessly critical mother into killing her (see "Patients with Antisocial Personality," Chapter Six). One of the abused women became a child molester as she entered her 20s; she would entice neighborhood children into her apartment and torture them. Another (see "Patients with Irritable Personality," Chapter Six) abused her own child and, after divorce, was prevented by a judge's restraining order from visiting the child. One man, who ended up living in the town next to his father's (each unaware of the other's whereabouts), had been abused physically by the father's second wife.

Sometimes bipolar illness in a parent was associated with irritability,

TABLE 7.6. Borderline Patients with a History of Parental Brutality

Patient no.	Sex	BPD?	Incest also?	Severity level[a]	Follow-up GAS score	Comments
				Patients were abused		
1	F	−	−	2	81	Father abusive; patient ran away
2	M	−	−	3	50	Father and stepmother abusive
3	M	+	−	4	2	Mother violent, later killed by patient
4	M	+	−	4	5	Both parents violent
5	F	+	+	3	55	Father abusive; incest with brother; mother urged her to commit suicide
6	F	+	−	4	30	Father threatened her with knife
7	M	+	−	2	56	Mother abusive
8	F	+	−	1	67	Father abusive
9	F	+	+	3	68	Mother abusive; incest with brother
10	M	−	−	3	Untraced	Father alcoholic, abusive
11	F	+	−	3	Suicide	Father often struck her in face
12	M	−	−	4	79	Beaten severely by parents
13	F	+	−	3	70	Father abusive
14	F	+	+	3	21	Father abusive; patient abused children
15	F	+	−	3	53	Father abusive
16	F	+	−	2	78	Father abusive
17	M	−	−	3	81	Mother alcoholic and abusive
18	M	+	−	3	85	Father alcoholic and abusive
19	F	+	−	4	Suicide	Stepmother violent
20	F	−	−	1	78	Father abusive
21	M	−	−	3	58	Mother abusive, then abandoned family
22	F	+	+	4	31	Father threatened with gun
23	M	−	−	2	61	Stepfather abusive to patient and mother
24	F	+	−	2	70	Father violent (worse to brothers)
25	F	+	−	3	75	Father broke her finger
26	F	−	−	2	71	Father gave her a black eye
27	F	+	−	3	82	Both parents abusive
28	F	+	−	2	63	Father abusive
29	M	+	+	2	41	Father abusive verbally more than physically
30	F	+	−	3	Suicide	Alcoholic, abusive parents
31	F	+	−	3	Suicide	Alcoholic, abusive parents
32	M	+	−	3	51	Father alcoholic, abusive
				Patients were witnesses only		
1	F	+	−		37	Father strangled brother
2	F	+	−		67	Father nearly killed mother
3	F	+	−		53	Father violent toward rest of family
4	F	+	−		71	Father abusive to mother
5	F	+	−		Suicide	Father violent toward brothers
6	F	+	−		84	Parents abusive toward each other
7	F	+	−		65	Father abusive to mother
8	F	+	−		80	Father violent toward mother, brother

[a]Severity levels: 1, mild; 2, moderate; 3, severe; 4, extreme.

133

explosive temper, and crude insensitivity to the feelings of others. One father with these characteristics used to place lit matches under the patient's hand "to teach him not to play with fire." On other occasions, this man (having divorced the mother and remarried) would taunt the (then adolescent) patient by lying naked with his new wife in bed and saying, "You wanna touch her tits, kid? Just come here and try it!" In some respects, "crazy" behavior such as this seems easier to deal with than cold malice; the PI-500 patients exposed to unpredictable outbursts of irrational violence, though damaged for life and still making only marginal adjustments, fared better than those exposed to calculated abusiveness and unrelenting hatred. The latter mostly killed themselves or others.

Effects of Combined Brutality and Incest

The BPD patients with a combined trauma history—parental brutality *and* incest—constitute a small group in the present series (see Table 7.6). Though meaningful statistical comparisons cannot be made, it is of interest that four of these five patients (all female) had follow-up GAS scores below 60 (21, 31, 55, and a suicide). If this kind of correlation were to hold up in other series, it would suggest that combined and severe abuse of this sort might be not only *causative* with respect to a certain proportion of BPD cases, but *devastating*. Perhaps the effects of abuse are particularly noxious where the emotional background is one of parental hatred, rather than of (exploitative) love—as is present in some cases of abuse and in many cases of incest. Children can forgive inappropriate love more easily than withering rejection.

The comparatively low rate of parental brutality among the psychotic-level patients (14 out of 238) provides another indirect clue as to the relevance of this factor for the pathogenesis of BPD. Years ago, the teaching staff at psychiatric training centers left their students with the impression that it was the schizophrenic patients who came from the worst homes. To be sure, the faculty placed greater emphasis on verbal "abuse" (e.g., the double-bind) than on physical abuse. But it was still surprising to note that, in the PI-500 at least, the borderline patients were considerably more likely to have been abuse victims than were the SZ patients, $\chi^2 = 3.82$, $p < .05$.

Effects of Verbal Abuse and of Witnessing Abuse

It has not been possible to enumerate all the cases in which verbal humiliation by a parent contributed heavily to the emotional disorder that precipitated hospitalization. Sometimes, as in the case of the man who ripped up his son's photograph, such an attack was the prime pathogen. But unless there was a similarly dramatic example of verbal assault, the PI records might contain only vague hints of verbal abusiveness. Cruelty of this sort figured in the histories of many of the PI-500, but only seldom in a way as quantifiable as instances of sexual or physical assault. There were other families in which emotional disorders were engendered not so much by what a parent did to the future patient, but by what the latter *witnessed* the parent meting out to some other member of the family.

One borderline woman became the captive audience of her father's chronic verbal and physical abuse of her three brothers, two of whom eventually attempted suicide (one succeeded). At PI, she was notably mistrustful and hostile toward men. At follow-up 10 years later, she had begun to make a good adjustment and had completed professional training. Another borderline woman saw her father beat both her brother and her mother; toward her, he was seductive and made open sexual advances, but she "got off easy" with respect to physical assault. During her adolescence she ran away from home, abused drugs, and lived as a street gamine—as did the man she married when she was 19. But after several difficult years she gave up drugs and made an excellent recovery (see "Drug Abuse," Chapter Nine).

In general (see Table 7.6), those who were *witnesses to* but not *victims of* parental brutality were more likely to do well at follow-up than were the victims.

General Comments

While it may be that the separation problems Masterson (1981) underlines, or the factors of loss and early deprivation mentioned by Volkan (1987), account for much of the pathological picture in certain ambulatory borderline patients treated in private practice, the array of etiological factors in hospitalized patients with BPD may be quite different in a large proportion of cases. In this section and the preceding one, I have concentrated upon parental brutality ("parental" in the broader sense of primary caretakers and close relatives in positions of responsibility and trust) and intrafamilial sexual exploitativeness. Their effects can hardly be overemphasized. In the PI-500, their effects seemed to loom larger in the causative chain culminating in a "borderline" condition than did the relatively milder stresses of loss or of a mishandled separation phase. One must also take into account sample variations. Some borderline (including BPD) patients have experienced rather little in the way of parental abuse, but the PI-500 are *nowhere near* the other end of the continuum. I suspect that the same is true of McGlashan's Chestnut Lodge sample. Our patients came most often from homes of professionals, successful businessmen, store proprietors, and the like; physical abuse was not the norm in these households. Most borderline samples I have encountered at other facilities—which I take to be more representative of borderlines here and in other countries—contain significantly higher proportions of abused children than were noted in the present study. To give just one example, the combined figure for sexual and physical abuse in the Australian borderlines I recently surveyed was 92% (Stone et al., 1988).

The other reason for emphasizing parental abusiveness, besides its sheer frequency, is its "heritability." I am not arguing here for some Lamarckian heritability of acquired characteristics; genetically, this does not happen. But *cultural* transmission of certain beliefs and personality traits is a powerful operator. Abused children go on to become abusing parents with a frequency that most likely exceeds the genetic transmission of, say, SZ or MDP (where perhaps only 10–15% of "children at risk" go on to manifest the corresponding classical psychosis). If my views about cultural transmission are correct, it means in effect that an impressive proportion of borderlines in any given generation are "made" borderlines (via parental cruelty or seduction), and that a proportion of these can be counted on to visit the same abuses upon their children, the "made" borderlines of the next generation. (Side by side with this contingent are the "born" borderlines—the children at risk for MDP, usually, whose impulsivity and anger are more biologically driven. See Chapter Five.)

For further comments on the pathogenic effects of abuse in all its forms (parental seduction, sexual overstimulation, rejection, verbal abuse, physical cruelty by parents), the reader should consult the papers of Beres, Eissler, Freud, and Glover (1951) and Spitz (1970), as well as the more recent publications of Jaffe, Wolfe, Wilson, and Zak (1986), who point out the special vulnerability of boys to parental discord (even if the boys themselves are not abused also), and of Straus, Gelles, and Steinmetz (1980), who comment on the high level of violence in American families.

Gender Differences and Factors Affecting Women's Outcomes

As I have noted earlier, women held a slight numerical edge over men in the PI-500 patient population as a whole (289 vs. 261). In some diagnostic categories, the female–male ratio approached or exceeded 2:1; for example, there were 145 women with borderline personality disorder (BPD) as opposed to 61 men, and 41 women with schizoaffective psychosis (SA) as opposed to 23 men (although males did tend to outnumber females in other categories of psychosis). It seems appropriate, therefore, to consider the question of whether there were significant differences in patients' outcomes according to gender, or to other factors that might have affected women's outcomes in particular. This chapter begins with a discussion of the issue of gender effects, and then considers a number of factors that either were limited to women by *definition* (children born out of wedlock, premenstrual mood disorders) or affected *primarily* women (eating disorders, the presence or absence of beauty, and rape).

GENDER DIFFERENCES IN BORDERLINES

Bardenstein and McGlashan (1988) reported recently on the influence of gender differences with respect to the natural history of the Chestnut Lodge borderline patients. Some differences existed already at the time of baseline evaluation: The females were more likely to have been married, more likely to have become dysfunctional in response to clear-cut precipitating events, and more likely to complain of certain depressive symptoms such as feelings of worthlessness or guilt. Their male borderlines were more apt to have been in trouble with the law and more likely to have left the hospital against medical advice. During the lengthy follow-up period, "the men surpassed [the women] . . . in quality of intimate relationships and frequency of social contacts" (1988, p. 74). The

137

women tended to decline in occupational and social functioning. The BPD women with poor outcomes sought heterosexual relationships, which they nevertheless tended to destabilize because of their continuing personality difficulties. As the authors concluded, "marriage for borderline women more often than not provided an arena for the enactment of psychopathology" (1988, p. 74). As the women entered their 40s, they frequently became increasingly symptomatic (depressed, irritable) and alienated their spouses or partners, further destabilizing their life situation. Some turned to alcohol in this setting. The men, in contrast, gradually improved in the area of work; they found strength more readily in attachment to job, treatment center (or therapist), or religious group than to a sexual partner. Alcoholics Anonymous (AA) often either took the place of or supplemented the religious group. But intimacy often eluded them. The poor-outcome males were particularly likely to abuse alcohol (and were perhaps less amenable to the kind of help offered by AA).

Bardenstein and McGlashan drew attention to the possibility of cohort effects. Women of the present generation, for example, more often have careers than did their mothers, the latter relying more on the traditional structure of husband, home, and children. Actually, many of the female patients in both the Chestnut Lodge and PI-500 studies were in transition: They were less oriented toward domestic life than their mothers, but less secure in alternate life structures than women born in the 1960s. Borderline women of certain cohorts, in other words, may be at special risk for recrudescence of symptoms during their premenopausal years, especially if they find themselves suddenly alone—partly because of poorer preparedness (fewer hobbies, fewer genuine work interests) for such eventualities.

In the PI-500, a number of gender differences also emerged, but these were not always the same as those observed in the Chestnut Lodge study. The borderline females, whether or not they also exhibited major affective disorder (MAD), were significantly more likely to be well (Global Assessment Scale [GAS] scores > 60) at follow-up than were the pure-BPD males (Stone, Hurt, & Stone, 1987). I believe this is a reflection of the greater proportion (11 of 28) of non-MAD male BPD patients who were comorbid for antisocial personality (ASP), compared with the BPD × MAD males (only 2 of whom had ASP), χ^2 = 9.97, df = 1, p < .01.

The male borderlines of the PI-500 were not more likely either to sign out against advice or to elope than were the female patients. If anything, the females were more apt to elope, χ^2 = 5.5, p < .05. But, having done so, the females were also more likely to have done well by the time of follow-up (see "Elopement," Chapter Ten). This difference, too, may stem from the overrepresentation of ASP patients—in this case, among the male elopees. Over the years, the female (and not so antisocial) elopees gradually improved; the males (who, if they were antisocial, were often severely so) did not improve.

In regard to alcoholism, the PI-500 female borderlines with poor outcome, whether or not one includes the suicides, were just as likely to have abused alcohol initially, or to turn to alcohol during the follow-up period, as were their male counterparts. Alcoholism was an accompaniment of about a third of the 22 female and 18 male BPD patients with follow-up GAS scores < 50.

The Chestnut Lodge borderlines were about 4 years older at the time of their index hospitalization than were the PI-500 patients. McGlashan and his coworkers have thus been able to observe a greater percentage of their patients as they cope with life in the fifth decade. My experience with female borderlines in my office practice is in accord with McGlashan's: As the borderline women enter their 40s, turbulence often increases; marriages may break up; substance abuse, suicidal ruminations, and even suicidal behavior intensify, and so on. Thus far in the PI-500 series, about a third (32.5%) of the BPD women who had married are divorced. Ten percent have divorced and remarried. The average and median age at this writing of the ever-married women is 40.0 (range = 30–56). Of the eight currently 45 or older, only two have gone through difficult divorces in their 40s that led to downturn in functioning (transient in both cases). One woman committed suicide at 40, shortly after her fourth divorce.

The DSM-III item "problems tolerating being alone" (or the DSM-III-R item "frantic efforts to avoid abandonment") was particularly noticeable in the borderline women who divorced in midlife. The men, as in McGlashan's series, married less often, found structure and solace in work or hobbies, and used their "obsessive" defenses quite effectively to cope with solitude. The women were caught in the conflictual situation of needing intimacy more than the men, but of being "programmed" (constitutionally, experientially, or both) to undermine the very ties upon which they so much depended. Some sabotaged their close relationships via inordinate clinging, others through hostility.

ANOREXIA NERVOSA AND BULIMIA NERVOSA

Both anorexia nervosa and bulimia nervosa have a long history. Accounts of unusual fasting in adolescent females go back at least to the time of the Venerable Lukardis (described in the hagiographic literature of the Analecta Bollandiana in the 13th century). Bulimia was recognized in the Talmud (Yoma 8, Mishnah 6) as a condition that excused one from the obligation to fast during Yom Kippur ("if anyone be seized with bulimy, he is to be fed even unclean things . . .").[1]

Most of the patients in the PI-500 who exhibited severe eating disorders functioned at the borderline level. An additional three had manic–depressive psychosis (MDP; two women with anorexia, one with bulimia). Three others were either schizophrenic (SZ; one woman with bulimia, one woman with anorexia) or schizoaffective (the one man with bulimia in the series).

---

[1] I am indebted to Dr. R. Winchel of the New York State Psychiatric Institute for this reference.

The same proportion of the eating-disordered borderlines showed the features of BPD as did the entire borderline subgroup (two-thirds). All but one were female. The anorectic/bulimic borderlines showed concomitant MAD less often (47%) than did the borderlines without an eating disorder (80%). MAD was present in 15 of the female borderlines with an eating disorder and absent in 17, whereas 116 of the 149 female borderlines without anorexia or bulimia had concomitant MAD, $\chi^2 = 12.6$, $df = 1$, $p < .001$. If we restrict our focus to the BPD patients, 14 of the 21 females with anorexia/bulimia had concomitant MAD. Among the *BPD* patients, that is, MAD comorbidity was not more common in those without an eating disorder.

Table 8.1 shows the actual distribution of eating disorders in this group: 16 of the women (50%) were anorectic only; 10 (31%) had "bulimarexia," with alternating periods of either anorexia or bulimia. Intentional vomiting followed binges in some of the bulimics (the exact proportion is unclear). Those with bulimia only ($n = 6$) accounted for the remaining 19%.

Table 8.1 also shows the follow-up GAS scores in these subgroups. The average GAS score for the 32 females was 68; for the 5 still-alive bulimics, 72; for the 9 still-alive bulimarexics, 65; and for the 16 anorectics, 68.4. Greater differences emerge if we compare those with BPD alone to those showing BPD × MAD: The latter group showed a trend toward poorer levels of global functioning. The two suicides, for example, belonged to this group.

I do not know how the balance between anorectic and bulimic symptoms noted in the PI-500 would compare with that in a comparable-sized contemporary sample of eating-disordered patients. How the absolute increase in anorexia/bulimia cases in North America and Western Europe might affect the ratio of eating-disordered to non-eating-disordered patients in currently hospitalized BPD samples is likewise unclear. In the PI-500, one female borderline in six had an eating disorder. Our unit did not specialize in the treatment of these conditions. In recent years, I have gained the impression that bulimic patients are more difficult to treat, especially those with bizarre habits (e.g., storing their vomitus in plastic bags until their homes or apartments gradually fill up with such material). They exhibit denial to a greater degree than do the "pure" anorectics, and they more often show the clinical features of bipolar II MDP (hypomania/serious depression). But the general fate of the PI-500 bulimics is not in line with this impression. We will have to wait for the follow-up results of the current generation to determine the prognostic implications of being bulimic as opposed to merely showing anorectic symptoms. Meantime, a few authors suggest that the outcome in bulimia *is* less favorable than in anorexia alone (Garfinkel, Moldofsky, & Garner, 1977; Hsu, Crisp, & Harding, 1979).

The recovery rate reported by Garfinkel and Garner (1982) for patients with eating disorders (bulimics and "restricters" combined) is in the range of 40%, with an additional 30% considerably improved at long-term follow-up. Of their combined sample, 20% were still seriously impaired; 9% had died, apparently as a result of their illness. These authors' data, pooled from a dozen studies, are quite in line with the results shown in Table 8.1 (44% recovered, 31% good, 19% impaired, and 6% dead among the 32 females). Garfinkel and Garner also mentioned that short-term follow-up showed a higher proportion of patients in the intermediate zones of outcome—an observation similar to mine concerning the borderlines (including those with eating disorders) at 5 years after discharge from the hospital, compared with 10 or 15 years after discharge.

Other reasons for suspecting that bulimics may have a less favorable life trajectory than "pure" anorectics are contained within the data Garfinkel and Garner (1982) provide concerning symptom patterns in the two populations. The bulimics, for example, showed significantly greater tendencies toward (1) vomiting, (2) use of alcohol or street drugs, (3) petty thievery, (4) suicide attempts, (5) mood lability, and (6) poor sexual history (pp. 46–47). Most of these attributes bespeak heightened impulsivity as well as greater irritability, either of which would predict (though not necessarily determine ineluctably) a worse outcome. Many bulimics are also given to compulsive rituals. These in turn may serve as mechanisms of containment, counteracting the impulsivity. Actually, therapy of impulse disorders depends upon adaptive, "healthy" rituals, whether these be in the form of attending Overeaters Anonymous (in the case of bulimia) or of attending AA (in the case of alcoholism).

A recent study by Herzog, Norman, Rigotti, and Pepose (1986) provides some evidence about the frequency of bulimia in a *non*patient population (specifically, female graduate students in law, medicine, and business): 12% met the criteria for bulimia. These women showed significantly greater levels of social impairment than did their non-eating-disordered peers. The authors did not, however, seek to compare the bulimics with a similar group of "pure" anorectics. The high and apparently increasing incidence of bulimia among college women was about 4 per 100 women per year in a recent Michigan survey (Drewnowski, Yee, & Krahn, 1988).

The only death attributable directly to anorexia nervosa in the PI-500 was that of a schizophrenic woman who starved herself to the point of cachexia, eventually dying in her weakened state (several years after signing out from the unit) of pneumonia caused by an "opportunistic" organism.

A number of investigators have drawn attention to the frequency with which anorexia and bulimia are associated with affective disorder in close relatives (Cantwell, Sturzenberger, Burroughs, Salkin, & Green, 1977; Morgan & Russell, 1975). Parallels of this sort occurred in the PI-500. One of the manic–depressive women with anorexia, for example, had a mother who had been treated with electroconvulsive therapy (ECT) for recurrent depression. But, in general, the proportion of first-degree relatives with MAD was not especially high in the present series: Among the 62 biological parents of the borderlines with anorexia and/or bulimia were only 2 with clear-cut MDP (unipolar in one case; bipolar in the other). Vandereycken (1987) feels that if an association between eating disorders and affective illness exists, it is more likely to be with bulimia than with "pure" anorexia. Laessle, Kittle, Fichter,

TABLE 8.1. Traced Patients with Eating Disorders at the Borderline Level

Patient no.	Sex	Follow-up GAS score	Anorexia?	Bulimia?	Family history		MAD	Suicidal acts?	Age at admission	Age at follow-up	Ever married?	No. of children
					Father	Mother						
					BPD patients							
1	F	70	+	−	−	−	+	+	16	38	−	0
2	F	68	+	−	(Adoptee)		−	+	22	38	+	0
3	F	Suicide	−	+	−	−	+	+	19	−	−	0
4	F	72	−	+	−	−	+	−	22	39	+	0
5	F	69	+	+	−	−	+	−	17	33	+	4
6	F	75	+	+	Depression	−	+	+	25	39	−	0
7	F	74	+	−	Alcoholism	−	−	+	14	36	+	1
8	F	91	+	a	−	−	+	+	15	32	−	0
9	F	85	+	+	−	−	+	−	17	37	+	0
10	F	62	−	+	−	−	+	+	28	46	+	1
11	F	73	−	+	(Adoptee)		−	−	29	40	−	0
12	F	70	a	+	−	−	+	+	27	38	+	0
13	F	64	+	+	−	−	−	+	17	31	−	0
14	F	54	+	+	−	−	+	+	20	35	−	0
15	F	21	+	−	Alcoholism	−	+	+	24	43	+	1
16	F	31	+	+	−	−	+	+	24	39	−	0
17	M	51	+	−	−	−	−	+	14	27	−	0

		Suicide										
18	F		+	+	−	−	+	+	24	−	+	0
19	F	58	+	−	−	−	−	−	21	36	−	0
20	F	74	+	a	−	−	−	+	14	37	+	2
21	F	65	+	+	−	−	−	−	15	26	−	0
22	F	70	+	−	−	−	+	+	20	35	−	0

D patients

| 23 | F | 84 | + | + | − | − | + | − | 28 | 50 | + | 2[b] |

Other BPO patients

24	F	52	+	−	−	−	−	−	30	52	−	0
25	F	68	+	−	−	−	−	−	19	30	−	0
26	F	83	−	+	−	−	−	−	19	40	+	1
27	F	61	+	−	−	−	−	−	15	30	−	0
28	F	78	+	−	−	−	−	+	26	48	+	2
29	F	60	+	+	−	−	−	−	19	35	+	0
30	F	75	+	−	−	−	−	−	20	38	+	1
31	F	90	+	−	Bipolar	−	−	−	15	28	+	0
32	F	76	+	−	−	−	−	−	15	36	+	0
33	F	68	+	−	Alcoholism	−	−	−	16	29	+	0

[a]Briefly or only to a mild degree.
[b]Adopted.

143

Wittchen, and Pirke (1987) agree with this, adding that depression in their series usually began *after* the eating disorder and may therefore have been "secondary."

Some of the PI-500 borderlines with eating disorders were completely asymptomatic at follow-up, even in the area of food intake. Several became "finicky" eaters but no longer felt compelled to starve themselves periodically, nor did they any longer oscillate between bingeing and restriction as they did during the active phase of their condition. Their life trajectory patterns (see Chapter Thirteen) did not differ from those of the borderline patients in general: About a fifth showed the ladle-shaped outcome pattern, characterized by 5 or 6 years of impairment followed by a "turning point" and rapid recovery at about age 30. Many improved dramatically shortly after leaving the unit and had remained well for years by the time of follow-up. One, with concomitant bipolar II illness, fell ill again in her late 30s after the breakup of a romantic relationship. At follow-up, the illness was chiefly affective; the eating symptoms were relatively quiescent. The two suicides had nothing to do with inanition, but rather with scandalous sexual affairs that led to a sense of entrapment.

Many of the eating-disordered borderline women expressed a desire to avoid having children (cf. Jeammet, Jayler, Terrasse-Brechon, & Gorge, 1984). Relations with their own mothers had often been strained—not always because of emotional disorders in the mothers (though some were extremely intrusive and controlling). In some instances, the daughters had been tantrumy and difficult from earliest childhood, trying their mothers' patience beyond the latter's flexibility. Either way, mothers and motherhood for these patients were troubles to avoid. The rates at which they eschewed the life tasks of marriage and motherhood did not exceed, however, the already high rates of remaining single (50%) or childless (75%) noted in the borderline women as a group (see Table 8.1).

Pope, Frankenburg, Hudson, Jonas, and Yurgelun-Todd (1987) have recently raised this question: Is bulimia associated with BPD? They answered it in the negative, although their study concentrated on ambulatory bulimics and used the revised (and more restrictive) Diagnostic Interview for Borderline Patients (see Kolb & Gunderson, 1980) as their instrument for diagnosing BPD. Whether a group of hospitalized bulimics, rated blindly as in Pope et al.'s study, would also fail to show a heightened incidence of BPD by the somewhat less restrictive criteria of DSM-III-R is unclear. In the PI-500, 15 of 18 borderline-level patients with bulimia had BPD; 15 of all 21 such patients (even including the three with psychosis) had BPD. About 1 female BPD patient in 10 (15 of 145) was bulimic. Self-damaging acts were more common among the BPD females with an eating disorder (15 of 21) than among the remaining borderline-level females with an eating disorder (1 of 11). But those with bulimia were not more likely to commit such acts than were those with anorexia. I suspect that the degree of correlation between bulimia nervosa and BPD will vary sharply from sample to sample, depending on the diagnostic criteria used; on the severity of illness (ambulatory vs. hospitalized); and on regional, cultural, and cohort factors. Probably in some samples (viz., of hospitalized BPD females with MAD and bulimia or bulimarexia), the eating disorder is causally linked to an underlying neuroregulatory disorder affecting both mood and symptom choice.

The death rate in the PI-500 series appears lower among the borderlines with eating disorders (2 of 33, or 6%) than in the remainder of the traced patients (60 of 480, or 12.5%), but the figures are based on a relatively small sample. The death rate in the Danish study of Isager, Brinch, Kreiner, and Tolstrup (1985), based on 151 anorectics, was approximately 6% (0.5% per year) at an average follow-up time of 12½ years. Because the suicide rate in Denmark is somewhat higher than in the United States, we cannot use the Danish figures as a reliable index of the "true" rate here—part of which depends, in any case, upon the proportion of bulimics to anorectics.

Herzog, Keller, and Lavori (1988), in their review of 33 follow-up studies (in the United States and Western Europe) of anorexia nervosa and 7 of bulimia nervosa, mention a range of mortality figures from 0 (as in Jenkins's [1987] 3-year study of hospitalized anorectics) to 22%, with over half the studies reporting 4% or less. Half the deaths in the anorectics seemed attributable to the condition itself; another fourth, to suicide. The death rate in the bulimics appeared lower, or negligible, though the follow-up intervals were briefer (up to 6 years).

Whereas the PI-500 bulimics were not more likely to engage in self-injurious acts than the anorectics, some studies suggest that bulimics are more likely to make suicide gestures or self-mutilative acts (Swift, Ritzholz, Kalin, & Kaslow, 1987). Prognosis in the bulimic group is variable, depending on authors and samples: 40% of Abraham, Mira, and Llewellyn-Jones's (1983) mostly ambulatory patients were asymptomatic after 1–6 years of therapy, in contrast to only about 10% of the hospitalized bulimics in Swift et al.'s series. More similar to the fate of the PI-500 eating-disordered patients were the results of Toner, Garfinkel, and Garner's (1986) Toronto study, though again this was a study of ambulatory patients: About two-thirds of both the anoretics and bulimics "improved" or were "asymptomatic" in 5–14 years, with a death rate of 6–7%. Brotman, Herzog, and Hamburg (1988) expressed the view, based on their 1- to 5-year follow-up study of 14 ambulatory bulimics, that patients with comorbid affective disorders and personality disorders (e.g., BPD)—that is, those with Axis I and Axis II disorders simultaneously—had the poorest prognosis. This was borne out in the PI-500: Whereas anorectics and bulimics with MAD did about the same (see above), the eight bulimics with concomitant BPD, MAD, and suicidal acts did poorly as a group (three well, three marginal to fair, two suicides). If significant differences do emerge in future outcome studies of "pure" anorectic versus bulimic patients, they may relate to differences in prior history of abusive life events. Root and Fallon (1988), for example, noted high levels of four types of victimization in their large series of bulimic outpatients. Two-thirds of these had experienced, singly or in combination, physical abuse during childhood, sexual molestation, battery, or rape. Presumably, such histories would predispose patients toward a less favorable life course. In the PI-500, I noted only a trend toward greater abuse histories in the bulimics, compared with the anorexia-only group. Only two patients (both bulimic) experienced *both* incest and parental brutality; one committed suicide, and the other was marginal in her functioning at follow-up.

Though the anorectic and bulimic borderline women of the PI-500 did not, as mentioned above, marry less often or produce fewer children than the other borderline women, conflicts about these issues did seem especially intense in the women with eating disorders. This was so marked in some as to suggest a "dynamic" factor for anorexia—namely, that the accompanying amenorrhea served as a "cure" for the threats of pregnancy and motherhood. Similarly, several reported having experienced severe dysmenorrhea or else paramenstrual depression and irritability in their adolescence; amenorrhea also "cured" these symptoms, just as keeping perpetually pregnant (and hence free of periods) was the customary doctor's advice for premenstrual syndrome (PMS) in the 18th century (Pinel, 1799). In at least two of the young women, the decision to lose weight in order to obviate the recurrence of dysmenorrhea was quite conscious and effective. Herzog et al. (1988) mention the frequent reports of ambivalence or avoidance of sexual matters in various studies of anorectics; articles dealing with bulimics have not routinely dealt with this topic. Future follow-up studies of female eating-disordered patients should make more methodical assessments at the outset of attitudes toward sex and toward motherhood, since conflicts in these areas appear (at present, anyway) to be of greater significance in this group than were the dynamics concerning autonomy that were emphasized a generation ago (Bruch, 1978). By the same taken, restoration of normal weight is often of less significance as an index of improvement in these patients than is their overall psychosocial integration.

ATTRACTIVENESS

Suspecting that attractiveness in women might prove one of the unfair advantages that tilted its possessors toward a good outcome (see "Natural Advantages," Chapter Ten), I rated the female patients on a 10-point scale (where 1 signified "least attractive" and 10 "most attractive"). Because of the need to safeguard confidentiality, I relied on the administrative assistant in the hospital record room, whose position entitled her to examine the photographs in the old charts. I hoped that the opinion of a woman would help allay criticism against a most unpopular undertaking, given the current sociopolitical climate. Her ratings and mine never differed by more than 1 point.

The distribution of scores approximated gaussian expectations reasonably closely. If one considered those individuals scoring 1 through 4 collectively as the "least attractive" group and those scoring 8, 9, or 10 as "most attractive,"

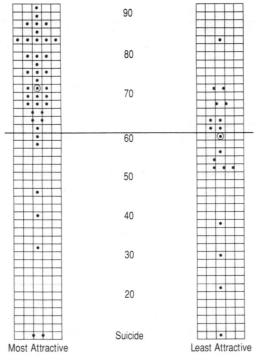

FIGURE 8.1. Outcome in borderline females in relation to attractiveness. The circled dot represents the median case in each group.

these extremes each accounted for approximately a sixth of the total population of female patients ("least" = 19%; "most" = 17%).

The diagnostic subgroups were not equally represented in these two compartments. The most attractive women consisted of some 50 patients, 41 of whom were borderline. The least attractive group consisted of 54 patients, of whom 19 were borderline. I am not sure what meaning to attach to this uneven distribution. Possibly the psychotic patients took fewer pains with their appearance, at least at the height of their illness.

Figure 8.1 shows the distribution of the borderline female patients at the two extremes of this variable. The median follow-up GAS score (72) for the most attractive patients in this group was over a decile greater than that of the least attractive patients (60). Although there was no significant difference between the proportion doing well (GAS scores > 60) between the two groups, the most attractive borderlines were more likely to be clinically recovered (GAS scores > 70), $\chi^2 = 8.1$, $df = 1$, $p < .01$.

The schizophrenic, schizoaffective, manic–depressive, and schizophreniform (SF) patients did not show significant differences with respect to attractiveness, either in global outcome or in their suicide rate.

The most attractive borderline women were more likely to have been married than the least attractive, $\chi^2 = 4.1$, $p < .05$, but did not prove more likely to have had a child, $\chi^2 = 1.2$. Two out of three of the most attractive patients had been married at follow-up, whereas at this writing one in three has had a child.

The raw data do not, of course, tell the whole story. With few exceptions, the most attractive patients, especially the borderlines, behaved as if possessed, like the cat, of a righting mechanism permitting them to land always on their feet. Many had led checkered existences before coming to the hospital and for varying lengths of time afterward, reeling from one crisis (romantic breakup, suicide gesture, etc.) to another. But another potential rescuer was always at hand ready to take up where a previous protector had left off. Or else a previous protector was willing to contemplate reconciliation after an outburst of hostility on the part of a borderline woman that would have led to a permanent rift had she been less attractive.

Incest figured prominently in the lives of the few most attractive borderline women with an impaired outcome. Three of the four with GAS scores ≤50 had an incest history. One of these women committed suicide. The fourth (also a suicide) had been caught up in a seductive father–daughter relationship just short of physicality. In effect, all the most attractive borderlines with an impaired outcome or suicide had experienced inappropriate sexuality in relation to a father or a brother. Incest had been a factor in five of the women with excellent outcomes (i.e., one in seven) in this most attractive subgroup. Not all the most attractive borderlines who had been incest victims did poorly, in other words, but the few who did poorly had all been incest victims. Apart from the incest factor, I can find no reason to explain why these four borderline women had bad outcomes: All were intelligent (IQs ranging from 119 to 130); only one had a family history of mental illness (depression), and she herself had no "endogenous" symptoms; none had lost a parent; and so on.

Some of the most attractive borderlines became immensely successful. Negative and positive factors were often so intermixed in these patients as to confound our original prognostications. One young woman, for example, went out of her way to be accommodating. The staff considered her a borderline of the "as-if" type (Deutsch, 1942). She was extremely shy and had made many serious suicide attempts since midadolescence, including several while at PI. We kept her for a long time on the unit, amidst serious ethical questions concerning the right to hospitalize a patient for years just to prevent a suicide (nullifying a possibly fuller life extramurally), versus her "right" to leave and kill herself (also nullifying a fuller life). Eventually she left, though continuing to work with the same therapist for many years. Following a certain turning point in her treatment (not identifiable except retrospectively), she gave up the habit of suicide threats. At follow-up, her life had been on a consistently high plane for over 20 years, enriched by a successful marriage, children, an advanced degree in one of the helping professions, and a gratifying career.

Another attractive borderline woman had made only some minor suicide gestures, but exhibited an abrasive and hypercritical personality during the months she spent on the unit. Later she eloped. Her prognosis seemed guarded, though less grim than that of the preceding patient. She immediately found an excellent position in the fashion industry. A few years later she married into a socially prominent family; at follow-up, she was devoting herself primarily to charitable work. In the 19 years since she left out unit, she had never sought further treatment. She did recall with fondness her therapist at PI, and asked me to convey to him her belated apologies for having been "difficult" with him when he had worked with her on the unit.

Whereas for the borderline women, attractiveness served usually to smooth the surface along their path to success, for the schizophrenic women attractiveness had more the effect of securing for themselves the devoted interest of a male protector. One such woman, whom we characterized as fée and bohemian while she was at the hospital, was still quite fragile when she was released a year and a half later. An avid guitarist, she met and married a man with similar musical interest. He encouraged her in her playing and placed no demands upon her to socialize or to engage in other activities for which her shyness would handicap her. In this protective atmosphere she has done well, and has never required rehospitalization.

In sum, attractiveness was a variable of some importance in determining outcome in the female borderline patients—a variable often overlooked and not easily disentangled from the multiplicity of other coexisting and interacting variables that also affect long-range outcome. I am also aware that, at its extremes, beauty may have ironic effects. Among the PI-500 borderlines, the 10 women with an attractiveness score of either 9 or 10 had been sexually exploited in three instances. Two had witnessed violence to their brothers at the hands of their fathers—the fathers, that is, who had at other times molested them. Their attractiveness, which had (in a manner of speaking) landed them in trouble when they were young, and which may have contributed to the misuse that made them "borderline," later helped extricate them from the borderline traits we saw during their hospitalization. One of these women committed suicide; another continued to function poorly. The other eight, however, recovered (average GAS score = 81; range 1 = 1 67–91).

CHILDREN BORN OUT OF WEDLOCK

Now that 96% of the females in the PI-500 have been traced, another of the gender-related issues we can consider is the number of female patients who bore a child out of wedlock. In the socioeconomic group of the PI-500, during the era relevant to the study, these events would have been uncommon. Altogether, there were 14 such patients (4.8% of the women in the study). One of the women (a schizoaffective) gave two children up for adoption; one borderline woman kept both her children and was raising them at follow-up. These 14 women represent about half the number of women in the PI-500 who had at least one pregnancy out of wedlock ($n = 29$), the remainder having terminated their pregnancies.

Ten of the 175 traced borderline women (5.7%) had a child out of wedlock (one had two such children). Three were raising these children; seven gave a child away for adoption. All 10 had BPD; none of the 34 dysthymic and other borderline-functioning women was ever pregnant out of wedlock, $\chi^2 = 5.43$, $p < .05$. Among the schizophrenic, schizoaffective, and manic–depressive women, one each gave at least one child up for adoption (two, in the case of the schizoaffective woman).

Females with BPD were not more likely than were those with a psychosis to have become pregnant out of wedlock or to have given up a child for adoption. The greater likelihood associated with BPD for both phenomena than is found with other borderline-function patients is presumably an expression of impulsivity—often noted in borderline-function patients generally, but almost *invariably* found in hospitalized BPD patients. The personality characteristics of the borderline women with at least one extramarital child varied from the mildly impulsive but predominantly conventional (seven instances) to the chaotic (seven instances).

One borderline woman gave a child up for adoption (this was a traumatic event for her and precipitated her hospitalization), but married another man shortly after leaving PI and had two children by him. As might be expected, the four borderlines whose out-of-wedlock babies were adopted and who never subsequently married were more impulsive than were those who have continued to bring up their children. One has remained very ill to this day and has been hospitalized many times. After eloping from PI, she led a "hippie" life for several years, joined a food-faddist commune, was rehospitalized elsewhere, eloped again, bore the child (who was then adopted away), was raped, and had an ectopic pregnancy. At follow-up, she was in and out of hospitals and halfway houses, living on public assistance. Her chaotic life exemplifies the extreme of *behavioral* as opposed to *cognitive* disturbance. Her speech was quite normal, and, as her relatives mentioned to me, "To talk to her, you wouldn't know she was ill."

Another borderline woman gave her child up for adoption the same year that her brother and sister-in-law, unable to have a child, adopted one. Two years later the patient killed herself. Her suicide seemed to have been triggered by a severe physical illness that added to the already crushing burdens of her barren existence.

A third had a child out of wedlock by the man she shortly thereafter married. The baby was given up for adoption, and no others were born of this union. This was perhaps fortunate, considering that the patient, herself the daughter of two alcoholics constantly at war with each other, was extremely impulse-ridden and had an explosive temper (with premenstrual exacerbation). She committed suicide a few years after her marriage.

Three of the children born out of wedlock to schizophrenic or schizoaffective mothers had been fathered by other schizophrenic patients in the hospitals (not PI) where they were under care at the time. One schizophrenic woman became acutely psychotic after terminating an out-of-wedlock pregnancy, but never recovered and had hospitalized for 25 years at follow-up.

Only one child was the product of two unmarried patients both from PI. In this instance, the father offered the (borderline) mother a sum of money if she would consent to an abortion. She declined and raised the child amid hard circumstances, relying on public assistance and some help from her mother. The child's father went in and out of the mother's life, adding to her burden because of his hostile and abrasive personality. Finally, she offered him the same sum of money he had once mentioned if he would just promise to stay out of her life. He took the money and, at follow-up, had kept his word.

Many of the patients with extramarital pregnancies, whether or not these were carried to term, exemplify some of the points made in the life events literature and in Chapter Seven, since a high proportion of them had been traumatized as children, mother-deprived, or both (see Crook & Raskin, 1975; Morrison, Hudgens, & Barchha, 1968; Murphy & Brown, 1980; Rutter, 1986). One woman with a dozen out-of-wedlock pregnancies was herself born before her parents' marriage. Pregnancy for these women was often part of an attempt to compel someone to remain with them, but in the end usually ended up as still another traumatic event superimposed upon the old ones. Not surprisingly, the suicide rate in the BPD women with at least one extramarital pregnancy (5 of 20, or 25%) was even higher than in the remainder of their group (4.1%).

PREMENSTRUAL SYNDROME

A number of studies suggest a correlation between premenstrual mood disorder (or, as DSM-III-R calls it, "late luteal phase dysphoric disorder") and psychiatric illness (Kashiwagi, McClure, & Wetzel, 1976), especially affective illness (Endicott, Halbreich, & Schacht, 1981; Hallman, 1986; McClure, Reich, & Wetzel, 1971). Wetzel and McClure (1972) reported on the correlation between suicide and the menstrual cycle. DeJong et al. (1985) caution against drawing firm conclusions about these correlations, unless one employs a prospective method for diagnosis: In retrospective studies, women tend to remember certain randomly occurring mood changes as having taken place premenstrually. This cautionary note aside, a large proportion of women complain of occasional premenstrual pain or dysphoria, though only about 4–10% suffer severe symptoms (Golub, 1985). The latter I refer to here as "premenstrual syndrome" (PMS; see Haskett, Steiner, Osmun, & Carroll, 1980; Parlee, 1973), though some prefer the term "*para*menstrual" ("around the time of. . ."), acknowledging that a proportion of cases occur during rather than the week before the menses. For the past 20 years, I have kept meticulous records (prospectively, with mood ratings once to thrice weekly) on my female office practice patients, paying particular attention to those with prominent mood fluctuations. I have found that PMS is more common in women with affective disorder than in those without; it occurs in about half of women with BPD, whereas women with schizotypal personality (STP) seldom complain of it (Stone, 1982, p. 337).

One might think that the 289 female patients of the PI-500—all in the reproductive phase of their life when first hospitalized—would, if carefully monitored as to mood changes, provide us with data that would help us enormously in answering some of the puzzling questions about PMS, BPD, and affective disorder. Unfortunately, and despite the unit's regulation requiring the charting of each menstrual period, this monitoring was carried out only haphazardly. Graphs with daily ratings were available for a few patients; for many others, all such information is lacking.

The possible connection between the menses and severe mood alterations became apparent to me early in my postgraduate experience, in relation to a young woman in the PI-500 who every so often and for no discernible reason became acutely suicidal—only to recapture her customary good spirits within 24–36 hours. Faced with this baffling situation, my colleagues and I took to charting her mood and behavior on a daily basis, in hopes some pattern would emerge. Figure 8.2 shows the results for the first 5 months of our observations.

The (nearly) 28-day cycle suggested a correlation with the menses, as turned out to be the case. We were then able to predict the next episodes with precision. The patient was at first so determined to destroy herself during a PMS attack that even on suicide watch she ran away from the nurse (during the late November episode) and hanged herself in the shower. She was cut down and rescued moments later by the nursing staff. Eventually, through a different course of medication (not indicated in the figure), we were able to bring the PMS under control. She did moderately well in the following 15 years, apart from a depressive episode precipitated by a loss in the family (two members of which suffered from recurrent unipolar depression).

Patients of this sort are puzzling diagnostically in another way as well: Their personality disorder is highly state-dependent. If their cycle is short (e.g., 24 days) and the PMS mood alteration is protracted (e.g., 8 or 9 days), they appear "borderline" and "dysthymic" for 40% of their (reproductive) life, and rather normal the rest of the time. They may pass so rapidly from irritability to tranquility and back again as to confuse both themselves and their intimates about which self is the "real" one.

Women with severe PMS, whether or not they have concomitant affective illness, resemble certain other affectively ill patients in the predictability of their

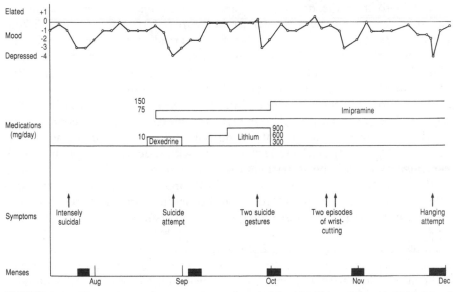

FIGURE 8.2. Observation results over a 5-month period for a PI-500 patient with PMS. Mood scale: +1, mild elation, overcheerfulness; 0, euthymia; −1, mild depression; −2, moderate depression, some suicidal ruminations; −3, severe depression with vegetative signs, suicidal preoccupations; −4, despondency, high suicidality. Menstrual periods are indicated by the black bars at the bottom of the diagram.

symptoms: those with seasonal affective disorder (Bick, 1986; Wehr, Jacobsen, & Sack, 1986; Rosenthal & Wehr, 1987), as well as rapid-cycling bipolar manic–depressives and the occasional male manic–depressive with episodes occurring at the full moon (Stone, 1976). The life course itself over a 10- or 20-year span may not be so predictable (other than that it would be turbulent if untreated), but the outbreaks themselves are as predictable as any condition in the whole domain of psychiatry. I recently had occasion to do a "psychological autopsy" in a legal case involving a woman who committed suicide in her mid-40s. A bipolar II manic–depressive, symptomatic since her 20s, she also exhibited all eight of the BPD traits, along with PMS. In addition, as I could reconstruct from hospital records, she had had annual "crises" characterized by extreme irritability and suicide attempts; one of these crises had occurred, over the last 8 years of her life, every March 15 (give or take 3 days). When the period of a periodic illness is long, it is easy to miss. Had the physicians in charge of this woman's care detected the annual rhythm, they might have been able to circumvent the crisis with lithium or other mood-regulating agents. But the 25- to 30-day cycle of most PMS cases is already long enough to be easily forgotten by both patient and therapist, so that it usually comes as a surprise.

Since the condition is remediable, it behooves the therapist or physician to detect the periodicity, to establish the (approximate) period by careful graphing, and then to treat the no-longer-mysterious syndrome. The predictability of suicidal intent in the case of the woman in Figure 8.2, once this was established, reached 100% before her condition was finally remedied. Compare this with the suicidality of the PI-500 BPD group as a whole: 17, or nearly 9%, have thus far committed suicide; 15 of the 17 did so within 6 years of admission. One BPD patient in 12½, that is, committed suicide within that time frame. This is a *fairly* good level of prediction, but not nearly good enough vis-à-vis the individual patient. Yet even "enriching" our high-risk sample by use of certain factors conducive to suicide (e.g., patients' being male, being in the third decade of life, having MAD, having ASP, etc.) still leaves us with little power to predict which *particular* patient will be at maximal risk.

As for the other known cases of PMS among the PI-500, one was a schizophreniform woman; the rest were borderline patients. Several of these women were chaotic in the storminess of their personality and life course (see "Chaotic Impulsivity," Chapter Five). The schizophreniform woman, for example, had abused marijuana, LSD, and cocaine; had been promiscuous; and had been raped and gotten pregnant before coming to our unit. After several difficult but less stormy years, she eventually recovered, having responded favorably to lithium. At follow-up, she was married, working, and largely asymptomatic. Two of the BPD suicides had severe PMS: the woman once jailed for shoplifting and later arraigned for child molestation, and an incest victim who had had rage outbursts premenstrually. Four other women with BPD × PMS are now doing well. One had episodes of vomiting with each period, which continued every 28 days even when she became temporarily amenorrheic through fasting. These seven BPD × PMS cases constitute 5% of the female BPD patients—a figure that grossly underestimates the true conjunction of these conditions. Future follow-up studies of borderline patients should pay much closer attention to the PMS factor than we did during the 1960s and 1970s. Such studies may shed further light on the question whether PMS is associated with primary affective disorders, in the classical sense, or whether PMS is instead (as Rubinow, Hoban, & Grover, 1987, suggest) a model for "cyclic mood state disorders."

RAPE, RAPE VICTIMS, AND THE HIERARCHY OF STRATEGIES

In the unequal struggle for the good things of the world, strategies that work well for some people are quite ineffectual in the hands of others. A man who is sensitive, tender, charming, patient, and comfortably off may earn the love of a good woman, and thus win for himself what is most valuable to his security over the longest span of time and without any display of force. As one descends the ladder of intrinsic appeal, there comes a point where the strategy, ethologically speaking, of "being nice" is no longer effective. The man who is insensitive, impatient, and unappealing must resort to cruder strategies, such as enslavement.

A woman enslaved may not be as spontaneously ardent as a woman in love, but at least she will stay. This approach worked well (temporarily) for the possessive R. Gene Simmons, who in effect imprisoned his family, 14 of whom he killed when some threatened to escape (*New York Post*, December 30, 1987). A man so low in the hierarchy of appeal that, to his way of thinking, the strategy of enslavement is beyond reach, may forgo even the hope of enforced permanency and settle for the more transitory gratification of rape. Incest, especially the sexual exploitation of a daughter, is at the crossroads of these latter two strategies: Here a father attempts to create a woman sexually addicted to his person (thus guaranteeing permanency of erotic love) by banking on the assumption that a child's natural love of its father will minimize, if not altogether obviate, the need for force. Indeed, Russell (1986) reported that 71% of the incest victims in her large series stated that no force had been used.

In the unrepresentative world of the PI-500, some of the fathers were capable and tender; some of the mothers were clearly "good enough" by Winnicott's (1965) yardstick of maternal effectiveness and warmth. Curiously, these were often the parents of the schizophrenics—bewildered by the sorry outcome of their parental efforts and humbled by the criticism heaped upon them by the mental health profession, according to whose then-prevailing wisdom the "schizophrenogenic" mother and the aloof father lay at the etiological foundation of their offspring's illness (Parker, 1982). But many of the parents, especially of the borderlines and the schizoaffectives, fell far short of the ideal, in ways so diverse as to recreate the entire taxonomy of parental failure. I have tried to outline this taxonomy in hierarchical form through Figure 8.3, organizing its "genera" by levels of force ("no force," "coercive," "abusive") and showing some of the "species" within each genus. Of the parents who were abusive, some were irritable manic–depressives with a penchant for violence; others were alcoholic or "character-disordered" for reasons that stemmed more from abnormal rearing than from faulty constitution. The more *immature* the parents (as in Vaillant's [1986] hierarchy of defensive patterns), the more desperate the strategies they employed, both inside and outside the domain of child-rearing. I have shown the correlation between certain traumatic childhood experiences and eventual outcome in the sections on "Parental Brutality" and "Incest" (see Chapter Seven). In some instances, these appeared to have causal, not merely correlative, significance. Admittedly, to claim cause is hazardous in a retrospective study. Still, one can sometimes detect at least the aroma of causation, as in the case of a schizoaffective woman who was forcibly raped by her father; she made a suicide attempt a few days afterward, was later admitted to our unit, and not long thereafter killed herself.

A similar connection between past and recent traumata was usually discernible in the lives of the PI-500 patients who had been rape victims. Table 8.2 outlines the history of traumatic events in those who had reported being

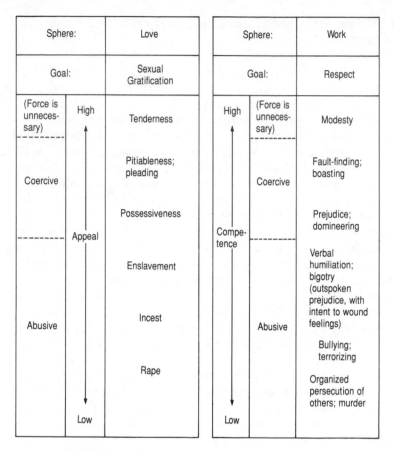

Sphere:	Love			Sphere:	Work		
Goal:	Sexual Gratification			Goal:	Respect		
(Force is unnecessary)	High	Tenderness		High	(Force is unnecessary)	Modesty	
Coercive	Appeal	Pitiableness; pleading		Competence	Coercive	Fault-finding; boasting	
		Possessiveness				Prejudice; domineering	
Abusive		Enslavement			Abusive	Verbal humiliation; bigotry (outspoken prejudice, with intent to wound feelings)	
		Incest				Bullying; terrorizing	
	Low	Rape		Low		Organized persecution of others; murder	

FIGURE 8.3. Hierarchy of strategies for goal satisfaction.

raped. For the most part, these were not entirely "random" cases, such as the unsuspecting women who make up the majority of rape victims alluded to in crime statistics. Antecedent traumata had usually set our patients up for rape. Abandonment by the mother, sexual misuse by the father, frank incest on occasion, being either victim or witness of a parent's violent rage outbursts—a string of events such as these had led some of the younger women to flee home and place themselves at the mercy of strangers (with the usual result), or else to drift into a life of promiscuity, drug abuse, and rootlessness (and thus to become easy prey for unscrupulous men). Graduates of the school of sexual exploitation—their fathers had carefully taught them that "men only want one thing"—these borderline women gravitated toward rape as though by a homing instinct.

Interestingly, the schizophrenic women in this series, though their reality-testing was by definition worse than that of their borderline counterparts, did not become rape victims. Their homes apparently had not programmed them to

TABLE 8.2. Rape Victims in the PI-500

Patient no.	Diagnosis	Life events								Follow-up GAS score	Comments
		Parental abandonment?	Death of a parent?	Parental suicide?	Parental alcoholism?	Parental psychosis?	Parental divorce?	Parental brutality?	Incest?		
1	BPD × MAD	+	+	–	+	+	–	–	–	55	Raped by a "guru" from whom she sought advice
2	BPD × MAD	–	–	–	+	–	–	–	–	60	Two suicide attempts. Became bipolar II. Raped by a stranger after she got into his car
3	BPD × MAD	–	–	–	–	–	–	–	–	40	Chaotic impulsivity
4	BPD × MAD	+	–	–	+	+	+	+	+	53	Raped by men in neighborhood
5	BPD × MAD	+	Both	Both	Both	Both	+	–	–	Suicide	Raped by neighbor
6	BPD × MAD	–	–	–	+	+	–	+	+	58	Father hit her on the head as if to make her forget his sexual molestation of her
7	BPD × MAD	–	–	–	+	+	–	a	+	Suicide	Chaotic life of promiscuity and addiction
8	BPD	–	–	–	–	–	–	–	–	83	Raped several times during a time when she was promiscuous and abusing drugs
9	SZ	–	–	–	–	–	+	+	–	34	Raped twice; abused drugs
10	SZ	–	–	–	–	–	+	–	+	50	Raped twice; lived as a "squatter" in run-down apartment
11	SA	–	–	–	–	+	–	–	Probable	68	On drugs; raped by a stranger at knifepoint
12	SA	–	–	–	–	–	–	–	–	35	Raped while in the hospital
13	SF	–	–	–	–	–	–	–	Possible	82	Extramarital pregnancy

aThis patient was a witness to brutality on the part of her father toward her brothers.

the same extent to lead the sort of life and to seek the kinds of men that multiply one's chances of being sexually victimized in this way. The percentage of 175 traced borderline women in this study who experienced incest (19.5%), for example, well exceeds that of the 37 traced schizophrenic women (5.4%). Though eight BPD females experienced rape, as against two of the schizophrenic females, the numbers are not statistically significant. Only one of the borderline rape victims is doing well, however. The other seven had early lives beset with the various untoward life events alluded to above. The rape, of course, became another traumatic event, further weakening their self-confidence and their zest for intimacy with men. All remained single, except one who married—and killed herself a few weeks later.

Substance Abuse and Its Effects on Outcome

As I write this book, the issue of substance abuse in the United States is assuming greater importance by the day. In this context, the effects that substance abuse had on patient outcome in the PI-500—which were substantial—appear to be of particular significance. This chapter discusses the incidence of alcoholism and drug abuse in the PI-500; the changing patterns of substance abuse over the period covered by the study; and the effects on outcome when substance abuse either went unchecked or was brought under control (usually through membership in one or another "Anonymous" organization). The chapter concludes with a look at a particularly negative combination of circumstances among the borderline patients: alcoholism, drug abuse, and antisociality.

ALCOHOLISM

Reliable statistics about the prevalence and incidence of alcoholism are difficult to come by, since, as Warheit and Auth (1985) point out, the data are often "fragmented, ambiguous and imprecise" (p. 3). These authors mention prevalence rates of heavy alcohol consumption as 12–18% for males and 2–5% for females. But these rates would be affected by a host of other factors: age, socioeconomic status, ethnicity, cohort, and geography. The PI-500—comprised of young, middle- to upper-middle-class patients raised in the Northeast during the 1950s and 1960s, more than half of whom were Jewish—would be expected to show lower rates than those just cited. Among the psychotic-level patients, this appears to have been the case. Two of the manic–depressives were alcoholic as well (one of each sex), along with two mildly alcoholic schizophrenics and one alcoholic patient with a schizophreniform illness (SF). The Jewish patients were rarely alcoholic unless they were manic–depressive themselves or had close relatives with this condition. The female manic–depressive/

159

TABLE 9.1. Alcoholism in the PI-500

Diagnostic category[a]	Severity level[b]				Total	Suicides	
	2	3	4	5		n	%
Borderlines							
BPD							
Males	2	6	5	0	13	2	15
Females	7	11	5	1	24	5	21
D							
Males	0	1	1	0	2	0	0
Females	0	0	0	0	0	0	0
Other BPO							
Males	0	2	1	2	5	1	20
Females	0	0	0	0	0	0	0
Psychotics							
SZ							
Males	0	3	1	0	4	1	25
Females	1	0	1	0	2	0	0
MDP							
Males	1	1	1	0	3	0	0
Females	0	0	1	0	1	1	100
SF							
Males	2	2	0	0	4	0	0
Females	0	0	0	0	0	0	0
Totals					58	10	17

[a]Diagnostic groups included here are only those in which there were alcoholics of the levels of severity noted.

[b]This table includes only moderately severe (2) to extremely severe (5) cases; 27 "mild" cases (severity level of 1) were excluded.

alcoholic led a chaotic existence and committed suicide 10 years after her index hospitalization.

One of the schizophrenic alcoholics was working at follow-up, but was still drinking and had done little in the way of social recovery. The other remained ill for many years but eventually worked part-time; she later married and had a child. At first she was unable to care for the child, but she became a more effective mother in later years. At follow-up, she no longer abused alcohol.

Among the borderlines, the alcoholism comorbidity was considerably more pronounced, and probably exceeded the population norm for males (20 of 118, or 16.9%); it certainly exceeded these norms for the females (24 of 181, or 13.3%). Their distribution is shown in Table 9.1.

Only 4 of the 44 borderlines with significant degrees of alcoholism were known to be problem drinkers at the time of admission. One was a girl of 16

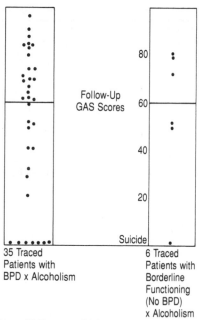

FIGURE 9.1.   Distribution of follow-up GAS scores among the traced borderline alcoholics.

who had begun to abuse alcohol the year before. Three would be considered alcoholic by conventional criteria and would thus have been excluded by Gunderson and Singer (1975) as examples of borderline personality disorder (BPD); they would simply have been diagnosed as cases of alcoholism. Two others had been drinking heavily during adolescence, but had never revealed this while at PI (they revealed this to me during our follow-up contacts). All the others developed alcoholism after leaving PI.

Compared with the ratios for the PI-500 as a whole, there was an overrepresentation of patients from Protestant backgrounds among the 58 alcoholics (such patients comprised 22% of the total sample, but $n = 24$ or 41% of the alcoholics) and an underrepresentation of patients from Jewish backgrounds (they constituted 53% of the total sample, but $n = 16$ or 28% of the alcoholics), $\chi^2 = 20.03$; $p < .001$. In the current generation, these differences would not be so marked.

Five out of six alcoholic borderlines had BPD. Among those still alive, no differences were noted in the average follow-up Global Assesement Scale (GAS) scores for the BPD versus non-BPD groups (64.8 for the BPD patients, 65.4 for the other borderlines). Figure 9.1 shows the borderline alcoholics' follow-up scores. The old maxim about outcome—"A third get better, a third stay the same, and a third get worse"—seems applicable to this population: Of the 41 borderline alcoholics who were traced (95%), 14 were clinically recovered (GAS scores > 70), 15 were either dead from suicide or had GAS scores below than

51, and 12 were mildly symptomatic. There were nine deaths in all at an average follow-up interval of 161/2 years. One man had been doing well, having finally conquered his drinking problem after 6 or 7 years; 12 days before his wedding date, he died of an aneurysm. The other eight deaths were all suicides. This yields a suicide rate thus far among the traced borderline alcoholics of 19.5% (8 of 41), about four times the rate noted in the 233 traced non-alcohol-abusing borderlines (11 suicides, or 4.7%). The subgroup of BPD alcoholics had a suicide rate similar to that for the borderline alcoholic group as a whole (7 of 35, or 20.0%).

The most striking observation vis-à-vis suicide concerns the female BPD patients with major affective disorder (MAD) comorbidity. These were among the most chaotic and impulsive patients in the entire sample. There were 13 such women; 5 had committed suicide by follow-up (38%). This subgroup and the ever-jailed patients (see "Jail," Chapter Ten) were thus the two most suicide-prone groups within the PI-500. Of the eight who survived, four were sober and doing reasonably well at follow-up (one was more depressed than alcoholic, had been "dry" for years, and had recently had her first child). The other four were an impaired and no longer employed physician; the woman prevented by the courts from visiting her child (see "Parental Brutality," Chapter Seven); a woman who lived for several years at the brink of suicide following the breakup of a love relationship; and a woman leading a marginal life in a hostile–dependent relationship with her mother.

Whereas the follow-up GAS scores for the surviving alcoholics were essentially the same as for the borderline group as a whole, those who achieved sobriety through, and who remained with, Alcoholics Anonymous (AA) had outcome levels a decile higher: These 10 borderline patients had a mean GAS score of 76.8. One might speculate that had we somehow been able to convince all our alcoholic patients to join AA, they could all have been salvaged. But I suspect that the decisive factor is not merely joining AA (which in itself has a success rate of about 60%), but having the personality traits to begin with that conduce to steadfast membership, rather than the mixture of impulsivity, immaturity, and contemptuousness that conduces to turning up one's nose at AA. In the favorable cases, in other words, certain personality factors interact synergistically with the group solidarity and symptom containment offered by AA.

Female alcoholics often pose a special problem, because of the apparent (and deceptive) mildness of their condition. Many female alcoholics are "problem drinkers" who abuse alcohol only episodically, especially during the paramenstrual part of their cycle, and who become violent on "only" two drinks. (This was true of the five BPD × MAD female suicides, just mentioned.) Clinicians find it more difficult to persuade such women (and their number is increasing in the current generation) that they (1) have a serious alcohol problem and (2) should enroll in AA to help prevent the destructiveness that, albeit emerging only once or twice a month, may do permanent damage to the central relationships in their lives.

Two of the PI borderlines rescued by AA have gone on to become alcohol rehabilitation counselors. Like many of the now-recovered alcoholics, they had been ill, skirting death and landing in disaster many times, for periods of 5 or 10 years before finally meeting someone who persuaded them to join AA.

Since all five of the female alcoholic suicides with BPD × MAD had been victims of parental abuse (incest in three, seductiveness just short of incest in one, assaultiveness in three), we must also hope that some of the new "Anonymous" organizations designed to help persons with this background become as respected and popular as AA.

A family history of alcoholism was common among the alcoholic borderlines: At least one first-degree relative was alcoholic in 11 of the 35 nonadopted BPD patients (31.4%) and in 2 of the 7 (28.6%) non-BPD patients. Though in general the denser the family pedigree for alcoholism, the worse the outlook, this maxim does not have much predictive value vis-à-vis the individual patient. In the eight cases where *both* parents were alcoholic, for example, one patient became alcoholic and eventually committed suicide; two did not drink but did commit suicide; and a fourth was the best-functioning patient in the PI-500 at follow-up (GAS score = 95). Of the remaining four, one was a fragile woman with BPD, both of whose parents committed suicide. After several difficult years, she was stable at follow-up, functioning well in the running of her home and in the raising of her four children. Another borderline woman was living in straitened circumstances, raising a child born out of wedlock to a man who had been hospitalized on a different unit during the time she was at PI. Yet another woman was leading a marginal life; she was rehospitalized many times and only became able to work part-time shortly before follow-up. The last patient, a man with borderline functioning but not BPD, had been well for 10 years, was married, and was working consistently; he was only troubled occasionally by suspicions of ill will on the part of his coworkers.

DRUG ABUSE

By coincidence, the era of the PI-500 begins with 1963 and ends with 1976— years that put parentheses around the Vietnam war. During these years our country had not only to grapple with a disaffected populace (the disaffection was especially pronounced in those of draft age), but with a populace able as never before to express its disaffection through "tuning out" by means of an expanded array of mind-altering drugs.

In the section on "Cohort Effects" (see Chapter Ten), I describe the rapid shifts in the patterns of drug abuse that we witnessed in the 1960s and the impact of these drugs upon our patient population. To give the reader a better

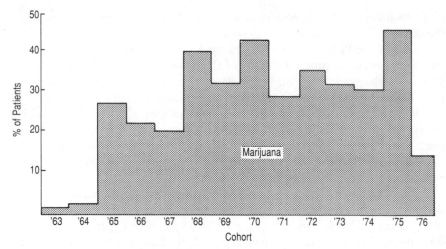

FIGURE 9.2. Percentage of patients in each PI-500 cohort who used marijuana at some point before index hospitalization.

idea of these shifts, I have charted the percentage of each cohort that used one or another substance. Marijuana is the bellwether in this regard, since many patients who began using it turned to other drugs as well, and a higher proportion of the PI-500 patients abused marijuana than any other substance. LSD and amphetamines provide less useful indices of overall abuse: They were used in only about half as many cases, and were rarely used exclusively. Figure 9.2 shows the percentage of patients in each cohort who had used marijuana at some time before the index hospitalization.

General Levels of Drug Abuse in the 14 Cohorts

Through review of the records, I reconstructed an outline of substance abuse for each patient and each cohort. The catalog of substances included alcohol; barbiturates; chloral hydrate; over-the-counter sleeping compounds; marijuana; LSD; peyote; mescaline; psilocybin; STP; DMT; Quaaludes®; amphetamines; opiates (including heroin, morphine, Demerol®, and codeine); cocaine; meprobamate; morning-glory seeds; and glue. Apart from (and soon overshadowing) alcohol, marijuana, LSD, and amphetamines were the most important items.

As Figure 9.2 makes clear, marijuana abuse was negligible in the first two cohorts. But by 1965, one patient in four was using marijuana, hashish, or some related tetrahydrocannabinol compound. By 1968, the rate had risen to one patient in three. The level exceeded 40% in 1970 and again in 1975. I cannot tell whether the precipitous drop in 1976 to 15% was a reflection of some real change in the body social or was merely an artifact of the selection process. Because the unit closed at that time, there is no way of learning what 1977 or 1978 would have shown. Peak usage, at all events, coincided with the student revolution of 1968–1969—the period of maximal frustration (on the part of the younger generation) with the "Establishment."

Table 9.2 plots not only the percentages of marijuana abuse (with or without concomitant abuse of other drugs), but also the percentages of patients in each cohort who abused *only* amphetamines, *only* LSD, or *only* alcohol. These three groups existed over and above the larger group of marijuana users. Taking all four together gives us a good idea of the *total* substance abuse in the entire series. These four groups accounted for five-sixths of all the drug abuse in the PI-500, since, as noted in Table 9.3, only 7.4% of the entire series remains when the 36.2% abusing marijuana, amphetamines, LSD, or alcohol is subtracted from the 43.6% of the series who ever abused *any* substance (7.4/43.6 = 17%). The 41 patients constituting this 7.4% included those who, though never abusing the "big four," used one or another of the substances alluded to in the catalog mentioned above. Some, such as glue, morning-glory seeds, or Quaaludes®, were used rarely. Barbiturate abuse was more frequent and did not

TABLE 9.2. Substance Abuse in the PI-500

Cohort	*n*	I. Marijuana (with or without other drugs) %	*n*	II. Alcohol only[a] %	*n*	III. LSD only[b] %	*n*	IV. Amphetamines only[c] %	*n*	% of cohort using any of three psychotomimetic drugs (I + III + IV)
1963	31	3.2	1	16.1	5	0	0	0	0	3.2
1964	55	3.6	2	12.7	7	1.8	1	1.8	1	7.2
1965	49	26.5	13	6.1	3	4.1	2	2.0	1	32.6
1966	37	21.6	8	2.7	1	2.7	1	0	0	23.3
1967	35	20.0	7	0	0	2.9	1	2.9	1	25.8
1968	38	39.5	15	5.3	2	0	0	0	0	39.5
1969	49	32.7	16	4.1	2	0	0	0	0	32.7
1970	68	41.2	28	2.9	2	2.9	2	2.9	2	47.0
1971	25	28.0	7	4.0	1	4.0	1	0	0	32.0
1972	38	36.8	14	2.6	1	0	0	2.6	1	39.4
1973	38	31.6	12	0	0	0	0	2.6	1	33.2
1974	42	31.0	13	4.8	2	0	0	0	0	31.0
1975	19	42.1	8	0	0	0	0	0	0	42.1
1976	26	15.4	4	0	0	3.8	1	3.8	1	23.0
Totals	550		148		26		9		8	

[a]*All* who ever abused alcohol: *n* = 85 (15.5% of sample).
[b]*All* who tried LSD, with or without other drugs: *n* = 102 (18.5% of sample).
[c]*All* who tried amphetamines: *n* = 81 (14.7% of sample).

TABLE 9.3. Incidence of Drug Abuse by Drug Category

A.		Percentage of patients abusing any substance(s)	43.6
B.	1.	Percentage abusing marijuana, with or without other substances	26.9
	2.	Percentage abusing only LSD	1.6
	3.	Percentage abusing only amphetamines	1.5
	4.	Percentage abusing amphetamines and alcohol (but *not* marijuana), plus percentage abusing peyote or mescaline only	1.5
C.		Percentage abusing alcohol only	4.7
D.		Percentage abusing the psychotomimetics (B; 31.5) plus percentage abusing alcohol (C; 4.7)	36.2
E.		Percentage abusing other substances (A − D)	7.4

always occur in conjunction with the four most popular drugs. The significance of fashion stands out clearly in relation to cocaine, which was used only by 14 of the PI-500 patients and never as their exclusive drug. One could not have guessed at the magnitude of the current cocaine problem in similar patient populations, judging only from our experience in the two decades preceding.

As might be expected in a unit devoted to analytic psychotherapy, we did not knowingly select heroin addicts for admission. Even in that era we recognized the superiority, in the treatment of opiate abuse, of specialized groups in self-contained environments. Places like Renaissance House and Odyssey House had begun to build their reputation; the Narcotics Anonymous organizations would make their appearance a decade later. Still, there were some 25 patients among the PI-500 who used heroin sporadically or (in a few instances) with some regularity.

Throughout the 14 years of the study, the *average* percentage of patients abusing drugs in any one cohort was 43.6%. But the actual figure for each year varied, as Table 9.4 shows, from a low of 29% in the first cohort to 54% or 55% in the early 1970s. In the 1963 and 1964 cohorts, when hallucinogen abuse was scarcely present, those inclined to use substances as anodynes for their mental discomfort resorted to alcohol—which was, for them, the only game in town. These were the "pharmacothymic" (drug-desiring) patients of whom Sandor Rado (1956) had spoken a decade earlier. Already by 1966, alcohol had lost its popularity to nonspiritous drugs; thereafter, the patients rarely used it exclusively (see Table 9.2).

Drugs and Suicide

Patients who presented with acute SZ-like reactions, where the course was transitory and the family history was negative for SZ, had precipitated their psychosis in three cases out of four through drug abuse. Next to these "schizophreniform" patients, the most substance-abuse-prone group was that of the male borderlines, followed by the manic–depressives, the female border-lines, and those with SZ or schizoaffective psychosis (SA). The percentages are set forth in Table 9.5.

The suicide rates were not significantly different in schizophrenic or in schizoaffective patients, whether or not they abused drugs. The tendency to commit suicide seems to have been higher in the schizophreniform and manic–depressive patients who did not use drugs than in those who did, but the numbers are not large enough to permit meaningful distinctions. Among the borderlines, the picture is clear: Suicide rarely occurred in the non-drug-abusing patients (2.5%) and was common in those who did abuse drugs (15 of 136, or 11%).

What is not so clear is the matter of etiology. Was the correlation one of causative significance? In other words, did the drugs destabilize the emotional controls of these borderline patients, propelling certain ones toward suicide who might have resisted the temptation otherwise? Or was the drug abuse a mere accompaniment to suicide that was preconditioned by factors (e.g., parental brutality or loss of all supports through death of loved ones) long antedating the first dalliance with alcohol or marijuana? Embedded within these questions is another: In the drug-abusing group, would suicide have occurred had the patients refrained from using the drugs, despite the abysmal home environment in which they had been reared?

To these important questions I can offer, unfortunately, only impressions, though these impressions are supported by some "hard data" from the old records. I attempted to measure the stressors impinging upon the patients' lives

TABLE 9.4. Proportions of Drug-Abusing Patients in the 14 Cohorts

Cohort	Cohort size	*n* with no substance abuse	% with no substance abuse	% abusing any substance
1963	31	22	71	29
1964	55	38	69	31
1965	49	34	69	31
1966	37	25	68	32
1967	35	20	57	43
1968	38	21	55	45
1969	49	26	53	47
1970	68	31	46	54
1971	25	15	60	40
1972	38	17	45	55
1973	38	17	45	55
1974	42	28	67	33
1975	19	8	42	58
1976	26	18	69	31

TABLE 9.5. Suicides in Various Diagnostic Groups According to Presence or
Absence of Drug Abuse

| | Borderlines | | | | | |
	Male	Female	SZ	SA	SF	MDP
	Non-drug-abusing patients					
Total n	60	103	69	45	10	22
Suicides, n	1	3	6	9	1	3
Suicides, %	1.7	2.9	8.7	20.0	10.0	13.6
	Drug-abusing patients					
Total n	58	78	30	19	26	17
Suicides, n	7	8	3	5	1	1
Suicides, %	12.1	10.3	10.0	26.3	3.8	5.9

Note. The drug-abusing patients (male and female taken together) had a greater suicide rate than their non-drug-abusing counterparts, $\chi^2 = 8.6$ with Yates's correction, $df = 1, p < .01$.

by comparing the approximate weights of these stressors in the two groups: borderline suicides who abused drugs, and those who did not. Eight factors seemed of special relevance: (1) death of a parent, (2) incest or molestation, (3) parental brutality, (4) chaotic home, (5) being adopted, (6) divorce of parents before the patient was 16, (7) parental abuse of alcohol, and (8) family history of severe depression. Re-examination of the records along these lines suggests that the eight variables were less often present in the borderline suicides who were *not* drug abusers and were more often present in those who *did* abuse drugs. This does not emerge as clearly from the percentages of patients in either category who had at least one such life event as it does from comparison of the total numbers of events in the two groups. As Table 9.6 shows, the borderline suicides who abused drugs had experienced about twice as many adverse events, collectively, as had the small group of non-drug-abusing suicides.

None of the homes of those who did not misuse drugs could be called chaotic. One male patient, aged 20, had lost his mother through suicide the year before admission and took his own life the year after discharge. The three female patients came from homes depicted as innocuous or only mildly disturbed. There were strong hints of incest in one, fainter indications of paternal seductiveness in the other two. Instead of facts in these cases, I had only clues, such as the following: An adolescent girl from a well-to-do family became promiscuous at 14, had two pregnancies out of wedlock by 18, was seduced by one of the attendants at the hospital, and in the meantime made five serious suicide attempts. She pictured herself as "evil," "worthless," "sinful," and deserving to die. Her sixth attempt, using materials belonging to her father, was successful. Having encountered this profile again and again in known incest victims, I strongly suspect that this patient had been caught up in some form of seductive relationship with her father. Oedipal fantasies by themselves are scarcely lethal. Paternal *rejection* may drive some young women to despair, but seldom to suicide. Seductiveness and incest carry much more risk.

Among the 15 borderline suicides who did abuse drugs, chaotic family life was the rule. Four of the eight women were incest victims; another had been raped by a neighbor. In the latter case, both parents had been alcoholic and had committed suicide within 2 years of her hospitalization. In two other cases, the patients' fathers had been alternatively seductive and assaultive; the seductiveness may have reached the level of incest, though this is unclear. The home environment had been chaotic (violence, loud arguments, periodic abandonments, drunkenness) in 9 of these 15 cases.

Abuse of alcohol had catalyzed the final suicide act in at least seven of the borderline suicides. In several instances I believe that abstention (achieved

TABLE 9.6. Life Events in Borderline Suicides with and without Drug Abuse

Patient no.	Stressors[a]							
	1	2	3	4	5	6	7	8
Borderline suicides who abused drugs								
1		+				+		
2								+
3					+			
4	+							
5								
6			+	+				
7	+			+			+	+
8			+	+	+			
9								
10		+	+	+			+	+
11								
12								
13		+	+	+			+	
14								
15			+	+			+	
Borderline suicides who did not abuse drugs								
16								
17								+
18	+	+						+
19								

[a]Stressors: 1, death of caretaker; 2, incest; 3, parental brutality; 4, chaotic home; 5, adoption; 6, divorce of parents; 7, parental alcoholism; 8, severe depression in a parent.

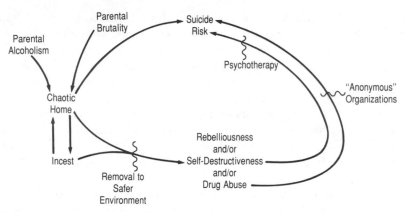

FIGURE 9.3. Suicidality in drug-abusing borderlines. Wavy lines indicate therapeutic interventions that might reduce the risk for suicide.

through AA, for example) would have been life-saving, and that the lives thus saved could have been gratifying and productive. But in perhaps seven instances, the damage had been too severe. These patients had no template for normal life, having witnessed nothing but cruelty, exploitation, and meanness from their earliest days. The horror movies into which their lives had degenerated were simply speeded up by drug abuse. Lives that could not have gone past 30 ended instead at 20 or thereabouts. Parental alcoholism may have fostered the predilection to substance abuse in the six homes where one or both parents drank to excess. But in all these homes, the suicide risk stemmed, as far as I can tell, not merely from seeing the parents drink, but from registering the effects (in the form of physical and sexual violation) unleashed by the alcohol.

The fatal sequence of events may be portrayed according to the schema depicted in Figure 9.3. In this schema, the worse the home (the greater the rejection, violence, or duration of sexual abuse), the greater the self-destructiveness and tendency toward drug abuse. The substance abuse acts synergistically to heighten suicide risk. If the factors are powerful enough and remain unchecked, a fatal dénouement may be inevitable. Removal from the home (e.g., hospitalization) may be life-saving in some cases; therapy may attempt to diminish the self-destructiveness that stems from the shattered self-image (the regular accompaniment of being reared in this environment); the "Anonymous" organizations may lower suicide risk through sobriety. Many of the PI-500 patients who came from abusive homes but who were well at follow-up were saved by one or all three of these interventions. Why were they able to pull out of the nose dive, while the others crashed? Some came from homes that were clearly less violent, had experienced incest tinged only slightly with sadistic overtones, and so on. Others came from environments every bit as malignant as those that toppled their dormitory mates who committed suicide; unlike the latter, however, they had more perseverance, better self-regard, *something*, that enabled them to survive. These positive factors are subtle (and clinicians seldom record them in their notes). Someone reading the old records who was "blind" to the patients' outcomes could seldom pick the survivors from the suicides.

THE RELATIONSHIPS AMONG ALCOHOLISM, DRUG ABUSE, AND ANTISOCIALITY IN BORDERLINES

Antisocial personality (ASP) has been discussed at some length in Chapter Six; however, the interrelationships among alcoholism, drug abuse, and ASP in the PI-500 borderline patients merit a separate discussion. Cadoret, Troughton, O'Gorman, and Heywood (1986) reported recently on their adoption study of gene–environment interactions in drug abuse, mentioning that "Antisocial behavior has been implicated as a factor in alcohol abuse and is also related to drug abuse" (p. 1131). Further on, they suggested that "some underlying biochemical foundation [is] involved in all of the substances abused or [there is] some common psychosocial factor leading to multiple types of abuse" (p. 1136). Cadoret et al. felt that antisocial behavior might constitute such a psychosocial factor, since it seems to intensify the predisposition to abuse substances. All three conditions are also overrepresented in populations of borderline patients, irrespective of diagnostic definition.

Figure 9.4 is a Venn diagram showing the areas of overlap and disjunction of these three attributes among the PI-500 borderlines. The alcoholic border-lines showed less of a tendency also to have ASP (10 of 52, or 19%), compared with the antisocial borderlines' tendency also to abuse alcohol (10 of 23, or 43%). The tendencies for the alcoholic and for the antisocial borderlines also to abuse drugs, however, were equal (54% and 52%, respectively).

The *suicide* rates in the nonantisocial alcoholic borderlines who either did or did not abuse drugs (9.5% in both groups) and in those who abused drugs but not alcohol (9.4%) resembled that of the BPD patients (8.9%). By contrast, borderlines who abused *neither* alcohol *nor* drugs had a lower rate (4 of 152, or 2.6%). Of interest is the fact that the antisocial but non-substance-abusing borderlines, admittedly a small group, had a zero suicide rate. Two in that all-male group died—one in a motorcycle accident, another while in jail. Two others committed murder. The small group with a three-way overlap (alcoholism × ASP × drug abuse) fared particularly poorly: Three were suicides (43%), and two were still grossly impaired at follow-up. One of the two recovered patients had been in AA for many years. The smallest group, that of patients with ASP × alcoholism, consists of one recovered patient (also in AA), one suicide, and one missing (for about 20 years) and presumed dead.

The antisocial borderlines, if one includes those who abused substances, had a strikingly high death rate (from suicide and other causes) compared with

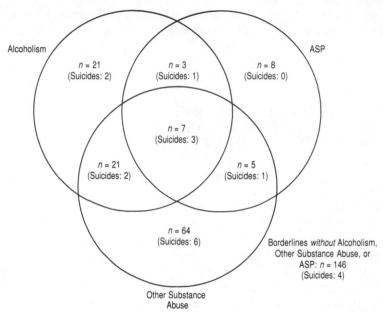

FIGURE 9.4.   The relationship among alcoholism, other substance abuse, and antisocial personality (ASP) in traced borderline patients (BPD, D, other BPO).

the nonantisocial borderlines: 35% (8 of 23), as against 6% (16 of 258). The
latter figure includes a small number of patients known to be alive as of this
writing, who have not yet been interviewed.

Though the alcoholic borderlines were more apt to show concomitant ASP
(19%) than were the nonalcoholics (5.4%), the nonantisocial alcoholics were not
significantly less likely to be well (GAS scores > 60) at follow-up than were the
nonalcoholic borderlines. Even the 21 nonantisocial alcoholics who *had* also
abused drugs were well in two-thirds of the cases (14 of 21). All the alcoholic
borderlines who joined and stayed with AA were doing well at follow-up;
another was in AA for a brief time, but still abused marijuana heavily and was
functioning only marginally. A few of the adolescents who abused alcohol
transiently during the extended crises that preceded their hospitalization
recovered and remained well without the help of AA.

CHAPTER TEN

Other Variables Affecting Outcome

AGORAPHOBIA

Agoraphobia was one of the more common secondary diagnoses among the PI borderline patients; for several, it was the condition necessitating hospitalization. In the patients admitted with a psychosis, agoraphobia was a less frequent accompaniment (the schizophrenic [SZ], schizoaffective [SA], and manic–depressive psychosis [MDP] groups contained one each). Anxiety/panic disorders and primary affective illness appear to be overrepresented in close relatives of agoraphobic (Fyer & Klein, 1985); similarly, the incidence of the syndrome in cotwins of monozygotic agoraphobic twins is more than double the incidence in dizygotic cotwins (Carey & Gottesman, 1981). Koehler, Vartzopoulos, and Ebel (1986) believe agoraphobia and panic disorder to be subcategories of a core endogenous anxiety illness.

The eight borderline agoraphobic in the PI-500 had 26 first-degree relatives, of whom 9 had a psychiatric disorder (depression in 6, alcoholism in 2, irritability and abusiveness in 1); 1 had a concomitant phobic disorder. As for the type of borderline condition in our eight patients, five fulfilled DSM criteria for borderline personality disorder (BPD; three of these had concomitant major affective disorder [MAD]), and three were borderline by Kernberg criteria only (two of these were also dysthymic [D]). There was no consistent relationship between the presence of MAD in patients and a similar occurrence in their relatives. (A ninth borderline developed agoraphobia *after* leaving PI and later still committed suicide; she is not counted among the cases in this section.)

All the agoraphobic patients have been traced. There was one suicide in a borderline woman whose life had been very chaotic (drug abuse, alcoholism, promiscuity, molesting children) and who had herself been the product of a violent family. (This woman is also described in "Parental Brutality," Chapter Seven.) Another, a schizoaffective woman, is also dead—of cardiac complications stemming from severe obesity.

The average GAS score at follow-up in the remaining seven borderline patients was somewhat lower (62) than the average for the whole borderline group (67); more importantly, three remained significantly impaired. Two remained housebound to the day of follow-up (21 years later), although one was briefly married before returning to the home of her parents. The other I located, having learned that she had an unlisted number in the town she grew up in, by driving to the old address in that city. She was still there. One of the males (who was only mildly agoraphobic) was married with two children at follow-up; one of the female patients married and had two children, but was divorced by follow-up. Three of the women remained unmarried in their 40s.

Several of these patients found great consolation in keeping pets (dogs in particular), which served, as they themselves mentioned, as "transitional objects." Such "objects" are of especial importance in the adult lives of many borderline patients (Morris, Gunderson, & Zanarini, 1986), especially those with problems in the area of dependency and separation typical of agoraphobic. One of the borderline patients, with whom I have kept in contact over the past 25 years, had a brief course of therapy after she left PI, married, and acquired a dog to keep her company both at home and on walks to the neighborhood stores. Hers was a steady uphill course; eventually she overcame her phobia completely and became active in community concerns, especially those relating to her children's school.

Another BPD patient had been a "symbiotic dependent" girl who kept a stuffed lion with her at all times, including during the year she spent with us. During her adolescence she had been sexually abused by an uncle. Eventually she did quite well; at follow-up, she was married and raising two children.

One of the patients who made a moderate improvement had been on tricyclic antidepressants for many years by the time of follow-up. For the most part, however, our treatment of the agoraphobics consisted of psychotherapy (expressive, mainly, in the case of the successful woman mentioned above) and occasionally some rudimentary behavioral technics. The more systematic use of tricyclic antidepressants and monoamine oxidase inhibitors, and of behavior modification technics, in the treatment of agoraphobia was just being pioneered during the era of the PI-500.

COHORT EFFECTS

A follow-up study of sufficient length can answer many questions in psychiatry concerning the stability of symptom pictures over time and the natural history of various conditions. One can also approach questions relating to changing fashions in symptom pictures from one generation to the next, if a long succession of cohorts is available for study. The PI-500 spanned 14 years; unfortunately, this time period is not quite a generation, but it does provide 14 cohorts within which to look for possible differences in patterns of illness.

Cohort study, for example, has established the absolute increase in incidence of bulimia over the past 20 years in Switzerland (Willi & Grossman, 1983). Within the PI-500, abuse of substances other than alcohol was noted with particular frequency (two patients out of three) in 1970, the upswing having commenced in the late 1960s. Few of the patients admitted in 1963–1967—only about 1 in 12—had such a history.

Various sociological phenomena might underlie the resurgence of drug use in the 1960s. The commercial production of LSD, founded partly on hopes that LSD could free up obsessional neuroses (Leuner, 1962), still required a receptive public. Availability met desirability in the form of a psychoanalytic community discouraged about the slowness of resolving obsessional symptoms through psychoanalysis, coupled with a lay community more likely to accept "alloplastic" measures than was the generation of the 1930s and 1940s. The success and popularity of psychoanalytic treatment at midcentury may have helped prepare the public to feel less shame over sexual impulses, with the (possible) result that the inhibitory neuroses of Freud's day became replaced to an increasing extent by syndromes of disinhibition and entitlement.

Other contributory factors may have included changes in patterns of affluence (affecting the affordability of drugs) and family structure (an increased divorce rate, leading to increased anomie and susceptibility to the blandishments of psychoactive drugs among young people). At all events, in place of the classical psychoneuroses (obsession, phobias, etc.) in patients utilizing chiefly autoplastic defenses, we began to see patients who resorted to predominantly external mechanisms, including substance abuse. Morphine and cocaine were no longer frightening to young people growing up in the 1950s and 1960s. They could have had no firsthand experience with the devastating effects of these drugs before World War I, reaction to which had led to the Harrison Act and to a less drug-abusing society for many years (Delpirou & Labrousse, 1986).

Viewed in this light, the PI-500 represents the tail end of a more inhibited generation, followed by the "student revolution" and a new and much less inhibited generation. Intense guilt over masturbation, premarital sex, homosexual impulses, and "unconventional" sex figured importantly in the histories of the PI-500, especially those admitted between 1963 and 1968. Obsessional handwashing, "germ phobias," and related syndromes were common in the generation still susceptible to inordinate guilt over these matters; they were less common in the last few cohorts. Already by the mid-1980s as I was compiling this book, sexual guilt and the syndromes it spawned have taken on some of the quaint, almost antediluvian, aura that now attaches to neurasthenia, chlorosis, and fainting spells. In their place are narcissism, bulimia, and cocaine abuse. In saying this, I do not mean to suggest that ours is necessarily a "worse" generation; merely a *different* generation. The absolute percentage of young persons suffering from definable emotional disorders probably does not change appreciably from one decade to the next. But the most popular configurations of symptom type and abnormal personality do shift over time. As one of my patients put it, with a wisdom beyond her years, "I guess there's just as many of us going downtown as there ever were, only we're getting there on different tracks."

CRUELTY TO ANIMALS

Of all the creatures that boarded the ark, man alone is capable of malice. And even in the ideal home, the most nurturing parents must still, with some regularity, frustrate and thus infuriate their offspring. If we would love unambivalently, we must turn to animals, especially to those with the most appealing characteristics, such as a puppy or a kitten. For reasons of this sort, many might prefer to believe that children who torture animals will come to a bad end. Much as it may offend our moral sensibilities, I cannot report that this was the regular fate of the 12 PI-500 patients who were cruel to animals at some point before their hospitalization. The phenomenon itself has, of course, a long history. Haslam of Bethlem Hospital (1809), for example, mentioned a 9-year-old boy who "oppressed the feeble, and avoided the society of those more powerful than himself" (p. 204). He was cruel to his cat,

> . . . and whenever this luckless animal approached him he plucked out its whiskers with wonderful rapidity. . . . After this operation, he commonly threw the creature on the fire, or through the window. If a little dog came near him he kicked it, if a large one he would not notice it. (p. 204)

Haslam, "being ignorant of any means by which he was likely to recover," did not retain the boy, who was thus lost to follow-up.

Although cruelty to animals is considered a bad prognostic sign in child psychiatry, the data necessary to work out the conditional probabilities that might validate this assumption are lacking. Because jails collect them, it is easy to survey those who have killed, in order to ascertain the percentage who had formerly tortured animals. But we cannot readily survey thousands of children and follow them to see how many (or, we may hope, how few) later injure persons.

The 12 animal-abusing patients in the PI-500 consisted of 6 borderlines, 3 schizophrenic males, 1 schizoaffective female, and 2 schizophreniform (SF) males. I succeeded in tracing all of these patients. One borderline woman was 15 when admitted, shortly after her mother abandoned the family. At that turn of events, she became cruel both to her cat and to her brother. She had become alcoholic during childhood, and did poorly until her late 20s, when she got into Alcoholics Anonymous (AA). At follow-up, she was clinically recovered. The other borderline woman was 14 when admitted, in the context of anxiety over incestuous relations with her brother. She kicked her dog at a time when she was in a dissociative state. At follow-up 22 years later, she was married, had two children, and was running a business. She had been asymptomatic and comfortable for most of the time since her release from the hospital.

One of the male borderlines came from an intact and caring family; his (relatively minor) cruelty to animals as a child could be seen as an epiphenomenon of his general hyperactive condition. As the hyperactivity was brought under control, the sadistic behavior subsided. Another male borderline, also cruel to animals only during his childhood, had been abandoned by his mother. He had made a "fair" adjustment at follow-up (GAS score = 58) and had avoided contact with his immediate family for many years. A more disturbing example of animal abuse was that of a borderline man manifesting considerable aggressiveness and depression throughout his early adult life. During a crisis in a personal relationship, he punched his friend's cat in the face. At follow-up 12 years later he was pursuing a constricted life; his behavior was much more subdued, and there had been no further violent outbursts.

One of the schizophreniform men had seen his father only once in his life; he was often angry with his mother, his dog, and life in general throughout his adolescence. He had two breakdowns, but at follow-up he had been well for 14 years. His relationship with his mother had mellowed, and he had worked steadily and proficiently since leaving the second hospital. The only oddities noticeable were a propensity to food-faddism and magical thinking. He had not been violent in his relations with friends of either sex. The other schizophreniform patient was doing quite well, having completed college and having embarked on a good career, when he was killed by a driver who ran a red light. One of the schizophrenic men grew up in an intact but argumentative home; his cruelty to animals was minor and confined to childhood. At follow-up, his adaptation was marginal, and there was a paranoid cast to his personality.

The schizoaffective woman, who during childhood squeezed her sister's turtle to death, was rehospitalized once but at follow-up was living alone and was self-supporting (GAS score = 52).

The most disturbing example was that of a male borderline with schizoid personality. His cruelty toward animals was confined to a solitary but gruesome act during his adolescence. As noted elsewhere (see "Homosexuality," below), the violence was closely related to murderous fantasies toward a parent.

The topic of childhood cruelty to animals is not without its paradoxes. The borderline man who was the most violent person in the PI-500, shooting three people to death in a killing spree shortly after joining the Marines, hated his (abusive) parents—hated all humanity, in fact—and loved only his dog.

There is a big difference between cruelty to animals as a *substitute* for murder and as a *prelude* to murder. It would represent a major advance in psychiatry if we could determine which such acts were truly predictive of violence against persons. I have only one such experience in my clinical practice: I predicted (unfortunately, correctly) that a patient who as an adult had killed an animal would later kill a family member.

Perhaps the later in life someone is cruel to an animal, the more ominous the implications are. Children are less socialized than adults and less able to modulate the expression of emotion. A (potentially) normal child in an abnormal situation (desertion or death of a parent, cruelty of a parent) may exhibit occasional cruelty to an animal, as may an abnormal child in a "normal" situation, such as the birth of a sibling. But by the time someone has reached the age of 20 or 30, cruelty to an animal, especially in response to the ordinary stresses of life, may indeed signify the kind of heartlessness and schizoid detachment that have predictive value for felonious behavior. Unusually *grotesque* torture of animals is probably a predictor of future violence, as suggested by biographies of notorious murderers. For example, Albert DeSalvo (the "Boston Strangler") tortured cats as a child, and Edmund Kemper decapitated first cats and later women (Leyton, 1986).

Felthous and Kellert (1987) have suggested that the contradictory findings in the literature concerning the implications of cruelty to animals may be resolved if one concentrates on direct interviews with patients and other study subjects. Reports based on such interviews do point to a connection between childhood cruelty to animals and later acts of violence against persons.

ELOPEMENT

Certain examples of clinical wisdom, repeated to each entering class of resident therapists, in time acquire the quality of conviction and eventually of unassailable truth. One such belief in the 1950s and 1960s held that patients who eloped or who signed out against medical advice had a bad prognosis. We clung to this belief, for its demoralizing alternative was that our judgment about the need to safeguard various patients within a locked unit had been overzealous or misplaced. Reason itself dictated that self-destructive persons (which most of our patients were) would be more at risk untreated than treated, and at greater risk still if they demonstrated the impulsivity, negativism, and denial of illness usually present in those who sought escape.

As it appears in the light of long-term follow-up, the clinical wisdom was both right and wrong. If we compare outcomes with respect to gender and diagnostic subgroup, we find that premature departure in male borderlines was indeed associated with a fate generally worse than that experienced by the majority of borderline males who stayed for the duration. Several attributes emerge as likely candidates in explaining this difference. If we focus with a finer lens upon individual case histories, we note that the 12 males who eloped or signed out were not only impulsive, but irascible and sociopathic in all but 2 instances. I have traced only 9 of these 12. These included a matricide (pressured by his parents to sign out); the elopee who, after joining the Marines, shot three people to death in a bar (see "Gradations of Antisociality," Chapter Six); a male prostitute; a hostile sociopath; a man missing for 18 years and presumed dead; an aggressive adolescent who eventually "straightened out" after leaving his violent family; and a once destructive and hyperactive boy who led a calm but only marginal existence after leaving the hospital. The two nonirascible males were schizoid loners who were on disability at follow-up. Two of the three untraced males were sociopathic. The courts remanded one of them to our facility as an alternative to placing him in a reformatory for juvenile delinquents; at follow-up, the other had skipped out on his wife and children, and even his sister and parents (I spoke with all parties) did not know of his whereabouts. We are dealing here, primarily, with whatever it is that makes males more prone than females to aggression and criminality. Similar factors operating elsewhere in mammalian life may explain such phenomena as "rogue males" (e.g., among lions), competitive struggles for the possession of a female, and the like (Wilson, 1975, p. 79). Wilson (1975, p. 248 ff.) also discusses the role of androgens in aggression, particularly in male–female differences within species.

Another example of clinical wisdom may be applicable here. Those who observed the PI-500 over the longest time span often remarked that our patient population represented an *Alice in Wonderland*-like antiworld, where the men were passive and the women aggressive. Whatever factors contributed to fashioning our patients in ways opposite to the prevailing societal stereotypes put them at greater risk, or so we speculated, for developing the kinds of difficulties requiring psychiatric hospitalization at some point in their life course. At all events, the 37 female borderlines who either eloped ($n = 29$) or signed out against advice ($n = 8$) did not differ markedly from those who remained: A few were unmotivated; many were impulsive, though not more so than some of the impulsive women who went along with the recommendations of the unit. Their outcomes did not differ, when averaged, from those of their more submissive or more cooperative counterparts. These impressions are pictoralized in Figure 10.1, which also shows, for purposes of comparison, the distribution of outcomes in the male and female borderline groups as a whole.

Though impulsivity by itself did not account for much of the variance among the already rather impulsive borderlines, immaturity, together with the impulsivity often prominent in immature persons, may have been an important factor. Adolescent borderlines, for example, were considerably more likely to elope than were those 18 or over. Of all 143 adolescent patients, 28, or 19.6%, eloped, whereas of the 92 borderline adolescents, 24, or 26.1%, eloped. The latter figures contrast with those for all borderlines (49 of 299, or 16.4%) and for borderlines aged 18 or over (25 of 207, or 12.1%). The contrast between the borderline adolescents and the borderlines aged 18 or over was significant, $\chi^2 = 9.12$, $df = 1$, $p < .002$.

The schizophrenic adolescents at PI numbered 18; not one eloped. They were more passive in general than the borderline adolescents. Elopement and signing out against advice were uncommon among schizophrenics of any age: Only 12 of 99 eloped (12.1%), the same rate found in the borderlines aged 18 and over. The distribution of outcomes among schizophrenics who eloped did not differ, as Figure 10.1 also shows, from the outcomes of the schizophrenics

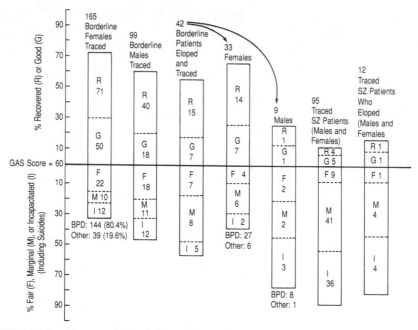

FIGURE 10.1. Outcomes in borderline and schizophrenic PI-500 patients who eloped from the unit and could be traced. Outcomes for all traced patients in these diagnostic groups are presented for purposes of comparison.

as a group (or of the 83 traced schizophrenics who did not elope). For schizophrenic patients, the illness itself appeared to dominate other factors in determining outcome, whereas for the heterogeneous group of borderlines, a number of nonspecific factors played the major roles (age, gender, personality type, etc.).

With respect to suicidality, the borderlines who eloped or signed out rarely committed suicide (1 of 42 traced, or 2.4%). The one who did was a depressed woman who had recently suffered the suicide of her father, as well as the death of her mother through the slow suicide of alcoholism. Review of the chart makes it clear that the staff took insufficient precautions with her—a rare lapse, actually, in a unit normally very conservative in the management of suicidal patients. What is not so clear is the matter of her long-range salvageability. In the absence of any external support system, her prognosis was poor, especially because she had few personality assets (talent, work skills, stamina). However, it appears that dysphoria—in particular, the predisposition to recurrent severe depression— weighs heavier in the balance regarding suicidality than impulsivity by itself. Paris, Brown, and Nowlis (1987) make a similar point. I hope that this comment does not lull mental health professionals into a false sense of security in the face of eloped borderlines. Their recklessness remains a cause for considerable worry.

It may be, however, that those *without* serious concomitant depressive disorders pose less threat of suicide than do those who show this comorbidity.

Some of the individual stories of the eloped patients are among the most moving in the entire series, the more so because they so often overturned our expectations. Of many, I can scarcely offer even the barest outline. In some instances, their protagonists have achieved prominence; in others, they have entered one of the healing professions. One of the borderlines, saddled with a rather insensitive therapist, eloped for reasons that appeared ominous to the staff but that were quite sensible when viewed retrospectively. This patient was eager to finish school and get on with a career, and felt unnecessarily held back by the hospital. The eventual outcome 20 years later—becoming a highly respected religious leader, without any further psychiatric help following the elopement— would seem to confirm the patient's judgment. Another elopee ran away from her adoptive home when she discovered (by looking in the mirror) that her roots were altogether different from those of her new parents. She later ran away from us. But instead of living out the gloomy prognosis we predicted, she was happily raising a family of her own at follow-up, having made her peace with her adoptive parents and with the initially unassimilable realities of her origins. Several of the borderlines had been incest victims as children, had become "wild" as adolescents, and had continued to lead "wild" lives of substance abuse and promiscuity after eloping from the hospital, only to settle down years later, after rescue by an "Anonymous" organization, into a middle age of productivity and comfortable intimacy with a partner. One of the schizophrenic elopees ended up in jail for murder, but another ended up a successful contractor and family man. One of the schizoaffective elopees, after a tortured existence of failed relationships and defeated projects, killed himself; another's story, however, was a success that deserves to be recounted in somewhat more detail. A maker of ceramics by trade, this young woman was probably made acutely "crazy" by an incest experience. She was alternately incoherent or mute on our unit, but gradually shook off the effects of what had befallen her, without further treatment. At follow-up, she was raising her children and pursuing her craft in a remote tropical rain forest (her brother was kind enough to arrange our phone call). She had eloped from PI because of difficulties in adjusting to a new therapist. Like the eloped borderline who suddenly quit using drugs and who thereafter made a remarkable recovery, the ceramist also relied predominantly on her own "true grit," with occasional encouragement from a religious adept from whom she later sought help.

FATHERS

I grew up hearing an expression that dealt presumably with the inscrutability of the child's mind: "It's a wise father who knows his own son." The reverse seems at least equally valid. Several of the PI-500 thought they knew their fathers but were mistaken. One patient assumed that the man who raised him was his father, but he was not. Another assumed that the man who raised her was not her (biological) father, but he was. There is a lesson here for students of hereditary/familial factors in psychiatric illness: It is a wise geneticist who knows his own fathers. The paradoxical situations just referred to were not discovered by the hospital staff, but were mentioned to me by various contactees in connection with my follow-up efforts years later. Needless to say, the original family trees in these cases, as portrayed in the old records, were inaccurate. A similar paradox cropped up in connection with some of the absent fathers: One, whom the patient had assumed was dead, was alive; another, whom the patient imagined was still alive, had (as I was told by a distant relative) died some years before.

I think it is fair to say that in the days of Freud and the pioneers, rather more attention was paid to the role of fathers in regard to pathogenesis. This was followed by an era in which mothers were stigmatized excessively (the "schizophrenogenic mother," etc.; see Parker, 1982). The PI-500, hospitalized during the tail end of this "matricentric" theorizing, were thought of as having dreadful mothers. A few of the mothers actually *were* dreadful. The fathers, unless flamboyantly violent, were pictured as "weak," "passive," or "absent"—not exactly exculpated, but guilty of lesser offenses. Re-examination in the light of contemporary knowledge suggests a more balanced view. In many of the families of the PI-500, the father's role was not merely important but determinative. The negative side of this is depicted in some detail in the sections on "Parental Brutality" and "Incest" (see Chapter Seven). Briefly put, a number of fathers literally destroyed their children through either abandonment, sexual molestation, or violence. Even here, they usually retained enough vestiges of chivalry as to beat only their sons. Sons deserted by a father often developed antisocial personality (ASP), as did several whose fathers died when they were young. Daughters who were the victims of both incest and assault committed suicide, regardless of favorable endowment with respect to attractiveness, talent, and social position. The self-esteem of several daughters was shattered by fathers' withering rejection; sometimes these fathers affected to "hate" their daughters as a defense against incestuous impulses. In general, assaulted sons became outcasts; the molested daughters, at best, experienced inordinate difficulties in intimacy, tending toward either promiscuity, homosexuality, or a global repudiation of sex and closeness. The personalities of brutalized children often solidified along paranoid or schizoid lines. One such borderline man became a vagrant and had not spoken to his father in 10 years by the time of follow-up; another became a loner, a practitioner in the martial arts, and had not spoken to his father in 20 years at follow-up.

On the positive side, I have found at least 10 instances in which the potentially ruinous effects of a mother's behavior were mollified by a father's protectiveness. In another three, a father made enormous efforts to compensate for the death of the mother early in the life of the patient. Of the first-mentioned group, seven of the mothers had been violent; two were given to verbal humiliation; the remaining mother was promiscuous and irresponsible.

FIRESETTING

Firesetting has understandably ominous overtures as a pathological trait (O'Sullivan & Kelleher, 1987). The effects of fire multiply quickly and geometrically; those of bricks and bullets remain linear. In addition, those who set fires often demonstrate a malice and a vengefulness that exceed the levels associated with other forms of violence. At the very least, they demonstrate significant social deficits (Geller, 1987). Whereas firesetters supposedly suffered from a specific brand of madness ("pyromania"), according to the 19th-century alienists (Ray, 1839, pp. 177–179), they may actually belong to any diagnostic category: SZ, alcoholism, personality disorder, and so on (Geller, 1987).

Of the 10 PI-500 patients I identified with this tendency, four had a psychosis; the rest were borderline. There was nothing noteworthy, that is, about the proportionality as to diagnostic groups. Despite the small numbers, a few generalizations are perhaps permissible. Among the borderlines, the family background in all but one case was unusually chaotic, eliciting at times such moralistic descriptions in the old records as "deplorable" or "vicious." Parental brutality, equally divided between mother and father, was associated in one patient (the Future Marine; see "Gradations of Antisociality," Chapter Six) with firesetting at a reformatory the year before hospitalization and with the murder of three people 4 years after his elopement. An adolescent male, having killed several people in an act of arson, set fires on our unit and pushed matches under the door of the seclusion room as if to aid an acutely suicidal patient in destroying herself. This young man, who was eventually transferred from our unit because of these incidents, remained a schizoid "loner," ambulatory but never well. A third, an incest victim during her adolescence, set fires at about the time of the sexual molestation; her life was characterized by chaotic impulsivity, suicide gestures, drug abuse, and promiscuity, and ended in suicide.

Sexual exploitation, in this instance homosexual, figured in the pyromania of another borderline adolescent (see "Episodic Dyscontrol," Appendix A). The other two came from violent homes, developed sociopathic tendencies, and later abused drugs and alcohol—but eventually made surprisingly good adjustments, after many difficult years, once they joined the appropriate "Anonymous" organization. One woman had set fire to her house following a violent family quarrel when she was a girl of 5, in the process destroying the roof and killing the family dog.

Many of these examples lend support to the common associations people have always made between fire and certain forms of violence. These associations are embedded in our language. We speak of "heated" arguments, "flames" of passion, "inflammatory" remarks, the "white heat" of jealousy, "seeing red," and so forth. These dead metaphors come alive in the histories of firesetters.

The same correlations were apparent among those admitted with a psychosis. One of the schizophrenic patients who almost committed suicide damaged his home with fire shortly after his failed attempt; another set a fire while at PI. Another schizophrenic man, an accomplished mathematician, had once set fire to his papers under the influence of command hallucinations. While at PI, he blew out his brains with a shotgun the day his therapist rotated off service. An adolescent admitted with a schizophreniform reaction set fires and engaged in homosexual activities after his father approached him sexually. A schizoaffective woman who was embroiled in a homosexual relationship while at another hospital set a fire there, hoping to disentangle herself by being transferred somewhere else. (She was.)

There was not enough information in the old records to examine whether firesetting and enuresis went together. The older literature on child psychiatry suggested such a connection (Hellman & Blackman, 1966; Felthous & Bernard, 1979); a recent study has challenged it (Showers & Pickrell, 1987). Wax and Haddox (1974) regarded these two phenomena, when accompanied by cruelty to animals, as predictors of assaultiveness in male adolescents. Of the firesetters mentioned here (all but one of whom was an adolescent), five of the six males (and none of the females) were either assaultive (three) or destructive (all six) at one time or another. In line with the impressions of Wax and Haddox, David Berkowitz ("Son of Sam") had been a chronic firesetter as a child and had begun to shoot dogs at about the time of his serial murders (Leyton, 1986).

HOMOSEXUALITY

Homosexuality, as we are coming to realize more clearly, is a complex taxonomy; it is in no way as unitary as the one-word label would suggest. Friedman (1988) has outlined four separate dimensions of psychological function regarding sexuality, all of which need to be taken into account in designating and defining groups of homosexual men and women: (1) consciously perceived erotic fantasy, (2) the nature of one's erotic activity with others, (3) gender identity, and (4) social role. Erotic activity may be analyzed further in relation to time, since patterns of sexual behavior may be lifelong or of lesser duration.

Established homosexuality of long duration was noted in 14 (12%) of the 118 male borderlines, in 1% of the 181 female borderlines, and only rarely in the other diagnostic groups. Another five borderline males were bisexual, meaning that altogether about one in six of the borderline males occupied, with respect to sexual preference, some position on the Kinsey scale (Kinsey, Pomeroy, & Martin, 1948) other than exclusive or nearly exclusive heterosexuality. Three of the exclusively homosexual (and none of the bisexual) men were effeminate.

Epidemiological studies bearing on this issue suggest population rates of about 5% for male homosexuality (Mihalik, 1988) and 1% for female homosexuality. Lifelong, exclusive homosexuality in males (Kinsey Type 6) is less common— approximately 0.5% to 1% (Friedman, 1988).

One might ask whether homosexuals are more apt to be psychiatrically ill than heterosexuals. There is no evidence that this is so from studies of the general population (Friedman, 1988). Furthermore, although there is increasing evidence for constitutional predisposition as a factor in male (and to a lesser extent in female) homosexuality (Eckert, Bouchart, Bohlen, & Heston, 1986; Ellis & Ames, 1987; Goodman, 1983; Lindesay, 1987; Money, 1980), there is no evidence that constitutional factors predisposing individuals to mental illness are in any way related to those governing homosexuality. In the meantime, older psychoanalytic theories about the causation of male homosexuality are being challenged from every quarter. Studies of males with low neuroticism in nonclinical settings, in contrast to the older studies based on those seeking psychiatric help, suggest "that disturbed parental relations are neither necessary nor sufficient conditions for homosexuality to emerge" (Hooker, 1969, p. 142). Siegelman (1974) found no significant differences in parental backgrounds between homosexuals and heterosexuals with low neuroticism. In neurotic and effeminate homosexuals, rejection by fathers was often reported; their mothers did not appear to be more often "intense, overprotective, indulgent," and so on, than the mothers in the heterosexual comparison group (Siegelman, 1974, p. 14). The overall impression is that, where paternal rejection was especially marked, this factor contributed greatly to the neurotic suffering of the homosexual sons, but little if at all to their evolving object choice.

The prevailing cultural attitude toward homosexuality during the era of the PI-500 was, if anything, more scornful than it is today. Ours is a particularly "homophobic" culture to begin with, considerably more so than certain other cultures (Whitam & Zent, 1984). This would help account for the bias of the therapeutic community when my colleagues and I were in training—namely, that homosexuals should be encouraged to become heterosexual. This, coupled with the notion that causation had only to do with unhealthy parental patterns, led to the further assumption that analytic treatment could (with some effort) effect such a conversion. Those of us who become the therapists of the PI-500 felt obliged to "change" homosexuals, as our analytic forebears seemed able to do with such alacrity and panache. Edmund Bergler (1957) was one of the chief culprits in this regard, but we had no way of knowing that his reports of "cures" on a wholesale basis were examples of either self-delusion or (more likely) prevarication. Working at cross-purposes with our homosexual patients, especially those admitted during the 1960s, we probably contributed more to the intensification than to the alleviation of their self-reproach and suffering.

To a certain extent, one can sympathize also with the parents of the homosexual patients: They were no more eager to contemplate "genetic death" (homosexuals, by definition, represent the terminus of a particular ancestral line) than parents in general. Also, the treating community lacked the knowledge that could have helped the parents understand that homosexuality will develop in a certain percentage of boys, irrespective of culture, era, or parental behavior (Mihalik, 1988). In the absence of controlled studies, the earlier psychoanalytic writers (e.g., Bieber, 1962) did not realize how common in anglophone society is the supposedly pathognomonic constellation that is hardly restricted to the families of homosexual males (Whitam & Zent, 1984). Had we been in a position to transmit such information, we might have helped these parents to develop greater objectivity and compassion and to overcome their guilt or animosity toward their homosexual sons. On this score, I can declare with conviction that had some of the parents been confronted during the mother's confinement by an angel bearing them advance word from the Almighty that they could have their choice of either a homosexual son who would be the next DaVinci or a heterosexual son who would be the next Al Capone, they would have opted unhesitatingly for Capone. There were several sets of parents who directed toward their sons an unending stream of derisive taunts, creating of their homes a manufactury of outcasts.

The adoptive mother of one of our homosexual patients, after some years of humiliating him through depreciatory remarks about his manliness, sought finally to resituate him along the path of heterosexuality by seducing him. Instead, he committed suicide. A farmer's son, ridiculed by both parents, was hospitalized at PI after sodomizing, then torturing to death, in animal. Though he remains a schizoid loner, he went on to make a remarkable recovery in other sectors of his life as a self-supporting professional. He was unmotivated for psychotherapy, being disposed more to "seal over" than to integrate (McGlashan, Levy, & Carpenter, 1975). Paradoxically, his depraved act may have rescued this man. We assumed, because what he had done was sadistic and shocking, that his prognosis was "zero." Besides, this animal sacrifice was a thinly disguised patricide. But murder it was not. He was spared both stigma and jail. The authorities saw to it that he was hospitalized, which automatically lifted him out of a noxious environment. Violence often had this salutary side effect among the PI-500 adolescents, but usually it was directed against the self. Three of the homosexual males, for example, had catapulted themselves out of intolerable family situations via spectacular suicide attempts so unusual in detail as not to permit description here for reasons of confidentiality. Two other males, both bisexual, did commit suicide. But the three near-suicides have largely recovered at follow-up: Two homosexual patients who are now working full-time, though their social life is constricted, and a bisexual patient who is now a professional, married, and raising two small children.

Outcome scores in the group as a whole were in a range consistent with that of the male heterosexual borderlines in the PI-500: At follow-up, about half were well (average GAS score = 62 for the 6 bisexual and 14 homosexual patients, all but 2 of whom were traced).

Alcohol abuse was no more common among the homosexual/bisexual males (20%) than among the heterosexual male borderlines (17%). There were too few females to permit meaningful comparisons.

The male homosexuals with good outcomes were more likely to come from homes where there had been paternal indifference rather than abusiveness. Neglect (unless it is particularly severe) is usually less wounding than cruelty. One of these men, in reminiscing with me over his days at the hospital, spoke good-naturedly about his well-meaning but rather silent therapist. There were five full sessions per week instead of the customary three. Yet throughout the 9 months of hospital care, the therapist rarely spoke. He modeled himself, the patient guessed, after the Freudian analysts of the 1920s rather than after Freud himself, who was often quite chatty with his analysands (see Ruitenbeck, 1973). But the patient had his therapist's undivided attention for 225 minutes a week. For this he was immensely grateful. His father had not listened to him that much in all the 20 years of his growing up. This man's course was not steadily uphill after leaving PI, however: He became alcoholic and spent 9 difficult years before joining AA. After that, he formed a stable relationship with another man, achieved a high position in his profession, and regarded his life at follow-up as fulfilling and happy. He expressed gratitude to PI for saving his life. Narrowly speaking, we could perhaps take some credit for that, since he had been grossly self-destructive beforehand. With respect to his overall *recovery,* I believe that PI was not instrumental, but contributory. AA was the necessary-but-not-sufficient factor. For the rest, the patient's own self-discipline deserves the credit.

INTELLIGENCE

Those who administered our unit, as well as the therapists directly in charge of the patients, assumed that intelligence would correlate well with amenability to expressive psychotherapy and ultimately with prognosis. The first assumption is probably correct, though its validity cannot be proven in a retrospective study such as the present one. The assumption concerning outcome was not, in the light of long-term follow-up, borne out—except in the stratospheric ranges of IQ. Apropos of IQ, the remarks that follow should be understood as relating primarily to IQ itself, since that is what we were able to measure on psychological testing of three-quarters of the PI-500. "Intelligence" is a more global and more elusive concept than "IQ." Strictly speaking, we can only approach this question: Does IQ correlate with outcome? In the schizophrenic group no such correlation existed, apart from the ironical negative correlation between high IQ and suicide (see Chapter Four). The other groups of initially psychotic patients were too small to permit us to test this assumption. (I have more to say about the psychotic patients below.)

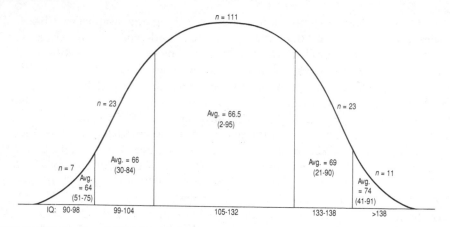

FIGURE 10.2. Traced PI-500 borderline patients who had not committed suicide: Average GAS scores ("Avg.") according to IQ compartment. (Ranges of GAS scores are given in parentheses.)

IQ Results for Borderline Patients

The large borderline group contained some 175 traced patients for whom IQ results were also available and who had not committed suicide. Figure 10.2 shows the distribution of average follow-up GAS scores in five segments of the gaussian IQ curve—that is, for those with IQs in the "average" range for the PI-500, and for the groups at one and at two standard deviations on either side. Since the mean IQ for the PI-500 was 118.2, the resulting compartments bear little resemblance to numbers representing the norms for the general population. The lowest IQs in the patient population (90–98) were the lower half of "average" in the general population. At the other extreme were patients with IQs in excess of 138 on the Wechsler Adult Intelligence Scale (WAIS).

Because the range of GAS scores within each compartment was broad, one may question the meaningfulness of the "average" scores for the five groups. The same result—namely, that outcome was similar in all groups *except* the group two standard deviations above the mean—emerges from inspection of Table 10.1, where the percentage of patients doing well (GAS scores > 60) versus not well (suicides included) is shown for each IQ compartment. Here again, only the group with IQs > 138 enjoyed better outcomes, on average, than the borderlines in the remaining four groups.

Because the PI-500 patients—like the patients of the Menninger study (Wallerstein, 1986), of McGlashan's series, or of Gunderson's Schizophrenia Psychotherapy Project at the McLean Hospital (Gunderson et al., 1984)—were skewed toward above-average IQs, the generalizability of the findings to the majority of borderlines is uncertain. Paris et al. (1987) noted outcome GAS scores in the same range (mid-60s) in their borderline patients at long-term follow-up; their series consisted predominantly of middle- to lower-class patients with IQs in the average range. If future follow-up studies of more representative borderline samples corroborate the observations of McGlashan and colleagues, Paris and colleagues, and my own group, our impressions about long-term outcome in borderlines may turn out to be reasonably accurate. Within the PI-500, 53 borderlines had IQs in the normal range (90–110); of these, 8 remain untraced, 1 committed suicide, and the remaining 44 had a mean outcome GAS score of 66 (range = 3–84). No fewer than 71% had GAS scores > 60.

Rather than doing "better," the high-IQ borderline patients differed from their average-IQ counterparts mostly in their chosen occupations. At follow-up, one of the average-IQ borderlines had PhD, a thriving career, a husband, and two children. Another became a highly successful decorator; a third shared with her husband the management of a restaurant; a fourth divided her time between teaching and raising her daughter. The outcome GAS score for each of these women was 84. Most of the average-IQ borderlines were in the business world or in occupations such as modeling, nursing, dancing, or ceramics. The borderlines with IQs one standard deviation beyond the group mean included two physicians, three social workers, a psychologist, a teacher, a laboratory manager, a financier, and an artist, but also a vagrant and an agoraphobic housebound for many years.

Only at two standard deviations from the mean did the PI-500 borderlines appear to have a real advantage. Almost all became professionals (two social workers, a psychologist, a lawyer, a systems analyst, a physician, a nurse, an accountant, and an engineer). All have done unusually well in other spheres of life also, except for two: one who committed suicide, and the gifted but self-defeating imposter (see Appendix A). For borderline patients, an IQ in the extremely high range may serve as a "natural advantage," along with talent and beauty; these may promote (even if they do not quite guarantee) a successful outcome. (See "Natural Advantages," below.)

Patients with high intelligence, unless they are hyperrational and concretistic (as some were in this series), usually work well with symbolism, are adept at unraveling their dreams, and in general accommodate well to the particularities of expressive therapy. As I examine the list of gifted borderlines one by one, I note that several had long and beneficial courses of expressive psychotherapy while at PI, and remember the hospital and their therapists

TABLE 10.1. Percentage of Borderline Patients with GAS Scores >60 or ≤60 in Five Compartments of IQ

	IQ range				
GAS scores	90–98 (*n* = 8)	99–104 (*n* = 23)	105–132 (*n* = 114)	132–138 (*n* = 25)	>138 (*n* = 12)
>60	62	69	66	68	83
≤60	38	31	34	32	17

fondly. But another felt that she was forced to stay far beyond the time during which she really needed residential care, and considered the hospitalization largely a negative experience. Judging from her outcome (GAS score = 91) and steady success from the day she eloped, she may well be correct. Still another had a disastrous experience at the hospital, but was able to marshal her ample resources in spite of it to make an outstanding recovery without further treatment.

These observations inspire me with a certain caution concerning not so much the efficacy of expressive therapy for borderlines (in properly selected cases it appears to work very well), but its essentiality. With hospitalized borderlines in particular, protection (e.g., during periods of high suicidality), role-modeling, problem-solving, and re-education seem paramount. Exploratory work for many of them is a kind of embellishment, strengthening the defenses and rounding out the treatment at a later phase, once the more supportive modalities have done their work. Extremely intelligent borderlines, like those with other natural advantages, get better for the most part—whether we fashion an ideal therapy for them or not. Many clinicians utilize an exploratory therapy with such patients, since this modality will often be congenial to both participants. This does not constitute proof that these patients could not have improved so markedly with any other approach.

IQ Results for the Psychotic Patients

The schizophrenic patients constitute the only other diagnostic subgroup large enough to permit statistical comparisons with the borderlines vis-à-vis IQ. Information on IQ was available for 64 of the 99 schizophrenics. Because so few had follow-up GAS scores in the good-to-recovered range, a more sensible cutoff score for the schizophrenic patients was 50. Even so, no significant differences emerged among the successive IQ deciles as to the proportion with better than marginal outcomes versus the proportion at or below this level. Of 10 schizophrenic patients with IQs > 130, for example, only one had a follow-up GAS score > 50. Similar ratios were discernible across the other deciles, with the possible exception of the 14 patients with IQs between 121 and 130; 4 of these 14 were clinically well. This difference was not significant. The only difference that did appear significant concerned the suicides. Of the 12 schizophrenic patients with IQs $\geq$ 130, 4 were suicides; by contrast, there were only 4 in the 52 with IQs < 130, $\chi^2 = 5.8$, $p < .05$.

This is admittedly a small sample on which to base an impression, but it may point to a heightened vulnerability on the part of particularly bright schizophrenics. They often do brilliantly in grade school or beyond, come from families of high achievers, and (inadvertently) foster parental expectations that they will continue to excel as they pass into adolescence and young adulthood.

It is during those latter phases, however, that their vulnerability manifests itself—leading in some cases to severe disappointment, humiliation, and suicide. This tragic sequence unfolded in the lives of all four of our schizophrenic suicides with "genius" IQs: the mathematician who shot himself the day his therapist changed service; the campus rebel (during the 1968 student revolution) who was never able to live up to his academic potential; the anhedonic and obsessional man whose sexual guilt took the form of a delusion that germs were crawling into his penis; and the mathematically gifted but tortured woman who complained on visiting day that her parents were "chunking" her—meaning that their comments were like so many unassimilable "chunks" of *their* egos dropping in, confusingly, amongst the disconnected elements of her own fragmentary identity.

Though the numbers are smaller still with the other diagnostic groups among the psychotics, the schizoaffectives seemed to escape this inverted relationship between high IQ and outcome. As with the borderlines, the schizoaffective patients with the highest IQs appeared to outperform their peers at follow-up. Of the eight with IQs ≥ 130, there was one suicide and one with marginal functioning; the rest had GAS scores of 50, 53, 62, 67, 70, and 77. Half, that is, were well (in contrast to the SA group as a whole, where 31% had follow-up GAS scores > scores 60).

JAIL

Though several other patients had close brushes with the law (their charges were dropped through the influence of their families), 18 of the PI-500 spent at least a night in jail for offenses ranging from drug possession to multiple murder. This figure represents 3% of the traced patients and is unexpectedly high, considering the socioeconomic background of the families. The males with borderline functioning were the most likely to commit an offense that led to incarceration: 8 of 100 traced (8%), especially if they met the criteria for BPD (6 of 52 traced, or 11.5%). Of the 18 untraced male borderlines, 6 had already been in trouble with the authorities—3 to an extent sufficient to have spawned a correspondence between the hospital and probation courts. At least 3 others, that is, were in jail at some point but are not counted in the 8% cited above, because I have been unable to contact either them or their relatives.

Most of these patients had lifelong histories of hyperactivity, extreme impulsivity, and defiance. This temperamental irritability was a more prominent factor than parental abuse: One of the males had been seduced by his alcoholic adoptive mother; the parents of another had screamed taunting remarks at the patient ever since he was born. The father of the imposter (see Appendix A) was similarly hypercritical. But in other instances the parents were calm persons faced with an irascible child, such as the adoptee who set fires and destroyed furniture at home after he was told that he had been adopted. The two female borderlines in this group—one jailed for burglary and drug possession, the other for shoplifting—came from incestuous and abusive homes. The shoplifter had additional run-ins with the authorities because of molesting neighborhood children, but was not sent to jail again.

Five of the seven patients in this series who killed someone spent varying periods of time in jail (two are still in prison at this writing and have been for many years). One died in jail from complications of neuroleptic medications.

The schizophrenic patients who had been in jail ($n = 4$) were impulsive, belligerent, and paranoid. Three had been imprisoned for murder; one was arrested for public exposure, although he had often tried to provoke fights in order to "prove himself." Their acts had a spur-of-the-moment quality, whereas some of the borderline patients were involved in illegal acts that required greater deliberation and planning (impersonation, check fraud). Arrests among the borderlines covered a wider range of infractions, whereas the schizophrenics were arrested less often, and then only for more serious charges.

As with most (and much larger) samples of ever-imprisoned persons (Wilson & Hernnstein, 1985), the ever-jailed group within the PI-500 was mostly young and mostly male. Table 10.2 outlines the relevant data.

One tends to think of a jailed population as composed in large part of sociopaths who, to the extent that they ordinarily take out their pent-up feelings on others, seldom kill themselves. As Table 10.2 makes clear, however, suicide is not the sole province of depression. The element of violence is central. Especially in the young, hopelessness without an admixture of violence leads more to tears and to inertia than to suicide. Hopelessness, even in those not habitually despondent, if admixed with a proneness to violence creates the chemistry of which many a suicide is composed. The incidence of suicide in the ever-jailed PI-500 patients was 37.5%, the same as noted in the other high-risk group—the female borderlines with BPD × MAD × alcoholism. Their stories were often ones of long-standing violence-proneness, triggered by transitory hopelessness (the sense of being "cornered," in some instances). The case of the borderline male who suddenly killed himself when warned he was likely to be rearrested (for arson) was typical of these. Only one of the borderline males had concomitant MAD; most of the seven who did not also had ASP. In this small series, none of the patients who had killed someone later killed himself, though one man tried (unsuccessfully) to kill his father and a few years later committed suicide. Another schizophrenic man, who does not appear in the table, had also made an attempt on his father's life and had later set fire to his house; the family did not press charges, however. At follow-up, the patient had been unemployed and reclusive for 20 years.

If one uses a GAS score of 60 as the cutoff point between the good-to-recovered group and those with fair outcomes or worse, Table 10.2 also makes clear that having been jailed, even overnight for something minor, was associated (in this white, middle-class sample) with a poor outcome in a remarkably high percentage (80%) of the cases. The only two who recovered

TABLE 10.2 Traced Patients Who Had Ever Been in Jail

Diagnostic group	Sex	Socio-economic category	Age on admission	Comorbidity, if any	Adoptee?	Killed someone?	Follow-up GAS score	Comments
Borderlines								
BPD	M	II	15	ASP	+	–	Suicide	Firesetting
	M	IV	13	–	–	+	5	Jailed for murder; hyperactive; extreme parental abuse
	M	III	26	ASP	–	–	41 [died]	Jailed for impersonation and other illegal activities; died in jail
	M	III	18	–	–	+	40	Jailed 1½ years for manslaughter; shot at in jail by an inmate and had to have colostomy
	M	I	16	–	+	–	Suicide	Briefly jailed for drug possession
	M	I	19	ASP	–	–	52	Stole cars; set fire to grandfather's house; vagrancy; male prostitution; alcoholism
	F	IV	16	MAD	–	–	80	Briefly jailed for burglary and drug possession; rehabilitated drug addict; incest victim
	F	III	36	MAD	–	–	Suicide	Check fraud; jailed briefly for shoplifting at 10; abuse victim; cruel to children
D	M	I	21	MAD	–	–	61	Jailed for car theft; later developed bipolar illness, treated with lithium
Other BPO	M	I	17	ASP	–	–	73	An AA-rehabilitated alcoholic
Psychotics								
SZ	M	III	19	–	–	–	Suicide	Arrested for sexual exposure in public; tried to provoke fights
	M	III	20	–	–	+	31	Paranoid, belligerent, killed someone in a bar; unable to adapt after prison; suicidal at times
	M	II	23	–	–	+	19	Jailed for murder; died in jail
	F	III	23	–	+	+	6	Jailed for murder
SA	M	III	22	–	–	–	Suicide	Jailed for auto theft (after argument with father)
	F	II	25	–	–	–	Suicide	Arrested for drug possession
MDP	M	III	27	–	–	–	58	Jailed briefly because of wandering in a psychotic state
	M	III	20	–	–	–	80	Jailed 3 days after arguing with father and stealing a car

(GAS scores of 70) were addicted patients who managed to overcome their drug habit.

NATURAL ADVANTAGES

A number of qualities confer unfair advantages on some people and unfair disadvantages on others. Some of these are predominantly innate attributes, such as beauty or brilliance (and their opposites). Talent perhaps also belongs in this category. Musical or artistic talent is often bolstered by perfect pitch or a gift for portraiture (mostly innate qualities), though discipline and prodigious amounts of work are indispensable ingredients. Other natural advantages are man-made and consist of social position (including positions of either power or aristocratic rank), fame, and wealth. It is possible to start out in life with all or most of these qualities and still end up in the scrap heap, if such heavy counterweights as parental brutality, high genetic risk for a psychosis, and the like are attached.

The reason I draw attention to this catalog of advantages relates to the observation all therapists make as they become seasoned: Some patients, though quite ill originally, succeed beyond our expectations and with only minimal efforts on our part; others fail despite "heroics." As a result, we must look beyond parochial controversies about the efficacy of this or that modality, this or that school of thought, if we are to account for these peculiarities. It is here, I feel, that the balance of the patients' pre-existing and seemingly extraneous balance of advantages verses disadvantages can explain some of the variance.

In the diminutive society of the PI-500, it was possible to categorize our patients according to the six aforementioned variables, and then to re-examine the outcome data by way of assessing what correlations there might be with the subsequent course. Leaving aside for the moment high intelligence, which is discussed in detail elsewhere (see "Intelligence," above), we see that some three dozen borderline patients showed at least one of the remaining natural advantages: social position, beauty, talent, or (in the parents' generation) fame or wealth. I have concentrated on the borderlines here, because this group showed the widest range of follow-up results and greatest chance of successful outcome. In the next largest group, the schizophrenics, the life course was so constricted by the illness itself that little effect of "natural advantages" was detectable.

The presence of these qualities in the borderline patients is outlined in Table 10.3. All the attributes vary on a continuum, but for purposes of simplicity the table is organized dichotomously. "High social position" usually refers to social class alone, since there is no hereditary aristocracy in our country. It is possible to enjoy enhanced social position in the absence of wealth or political power, if one is a descendant of the *Mayflower* settlers, the great-grandchild of a president, or the like; this was the case with several of the

TABLE 10.3. Traced Borderline Patients with at Least One Natural Advantage

Patient no.	High social position	Beauty 2 SD above mean[a]	Famous family	IQ 2 SD above mean[b]	Talent	Family wealth	Follow-up GAS score
1	+		+				Suicide
2	+					+	84
3	+						70
4		+		+			91
5	+		+			+	70
6	+		+			+	52
7	+		+				73
8					+	+	65
9		+					67
10	+						62
11	+					+	88
12	+					+	61
13		+					71
14	+						78
15		+					87
16						+	Suicide
17	+		+			+	64
18		+		+			70
19	+	+	+		+	+	Suicide
20	+		+				62
21	+	+	+			+	45
22						+	65
23	+						83
24	+	+	+		+	+	84
25						+	84
26			+			+	41
27	+		+			+	83
28		+					84
29		+					90
30					+		87
31					+		65
32					+		73
33					+		81
34						+	73
35	+					+	79
36					+		70
37	+		+			+	81
38					+		68
39	+						72

[a]This natural advantage is discussed in more detail in section on "Attractiveness" (see Chapter Eight).

[b]Those with *only* this natural advantage are discussed in section on "Intelligence," above.

borderline patients. The closest any of our patients came to actual "aristocracy" was a borderline adolescent whose self-indulgent mother had skipped out on the patient and his sister to marry a member of the European nobility.

"Beauty" was confined to females two standard deviations above the mean. The topic is discussed more fully elsewhere (see "Attractiveness," Chapter Eight). Likewise, only verbal IQs two standard deviations above the mean are indicated in the table, even though the "average" PI-500 patient was already well to the right of the general-population mean. The other measures were more subjective: For example, it was not possible to assign a dollar amount to the net worth of the "wealthy" families, since this information was almost never available.

Table 10.3 shows that half of the borderlines with *any* natural advantage were clinically recovered at follow-up (GAS scores > 70). The *average* outcome GAS score of nonsuicidal patients in four of the categories (high social position, beauty, talent, and family wealth) equaled or exceeded 70. Having a famous parent seemed, on average, to confer no particular advantage; here the mean GAS score was the same as for the entire group of traced borderlines.

Though the deviations from the mean for the borderline group as a whole were small, the average scores for those with talent or beauty marginally exceeded those for social position and family wealth. This is not out of line with expectations, however, since those with talent and beauty generally make their own way in life and carry their advantages with them. Those who come from families of position and wealth can easily fail if they have neither talent nor discipline.

Only two borderlines had five "advantages." One, who was deprived but not abused by her parents, did very well after many difficult years; at follow-up she was managing a large business she started herself, based on her artistic talent. The other, a multiple incest victim, committed suicide.

It would appear that talent can eventually offset a great deal of "borderline" psychopathology and can act as a strong predictor of favorable outcome. The woman just mentioned committed suicide, but the other eight with recognizable talent were all clinically well at follow-up (GAS scores > 60). They included a ceramist, two interior designers, and four artists. One of the artists, languishing in a municipal hospital before his transfer to our unit many years ago, had acquired an international reputation by the time of follow-up. The other talented borderline was, as an adolescent on our unit, an electronics "whiz." He could fashion all manner of ingenious devices from blueprints he designed himself, and could repair broken-down equipment of any sort.

In the entire group with at least one natural advantage, five borderlines out of six were well at follow-up. Their functioning was thus in the same range as those with IQs > 138 (two standard deviations above the mean) or the alcoholics who recovered via enrollment in AA.

The effects of family wealth were complex and not immediately evident from outcome scores alone. Some wealthy families were unstinting in their support of their emotionally ill children and made sure they were treated by good therapists at excellent facilities for as long as was necessary. The patients from these families got the best education and job preparation as they became more self-sufficient; they then had entrée into the best graduate schools, corporations, and so on before finally detaching themselves financially from their parents. But other wealthy families, made up of idle, narcissistic, and neglectful parents, were breeding grounds of trouble (see "Incest," Chapter Seven, and "Episodic Dyscontrol," Appendix A).

Family wealth was particularly helpful in the lives of several schizophrenic patients. There were two young men, for example, who improved enough at PI to leave the hospital, but were still scarcely capable of productive work. It is not clear what would have become of them if they had had to support themselves through their own efforts. At follow-up, both were living agreeable lives, playing their musical instruments, entertaining their small circle of friends, and maintaining themselves in their apartments—thanks to generous trust funds set up in their behalf by their parents. Two of the borderlines (both males) were also living on trust funds at follow-up, after first having tried (admittedly, without much enthusiasm) to get by without their parents' help. Where wealth did not serve as a catalyst to autonomy and genuine success, it at least provided a cushion.

POSTTRAUMATIC STRESS DISORDER

There are laws for everything except the harm families do.
—Grafton (1987, p. 50)

Posttraumatic stress disorder (PTSD) has begun to receive widespread attention. The definition of the disorder in DSM-III emphasizes the magnitude of the stress ("an event that is outside the range of usual human experience") more than host factors, such as the previous history and general resilience of the victim or the modifying influences of family and community. Breslau and Davis (1987) consider the relative omission of the latter factors as a serious flaw in the official definition, at the same time acknowledging that "If stressors are defined in terms of their subjective meaning, then their measurement is also inextricably entangled with the specific life experiences and circumstances of the individual" (p. 260). These authors are unimpressed with claims that certain stressors may be causally associated with a distinctive psychiatric syndrome, asserting (p. 262) that the literature provides no corroboratory evidence. The latter tends to focus on war experiences, both of combatants (e.g., shell-shock victims) and of civilians (e.g., Holocaust victims).

Despite the objections Breslau and Davis raise, PTSD appears to be a useful diagnostic entity, or at the very least a useful nosological concept. Kolb's (1987) approach seems particularly useful, lending itself to a definition applicable to

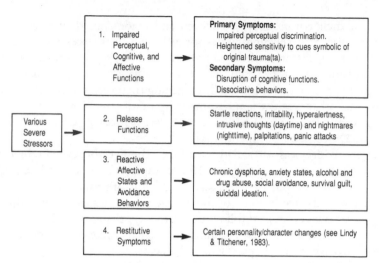

FIGURE 10.3. Kolb's model of PTSD. Adapted from Kolb, L. C. (1987) A neuropsychological hypothesis explaining post-traumatic stress disorders. *Am. J. Psychiatry 144*: 989–995. Adapted by permission.

many traumatic experiences in everyday life, not just in wartime. Drawing upon the experimental literature on animals, as well as upon his own clinical work with soldiers subjected to severe stress, Kolb offers a theoretical model that is portrayed schematically in Figure 10.3.

The key elements in PTSD, if we can accept the validity of this syndrome, are the lastingly altered excitation states in certain central nervous system (CNS) pathways (including those subserving the traumatic memories) and the hyperarousal or exaggerated irritability that stems from these "heated-up" excitation patterns (Stone, 1988b). The syndrome is not limited to combat victims or plane crash survivors. The patients within the PI-500 who best exemplified this condition had not experienced impersonal traumata of this sort, but rather the highly personal, intrafamilial traumata of incest or parental physical brutality—where the offending parties had added betrayal (of the trust children invest in their caretakers) to the shock and hurt of the abuse itself. In the worst cases, this betrayal, by undermining trust in future intimate relationships, created situations more traumatic (i.e., with more lasting or shattering effects) than rape by a stranger. The cases described by Goodwin, Cheeves, and Connell (1988) of extreme incestuous abuse also serve as examples.

I could not make a precise estimate of the population within the PI-500 to whom either the narrow definition of PTSD in DSM or the broader definition adumbrated in Kolb's (1987) article might apply. Deficiencies in the old records account for this: The therapists of those years did not make systematic inquiries about histories of sexual abuse, nor did they ask about "flashback" phenomena, state-dependent traumatic memories, or other long-term sequelae of childhood abuse. Future follow-up studies, we may hope, will include the kind of data that will permit more accurate identification of PTSD cases and more methodical appraisal of their natural history.

Brutality and sexual abuse both have the power to set PTSD in motion. The more severe the stress, the fewer the victims who can (presumably) resist development of the syndrome. The cases where this sequence was most visible in the PI-500 happened to be those of incest victims. In other series, the adverse conditioning effects of physical brutality or of war traumata are equally apparent (cf. Kardiner & Spiegel, 1947). Combined physical and sexual abuse are common antecedents in patients with multiple personality—so much so that one might understand the latter as a special form of PTSD (see Bliss, 1986, and Kluft, 1985; see also Appendix A). A child who witnesses one parent killing the other may also be at heightened risk for PTSD (Malmquist, 1986). Overwhelming traumata of these types apparently have a "kindling" effect on the CNS, setting in motion the symptoms (flashbacks, nightmares, startle reactions, etc.) that we subsequently diagnose as PTSD (Putnam, 1986; Ross et al., 1989).

One of the incest victims in the present series exhibited state-dependent memory of her father's attempts at anal sexual contact when she was 5 or 6. Hospitalized on several occasions for multiple suicide attempts during her 20s, she mentioned having no recall of the incestuous experiences—except when her fiancé's penis would brush against her buttocks during sex. When this happened, she would suddenly recall the scenes with her father. Both panic and fury accompanied these flashbacks; she would run out into the street naked, as if to save herself. These episodes often ended with a suicide attempt.

Another woman, also in her 20s, showed hypervigilance while on the unit, along with a marked startle response and irascibility to the point of "psychotic" rage outbursts. Her incest history did not come to light for many months (her father threatened to kill her if she related what had happened). Initially she presented with a catetenoid state (see Kolb, 1987, p. 989), misdiagnosed (in the light of subsequent events) as "schizophrenia" or "depression."

A third woman, described in the section on "Multiple Personality" (see Appendix A), decompensated after sexual advances by her therapist.

The PI-500 case *closest* to PTSD as delineated in DSM was that of a young manic–depressive woman hospitalized with recurrent nightmares, fears of death, and suicide gestures, following the traumatic death of a close friend (see also Chapter Fifteen).

A man with episodic dyscontrol (see Appendix A) may represent an instance of combined constitutional and environmental liability. Sexually molested by persons outside the immediate family, he had shown signs of mild neurological damage in his earliest years. Once traumatized, he behaved with the outbursts of rage and irritability Kolb (1987, p. 994) mentions as expressions of the excessive sympathetic nervous system arousal characteristic of PTSD. Any gestures by males that this patient could construe as a threat, especially as a homosexual "pass," led immediately to a startle reaction and to wildly aggressive actions in "self-defense."

The topic of PTSD is of special relevance to BPD. Among the 206 PI-500 patients with BPD, 51 (24.8%) were victims of incest (28 females and 6 males), parental brutality, or both. This figure does not include the man with episodic dyscontrol or several others whose abuse (molestation, rape, etc.) stemmed from experiences outside the family. In many of these patients, some of the symptoms (inordinate anger, emotional lability, etc.) that identified them as examples of BPD appeared to originate in the repetitive traumatic experiences of childhood and adolescence. The "incest syndrome" described by Molnar and Cameron (1975) and later by Alter-Reid, Gibbs, Lachenmeyer, Sigal, and Massoth (1986) contains many of the elements subsumed under the heading of PTSD. Not all manifested the prototypical picture of PTSD as depicted in DSM, but if one takes a broader view of this syndrome and includes less complete or less dramatic instances, then the overlap between BPD and PTSD would occupy an even greater territory. And, as I have mentioned elsewhere, the PI-500 constitutes one of the less traumatized series of hospitalized patients, compared with others around the country.

VIOLENCE TOWARD FAMILY

Threats of harming self or others are among the most common precipitants of psychiatric hospitalization, voluntary or otherwise.

Some of the violence done *to* the PI-500 patients by their parents has been recounted, and its effects have been analyzed, in the section on "Parental Brutality" (see Chapter Seven). Not all our patients took this abusiveness lying down. There were many more, however, who lashed out physically against family members who had done little or nothing to provoke attack. Perhaps the more usual scenario had transpired: A parent or sibling had been verbally abusive, teasing, or whatever, and the retaliation was physical.

The incidence of violence toward family across all the major diagnostic groups was 10.2% (55 of 537). Table 10.4 shows the breakdown according to group. Figures varied from 0 in the dysthymic group to 22.9% in the other males who met Kernberg criteria for borderline personality organization (BPO). Many of the latter were comorbid for ASP. The incidence was also high in the schizophreniform males (18.5%). Intergroup differences were not significant, however, with the exception of a trend toward greater violence in the BPD than in the dysthymic males, $\chi^2 = 3.64$, $df = 1$, $p \cong .06$. In the whole series, males were more likely to commit acts of intrafamilial violence than were the females, $\chi^2 = 10.2$, $p < .01$. Males between the ages of 18 and 30 are more likely to

TABLE 10.4. Patients Who Were Violent toward Family Members

Patient no.	Sex	Age	ASP?	Victim[a]	Follow-up GAS score	Patient no.	Sex	Age	ASP?	Victim[a]	Follow-up GAS score
BPD patients						SZ patients					
1	F	16		M, F	77	1	F	19		B	81
2	M	16	+	S	Suicide	2	M	26		F	Suicide
3	F	18		M	75	3	M	19		M, F, B	54
4	M	16		M	2	4	M	35		F	39
5	M	21		M	?	5	F	21		S	Suicide
6	F	14		F, B	73	6	M	29	+	M	19
7	F	17		M	69	7	M	24		F	58
8	M	13	+	F	5	8	M	28	+	M	6
9	F	21		M	?	9	M	18		M	32
10	F	18		M	80	10	M	18		M	20
11	M	14		M	56	11	M	15		M, F	24
12	M	16		F, B	72	12	M	16	+	M, B	45
13	F	19		M	68						
14	F	14		M	68	SA patients					
15	M	20		M	79						
16	M	14		M	50	1	M	25		S	Suicide
17	F	14		M	75	2	M	26		M	46
18	F	17		S	63	3	F	18	+	M	5
19	F	20		M, B	62	4	F	16		M	Suicide
20	M	17	+	M, F	Suicide						
21	F	14		B	80	MDP patients					
Other BPO patients						1	F	25		M	Suicide
						2	M	18		M	47
						3	M	20		GM	27
1	F	22		F	67	4	M	23	+	M	6
2	M	13		M, F	?						
3	M	5	+	A	72	SF patients					
4	M	15	+	M	?						
5	M	14	+	M	?	1	M	20	+	M, U	?
6	M	16	+	M	?	2	M	29	+	W	36
7	M	15	+	M	73	3	M	18		M	50
8	M	17		B	70	4	M	17		M, F	47
9	M	14	+	M	?	5	M	23		M, F	64

[a]Victims: F, father; M, mother; B, brother; S, sister; GM, grandmother; U, uncle; W, wife; A, aunt.

behave violently than at later ages (Wilson & Herrnstein, 1985). In the PI-500, the accent was definitely on youth: 29 of the 30 violent borderlines were, on admission, younger than the series mean age of 22 (see Table 10.4).

The usual victims of this assaultiveness were mothers (cf. Maqueda, 1988)—partly because more of a child's life is spent interacting with the mother than with the father; partly because many of the fathers had died, divorced, or otherwise abandoned their families; and partly because mothers, being smaller, are safer targets. Two families had to obtain restraining orders preventing their children from returning home (a schizoaffective daughter and a manic–depressive son). Some of the assaulted mothers had been truly provocative, including the one killed by her son (see "Gradations of Antisociality," Chapter Six).

Some patients had been violent toward more than one family member. All told, a mother had been the object of the assaultive behavior in 38 instances; a father in 13; a brother in 8; a sister in 4; and a wife, uncle, aunt, or grandmother in 1 instance each.

The only patient who actually attacked his therapist (a borderline male threatened to, but did not follow through) was a schizophrenic man who had also assaulted various members of his family. He had a particularly dismal life course: He was a "missing person" (see Appendix B) for several years, which he spent living as a street vagrant and "homeless person." Of two other schizophrenics (both male) who tried to kill their mothers, one has been hospitalized ever since; the other was killed while committing a crime (see Appendix B).

Outcome in the BPD group was essentially the same as for BPD patients in general (median GAS score = 68). Two of the males committed murder; another (who eventually committed suicide) was an arsonist. The rest largely overcame their aggressive tendencies. In some instances, their aggressive acts were limited to a period of time when they lived with abusive relatives. One girl, abandoned by her mother, was raised along with her brother by a distant—and physically abusive—relative. The patient assaulted her brother on a few occasions while living in this arrangement, but had been mild-mannered and tender toward this brother and toward her own children over the 21 years after she left the unit.

The "other BPO" group contained five untraced males, four with ASP comorbidity. The latter all came from chaotic homes. The fathers had abandoned the family in three cases; in the fourth, the mother was alcoholic and herself violent.

Among the psychotic patients, (all but one of whom I was able to trace), assaultiveness toward family was often an epiphenomenon of their intrinsic illness, whereas the borderlines' violent behavior was often a counterattack directed against parental cruelty. The psychotic patients seldom came from broken, much less abusive, homes; instead, they lashed out under the influence of delusional ideas about the "malevolence" of actually unexceptionable parents. Often one could discern an underlying dynamic involving a patient's irrational attempt to stake out an identity separate from that of the parent by killing the parent. As mentioned elsewhere, two of the mothers sought restraining orders in hopes of keeping their violent children off their premises. A schizophrenic man nearly strangled his mother to death; another also tried to kill his mother. One of the schizoaffective men assaulted both parents with a knife; another repeatedly struck and sexually molested his sister. These attacks were unprovoked. The assaultive schizophrenic men were all markedly paranoid.

Outcome in the 15 traced BPD patients without ASP comorbidity was mostly in the good-to-recovered range. The three who failed to reach this level were a man from a violent home, who eventually killed a parent; a hyperkinetic adolescent, who was still leading a marginal existence 25 years later; and a man, brutalized by his father, who in turn assaulted his mother. This last patient worked only sporadically at menial jobs over the 25 years after he left the hospital, and had only meager social contacts. At the other end of the spectrum was a patient who as an adolescent had struck her mother, but who at follow-up had gone on to marry, complete an advanced degree in one of the helping professions, and administer a facility for disturbed adolescents. Her own emotionality had been well modulated for the 20 years following her release. Her GAS score was 80.

Cases in which parental violence preceded the patient's violence toward the offending parent(s) or toward other family members encourage one to make the equation "violence breeds violence" (see Oliver, 1988). In the general population, where studies on a very large scale are possible, this equation is probably valid (Gelles & Straus, 1988). But the violence is not always visited upon the parents; many abused children somehow refrain from committing acts of violence against either family members or outsiders. Only 6 of the 21 BPD patients with a history of assaultiveness toward family had been the victims of parental abusiveness. Twenty-three borderlines who were victims of parental brutality were not violent toward anyone; an additional two were abusive toward children.

With regard to the present study, there is strong evidence that parental brutality had, on average, a deleterious impact upon the life course of the abused children. There is lesser evidence that this necessarily induced retaliatory violence against the offending parent(s) or that the life course of borderline patients who behaved assaultively toward a parent was poorer than the group average, unless the home environment was particularly chaotic or violent. In the latter situation, the factor determining poor outcome would appear to be the chronically destructive environment itself and not the mere fact that on occasion the child had struck a parent or a sibling.

CHAPTER ELEVEN

Outcomes for the Borderline Patients: Correlations and Case Vignettes

WHAT BECOMES OF BORDERLINE PATIENTS AS THEY GET OLDER?

To the practitioner treating borderline patients in the here-and-now, "border-line" is a clinical syndrome with reasonably firm boundaries (despite the inherent vagueness of the word); being borderline, that is, appears as a separate thing. To the natural historian of mental disorders, "borderline" takes on a different aspect. The *syndrome,* or even the functional *level* as defined in the language of object relations and structural theory, is seen as a way station along a path of development beginning with various mood and conduct disorders in children, and ending up in a variety of conditions—occasionally more serious, but often less serious, than the original "borderline" condition. Sometimes the borderline functional level remains detectable into middle life. But often enough it becomes attenuated into a neurotic-level disorder, especially after lengthy treatment. In place of DSM-defined borderline personality disorder (BPD), one finds any one of a dozen other "personality disorders." The latter are not evenly distributed over the spectrum of *true* personality disorders (i.e., those correctly labeled via constellations of personality *traits*). BPD is not an ideally defined personality disorder, since its diagnosis does not depend entirely upon personality traits, but also relies upon symptoms, aberrant thought patterns, and defenses (e.g., identity disturbance and suicide gestures are not "traits"). In middle life, however, borderline conditions may melt into "depressive–masochistic personality," "narcissistic personality," or "cyclo-thymic temperament," whereas during the third decade of life the diagnosis might have read "BPD (or borderline personality organization [BPO]) with depressive–masochistic/narcissistic/cyclothymic features."

There is a tendency, as noted earlier (see Chapter Five), for patients with BPD × major affective disorder (MAD) to remain borderline by DSM criteria into later adult life and to show with increasing definition the stigmata of manic–depressive psychosis (MDP). The latter may take on the coloration of bipolar or bipolar II illness, or else may take the path of unipolar, recurrent depression.

Patients who have been severely victimized as children but who do not show evidence of constitutional vulnerability to MDP would be much less likely to appear, years later, on the MDP track. Theoretically, they should not be at risk for MDP at all. They may remain as (DSM-defined) borderlines, leading tempestuous, impulse-ridden lives (mellowing somewhat with age as most people do); otherwise, they may develop (1) chronic alcoholism or other substance abuse, or (2) personality disorders of one sort or another. Identity disturbance usually grows less prominent with advancing age. One may be left with a patient who no longer "acts out" conflicts, but who is merely placid, form-conscious, and devoid of genuine interest. Many borderlines, nevertheless, truly conquer their adolescent wildness, become less dependent upon strong sensation, and the like; they grow with the years into highly productive persons with emotionally rich and rewarding lives.

Clinical recovery was common among the PI-500 borderlines; to emerge in one's 30s or 40s as either "good" (Global Assessment Scale [GAS] score of 61–70) or "recovered" (GAS score > 70) was the rule rather than the exception. But even here, it must be noted that some former borderlines who had a GAS score of 80 at follow-up were leading somewhat constricted lives, though seamless and symptom-free; by contrast, several with lower scores complained of periodic mood swings, bouts of gloom, premenstrual irritability, and the like, yet were living unusually productive lives. Perhaps Mozart would have had a lower GAS score than Salieri!

Nature and nurture influences, as they crystallize into this or that form during childhood, rearrange themselves into borderline conditions in early adult life and finally congeal into a condition even a biometrician would describe as "well defined," as depicted in Figure 11.1. The severity of the final constellation may be less than, the same as, or greater than the severity of the form observed during the chrysalis stage. Proper therapy, I believe, conduces toward a lessening of severity and toward the disappearance (into neurotic-level organization) of borderline structure. But, as several PI-500 case histories exemplify, a few borderlines get worse despite our best efforts; others get much better with no more than a passing nod from the therapeutic community.

CORRELATIONS BETWEEN VARIOUS FACTORS AND OUTCOME FOR ALL BORDERLINES

An important task in follow-up work is the detection of factors that correlate with outcomes distinctly better or worse than the average fate of the group in

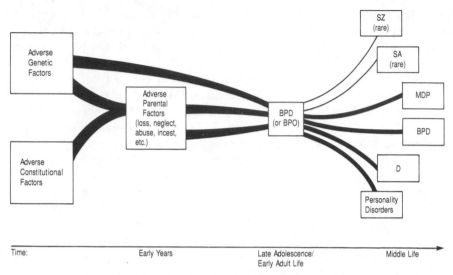

FIGURE 11.1.   Genesis and evolution of borderline disorders.

question. The greater the deviation from the average, the more "predictive" the factor in question. Ultimately, we would aim at the assignment of more precise *weights* in accordance with the relative predictive powers of each factor. Ordinarily, any given patient is an amalgam of many factors; some of these factors constitute assets and others liabilities with respect to life course and outcome at any fixed age. It is this immense array of interacting factors that defeats the clinician's attempts to predict "scientifically." The educated guess must take the place of accurate foreknowledge. Some crushingly negative factors can, I believe, outweigh any and all positive qualities. Borderline patients whose psychopathology is the outgrowth of unrelenting parental rejection, physical and sexual abuse, *and* malice—however appealing they may be outwardly, and however evocative of our sympathy—are usually, from a rehabilitative stand-point, damaged beyond repair. Others have such innate and acquired strengths as to permit them near-total recuperation, like cats who have lost only eight of their nine lives.

With most factors, examined singly, we see a spread of outcomes 10 to 25 years later. This spread may cover the whole range from suicide to recovery. But there will be an *average* result for each, and these averages may diverge rather widely. This already helps us distinguish the more important factors—that is, those associated with average outcomes well outside the grand average for all BPD patients—from the less important ones. In the PI-500, 63% of BPD patients had GAS scores > 60 at follow-up. Table 11.1 shows some two dozen combinations of associated factors as they relate to this grand average.

TABLE 11.1. Various Factors in Borderlines: Correlations with Outcome

Factor	*n* Traced	Follow-up GAS Scores > 60		
		n	%	
Borderline × alcoholism × AA	10	10	100.0	More than $1\frac{1}{2}$ GAS deciles above average
Borderline × artistic talent	9	8	88.9	
BPD × obsessive–compulsive personality	17	15	88.2	
Borderline × attractiveness (1 *SD* above group mean)	25	22	88.0	
Borderline × IQ (2 *SD* above group mean)	18	15	83.3	
BPD female; no MAD	37	28	75.7	
D borderlines	34	25	73.5	
Borderline × male homosexuality	13	9	69.2	
BPD × anorexia nervosa/bulimia nervosa	22	15	68.2	
BPD × MAD female	100	66	66.0	
All BPD	185	118	63.8	
Borderline females who eloped	33	21	63.6	
BPD × MAD male	27	17	63.0	
Borderline female × incest	35	22	62.9	
BPD → MDP	26	15	57.7	
BPD × alcoholism	35	19	54.3	
BPD female × incest	28	15	53.6	
Borderline × male/female homosexuality/bisexuality	23	12	52.2	
Borderline × parental brutality	30	15	50.0	
BPD female × incest with father/stepfather	22	10	45.5	More than $1\frac{1}{2}$ GAS deciles below average
Borderline × STP	14	6	42.8	
BPD × parental brutality	22	9	40.9	
BPD with all eight DSM items	15	6	40.0	
Borderline × firesetting	8	3	37.5	
BPD male; no MAD	24	9	37.5	
Borderline males who eloped	9	2	22.2	
BPD × ever raped	7	1	14.3	
BPD × ever jailed	8	1	12.5	
(Schizophrenia)	95	8	8.4	
BPD × ASP	13	1	7.4	

Although many acknowledge that scores over a decile higher or lower are significantly different from a given average, some may wish to apply a more rigorous test of statistical significance, asking for a minimum difference of a decile and a half. The size of the subgroup figures in the equation: The smaller the group, the more deviant it must be from the average before one can claim significance.

From the standpoint of chi-square comparison, significant differences only

TABLE 11.2.   Outcomes of Patients with BPD Exhibiting All Eight DSM Items

Sex	Concomitant MAD?	Alcohol abuse?	Follow-up GAS score	Comments
M	–	+	Suicide	ASP; committed arson
F	+	–	Suicide	Suicide occurred on the unit
F	+	–	68	
F	+	–	35	
F	+	–	37	Multiple subsequent admissions
F	+	Mild	69	Became unipolar
F	+	Mild	62	
F	+	–	53	Became SA
F	+	–	68	Drug abuse in adolescence
F	+	+	Suicide	Chaotic; child molestation
F	+	–	70	Parental physical abuse
F	+	+	88	Incest victim
F	+	+	Suicide	Incest victim
F	+	+	Suicide	Incest victim
F	–	–	Suicide	Both parents alcoholic

Note. Resumé of outcomes: recovered, 1 (7%); good, 5 (33%); fair, 1 (7%); incapacitated, none; suicide, 6 (40%).

emerged for factors beyond the range of a decile and a half (failing only in the case of the small group with artistic talent). Differences were most marked with the lowermost factors (e.g., BPD with all eight DSM items, $p < .05$, but BPD × antisocial personality [ASP], $p < .001$). Partly this is a reflection of there having been more room at the bottom, given a grand average of about 64% doing well at follow-up. Certain factors, analyzed in another manner, yielded more striking differences. The borderlines with artistic talent, for example, not only had GAS scores > 60; they were nearly all recovered (GAS scores > 70). The patients who had BPD with all eight DSM items did even worse than Table 11.1 suggests. As Table 11.2 shows, 40% of these patients were suicides.

The factor "ever in jail" was highly associated with poor outcome. In most instances this factor was an index of the even worse factor of ASP, though some of the ever-jailed patients were more reckless than antisocial, strictly speaking.

If we use the 10 most negative factors from Table 11.1 as a first catalog of poor prognostic indicators, we can isolate 85 traced BPD patients who showed at least one such factor. We may designate these factors for brevity as follows: jail, rape, ASP, eloped male, father–daughter incest, brutality, eight-item BPD, schizotypal personality (STP), male without MAD, and firesetting. Only 37 of these patients were well at follow-up, in contrast to 80 of the 100 patients *not* exhibiting any of these qualities, $\chi^2 = 26.3$, $p < .0001$. Only seven patients had three or more negative factors. Though six did poorly, this difference was not statistically significant.

The unequivocally positive factors, as noted in Table 11.1, may be designated for brevity as follows: Alcoholics Anonymous (AA), artistic talent, obsessive–compulsive personality, high attractiveness, and exceptionally high IQ. The BPD patients who had one or more of the especially positive factors made up a smaller group of 53, the great majority of whom (48) were well at follow-up, $\chi^2 = 24.2$, $p < .001$. The patients lacking one of these qualities were more evenly distributed as to outcome (59 were doing well, 56 doing poorly).

There were 11 "counterintuitive" cases, in which a positive factor failed to correlate with good outcome. Six of these patients also had one or more of the strongly negative factors (father–daughter incest in three, ASP in one). Another was chaotically impulsive. One of the incest victims also had severe bipolar II affective illness. Five were not burdened by such factors, yet still did poorly (one had a sadistic personality and later committed suicide; one abused marijuana for years; one developed severe unipolar illness and committed suicide; one had an extremely seductive father, though there was no incest). I have described in more detail a number of the "counterintuitive" cases in the chapter devoted to this topic (see Chapter Fifteen).

Equally of interest were the 11 BPD patients with both positive *and* negative factors who eventually did well. Six had an incest history, though of a kind less severe than experienced by the poor-outcome group.

Some factors, such as chaotic impulsivity, are difficult to qualify. In Chapter Five, I have noted that only 1 of 19 borderlines with this attribute is now well: a borderline woman with both alcoholism and attractiveness, who joined AA and recovered.

Figure 11.2 summarizes the results in the entire traced BPD group. Here, for reasons of homogeneity and clarity, I have omitted the dysthymic (D) and other BPO borderlines, though Table 11.1 refers to some of the latter patients (e.g., many of the borderlines with artistic talent did not have BPD and thus do not appear in Figure 11.2).

As Figure 11.2 demonstrates, BPD patients with one or more positive factors from Table 11.1 and none of the negative factors were 10 times as likely to have a good outcome as a poor outcome. The 47 patients not displaying either set of factors showed no special tendencies in either direction when compared with the BPD group as a whole.

The detection of prognostic factors and the assessment of their relative weights contribute to the determination of etiology. Within the borderline domain, many variables have the quality of aggravating factors. Marijuana abuse and early loss, for example, appear to intensify the psychopathological picture— not only in borderline patients, but in all diagnostic groups. A few factors seem more specific for the clinical picture of BPD. Transgenerational (especially

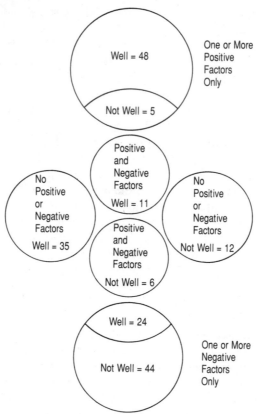

FIGURE 11.2. Current status of traced BPD patients in relation to certain positive and negative factors.

parent–child) incest and extreme parental abusiveness (either physical or verbal), though they would aggravate any psychiatric condition, may be more specific for BPD. In the PI-500 both phenomena were less common in the other disorders, with the exception of schizoaffective psychosis (SA), some examples of which could be viewed as instances of BPD with prolonged psychoticism in response to severe abuse. Some view separation–individuation problems as of etiological significance in borderline conditions (Masterson, 1981). This may be true in certain patients with BPO, especially ambulatory patients. In the hospitalized borderlines, especially in those with BPD, constitutional and traumatic factors (abuse, catastrophic loss, etc.) seemed more important. Future follow-up studies should clarify these issues further. As matters stand, we are already in a better position to create more sophisticated models of prognosis and of pathway analysis (cf. Harris, Brown, & Bifulco, 1987) than we were before the current wave of follow-up studies.

MULTIVARIATE ANALYSIS OF THE DATA ON BORDERLINE PERSONALITY DISORDER PATIENTS

With the help of Dr. Hans Stassen of the Psychiatric University Hospital (Bürghölzli), Zürich, I have begun to examine the data on the BPD patients via multivariate analysis. Our hope has been to establish a rank order of most to least significant factors bearing on outcome, and also to quantify the extent to which the whole set of identifiable factors accounts for the total variance.

Thus far, we have assessed the influence of 14 factors. These are gender; age at index hospitalization; MAD comorbidity; incest history; alcoholism; suicide gestures; suicide attempts; use of marijuana, LSD, amphetamines, cocaine, heroin, or hypnotics (each as a separate factor); and parental brutality. If we use a forward selection procedure for the dependent variable "GAS score at follow-up," a sequence of variables emerges in the order of their contribution to the variance. The bottom section of Table 11.3 the sequence relevant to the BPD group as a whole. The partial impact on the variance is greatest in the case of parental brutality, which accounts for nearly 7%.

The factors employed account altogether for 11.65% of the variance. The age factor refers to the tendency for patients who were older when admitted to have a better outcome than the adolescents. As noted in the top two sections of the table, this age effect is not demonstrable among the females, but is quite apparent among the males. This in turn would seem to reflect the disproportionate percentage of ASP comorbidity (with the associated generally poor outcome) in the young male subgroup. Drug abuse accounts for half the identified variance in the females (7.53%), but only a sixth in the males. MAD comorbidity is a recognizable, though modest, factor only in the males. This is consistent with the observation (about the global results) that the BPD × MAD males were a little less likely to have good outcomes than the BPD × MAD females, but considerably less likely, compared with the "pure"-BPD females (see Chapter Five). Alcohol abuse does not account for enough of the variance to be singled out in the multivariate analysis, possibly because the recoveries of some alcoholics (in AA) counterbalanced the marginal outcomes of others.

In Dr. Stassen's experience, the variable aggregate examined in multivariate analysis of long-term follow-up studies can seldom account for more than a sixth of the variance. The addition of more, and necessarily more subtle, variables to the analysis is not likely to add appreciably to the overall percentage of variance for which one can account. We can view this, via its inverse, as a measure of the great unpredictability of long-term outcome in samples of borderline patients. This is a quite different exercise in statistical analysis than we encounter in the task of predicting the fate of certain individual cases. As we have seen earlier in this chapter, some borderline patients who happened to harbor many of the known "worst" factors had outcomes that were all too predictable. Similarly,

TABLE 11.3. Multivariate Analysis of Factors Affecting Outcome in Patients with BPD (Forward Selection Procedure for Dependent Variable)

Variable	Partial impact on variance (%)	Cumulative impact (%) (1; 1 + 2; 1 + 2 + 3; . . .)
Female patients		
1. Parental brutality	6.44	6.44
2. Amphetamines	1.47	7.91
3. Other substances	3.23	11.13
4. Cocaine	0.79	11.93
5. Heroin	1.62	13.55
6. Incest	0.62	14.17
7. Marijuana	0.42	14.59
8. Suicide attempt(s)	0.49	15.08
Male patients		
1. Parental brutality	15.41	15.41
2. Age[a]	7.53	22.94
3. Heroin	5.25	28.19
4. Suicide attempt(s)	3.67	31.85
5. Incest	2.84	34.70
6. Suicide gesture(s)	3.31	38.01
7. Subsidiary diagnosis	1.97	39.98
8. Marijuana	1.30	41.28
9. LSD/mescaline	0.85	42.13
Combined BPD patients		
1. Parental brutality	6.76	6.76
2. Age[a]	1.54	8.30
3. Suicide gesture(s)	0.98	9.28
4. Marijuana	0.94	10.22
5. Other substances	0.40	10.62
6. Cocaine	0.53	11.15
7. Subsidiary diagnosis	0.50	11.65

[a]The tendency of patients who were older when admitted to have higher follow-up GAS scores.

those with a ''best'' factor and no worst factor had, at least in this series, a 90% chance of a good outcome.

GENERAL COMMENTS

Contained within any discussion of predictability in psychiatry is an ironical situation, akin to what one might call the ''pollster's paradox.'' People, unlike

tossed coins, pay attention to the results of a poll and often behave contradic-
torily so as to prove the poll wrong (e.g., a report that a Democratic candidate
is a "shoo-in" may inspire every Republican to go to the voting booth). My
assertion that 4 out of 10 hospitalized "eight-item" BPD patients, in their early
20s or younger, will commit suicide within 5 years may inspire the current
generation of therapists to exercise such caution with these patients that the next
follow-up study will show a much lower figure. For the patients' sake, I hope
the study has precisely that effect. If so, future investigators will ascribe my
"error" to a "skewed sample" or whatever.

Meantime, the strongest factor I have been able to identify is that of
parental brutality. This finding holds up irrespective of gender; however, it was
a more powerful operative in the male borderlines, even though males were not
overrepresented numerically among BPD brutality victims.

The important factor of drug abuse needs continuing study, particularly as
the current generation of borderline patients in the United States is showing a
different profile of abuse—using less heroin and much less LSD, mescaline, and
other "psychotomimetics," but much more cocaine, than the preceding
generation. It is not clear what these changing patterns portend for long-term
outcome.

Alcohol abuse remains an important factor, particularly because of the
synergism between alcohol and suicidality. Further efforts need to be made to
identify personality factors that predispose individuals to refusal or to acceptance
of AA, given the excellent results in alcoholics who join and remain.

Future follow-up studies should also focus on the BPD × MAD group. In
the 1960s, the range of available antipsychotics was narrower than at present;
for example, carbamazepine was not yet available as an alternative in lithium
nonresponders. Perhaps, also, the psychiatrists of that era were generally less
sophisticated about the use of medications than their colleagues of the current
generation. It remains to be seen, then, whether borderlines with prominent
affective symptoms will have a smoother life course than did the "comorbid"
group a generation ago.

Admixture with STP elements, in what is sometimes called a "mixed"
borderline personality, also does not by itself nudge prognosis in one fixed
direction or the other. Depending, probably, upon the particular STP trait that
is most prominent, a borderline patient may fail repeatedly to connect up closely
with other people and thus may lead a marginal existence (worse than that of
certain BPD cases), or else may lead a calm and measured (if somewhat colorless)
existence, free of the affect storms and upheavals of certain other BPD cases.
"Mixed" borderlines with strong paranoid trends are often particularly resistant
to therapy because of their propensity to lose faith even with the most
trustworthy of therapists. They are susceptible to pathological jealousy, if they
permit themselves any intimacy at all, and thus ultimately alienate and drive
away their partners.

The least predictable borderlines at present are those who demonstrate neither a "best" nor a "worst" factor among the factors outlined in Table 11.1 and in the text. Clinicians may in the next decades identify hitherto neglected variables that will help narrow the range of outcome in these "wild card" patients. Closer attention to associated personality traits, and especially to personality *assets,* may yield the most fruitful results in this search.

In the section that immediately follows I offer a number of clinical vignettes illustrating various levels of outcome within the borderline domain. Six of the eight concern patients with BPD. I hope the vignettes will bring more alive, in their human dimension, what I have hitherto been discussing mostly in a general and statistical way. Eight vignettes can give but a meager picture of the 500 and some patients whose individual, and often quite fascinating, stories make up the real substance of this study. I hope, in a later work, to sketch the life stories of several dozens of these former patients, drawn from all the pertinent diagnostic categories, not just from the borderline group.

CASE VIGNETTES

Recovery in a Patient with Borderline Personality Disorder

A 19-year-old woman, having spent most of the preceding 5 years in a succession of treatment facilities, entered our unit in hopes of receiving a "definitive cure" of her suicidal tendencies. These first came to the surface when she changed schools in ninth grade. Though an excellent student, she was extremely shy, did not fit in with the other students, and felt like an "outcast." Her parents had been having quarrels over the past year, some of them violent, since the mother was beginning to suspect that her husband was unfaithful. During these spats, the patient and her younger sister would cower in their bedroom. The patient began to have insomnia, nightmares, anxiety attacks during the day, and suicidal thoughts. She felt that her parents' disharmony was somehow her fault. Her father's behavior toward her intensified these feelings, since he favored her outspokenly and on occasion fondled her. (How much actually took place between them remained unclear.) She began to cut her wrists superficially, but so often—nearly once a week—as to make this practice noticeable to her teachers. This led to consultation with the school psychologist, to a meeting with the parents, and then to the first of the five lengthy hospitalizations (some in residential schools for disturbed children) that preceded the index hospitalization.

On our unit, where she remained an additional 2 years, she was at first evasive, almost mute, as though guarding secrets. She tolerated poorly even brief absences by her therapist and made suicide gestures in connection with each absence. Pharmacotherapy with tricyclic antidepressants was without benefit. During her thrice-weekly psychotherapy she formed an intense, sadomaso-chistically tinged attachment to her therapist: She filled up notebooks with amatory poems about him, only to push pins into her skin or burn her forearms with cigarettes in anticipation of his absence. At such times, her dreams contained vivid images of torture devices by which she "punished" him, though outwardly she remained reverential and uncritical toward him. Toward the end of her long stay, her tolerance of separation grew greater. She was able to get through several of the therapist's vacations without harming herself.

Though fragile, she was able to continue in treatment with her therapist as he finished residency training and began a practice. Their work together spanned 8½ years. Having graduated from high school at PI, she enrolled in college—part-time at first, then full-time. She developed an interest in the law (her father's profession) and later went to law school. There she met her future husband. They married, set up a joint law practice, and had three children. She never required rehospitalization and had made no self-injurious acts in many years by the time of follow-up. She did have a tendency to become depressed premenstrually, but controlled the symptoms with diuretics or anxiolytics. She was much more at ease socially than she had been upon leaving the unit, and no longer manifested the traits that once supported the diagnosis of BPD. Her GAS score at follow-up was 84.

Recovery in a Patient with Eating Disorder and Borderline Personality Organization

A young woman of 16 became severely anorectic in the summer of 1971. She entered our unit at the urging of the family physician, who grew alarmed over her having lost a third of her body weight. The youngest of three children, she was the envy of her two brothers because of her attractiveness and outgoing personality, but envied them in return because they got (slightly) better grades. Their parents had taken them on a vacation that summer, in the course of which her brothers had made cruel remarks about her figure, calling her "fat" when actually she was not. She went on a crash diet, and kept on losing weight; at the time of her admission to PI, she weighed 64 pounds.

Psychological tests done shortly after she came to the unit suggested that she had severe narcissistic and obsessional traits, along with problems in accepting her gender identity. Her parents were experiencing marital difficulties (and subsequently divorced); each turned to one of the sons as ally and confidant. The patient felt she had nowhere to turn. In her treatment, the task of restoring her weight to an acceptable level had highest priority. After 2 months, her weight returned to its usual level (98 pounds). She worked well with her therapist in an analytically oriented "expressive" therapy, exploring her fears of sex and pregnancy as well as her idiosyncratic views about food. The two sets of fears were interrelated, since normal weight meant the return of her periods and thus fuller awareness of her sex-role conflicts.

Because of the instability of the family, the staff permitted the patient to remain on the unit a year and a half until she matriculated at college. After her discharge, she began a four-times-a-week psychoanalysis, which she found most helpful in coming to terms with both sex-role conflicts and the issue of separating emotionally from her parents. In the following 15 years, her course was uniformly smooth and successful. She graduated from college with a *cum laude* in fine arts, took an advanced degree in this area, got a job as assistant curator in a museum, married 3 years prior to follow-up, and was planning to start a family of her own. Her weight remained stable. The only hints of her anorexia nervosa were a certain "calorie consciousness" and involvement in some of the currently popular diet systems. She maintained close ties with her original family, whom she saw in retrospect as having perhaps been "not very good" when she was an adolescent, but also as never very bad at any time (there was no abusiveness, neglect, molestation, alcoholism, etc.). Her follow-up GAS score was 90.

Recovery in the Modal Patient with Borderline Personality Organization and Antisocial Personality

A family requested hospitalization for their 15-year-old son because of his truancy and drug abuse. He had been a "model child," compliant, studious, sports-minded, and friendly, till "something got into him" at about age 13. His parents were undergoing divorce at that time, which also marked the beginning of his puberty. He became defiant, negativistic, and impulsive both at home and at school. He began to set fires in wastepaper baskets at school, which led to his expulsion. He then went to a stricter school but ran away, abused psychotomimetic drugs and alcohol, and on one occasion drove the family car while "under the influence." A policeman spotted him and gave chase. In the aftermath of his arraignment, the judge offered the family the alternative of psychiatric hospitalization.

On our unit, the admitting therapist noted the patient's "referentiality," "grandiosity," and gender confusion. He told no one of his year-long abuse of alcohol. Treatment consisted of thrice-weekly analytically oriented psychotherapy plus chlorpromazine in moderate doses. Neither had any discernible effect. Psychological tests revealed a large discrepancy between Verbal (120) and Performance (102) IQ, suggesting that depression was interfering with his mental functions. Clinically he was not depressed. He was popular with the other patients, but the staff distrusted him because he always seemed to be fomenting dissention and was perhaps secreting drugs on the unit. For these reasons, the staff arranged his transfer 6 months later to a residential facility specializing in the treatment of dyssocial adolescents.

His course over the 18-year interval between discharge and follow-up was tumultuous until the last 5 years. His alcohol abuse continued unabated. He worked sporadically at odd jobs, never settling in any one community for more than 1 or 2 years at a time. Often he would be "on the lam" because of accumulated speeding and parking violations and would be just a step ahead of the authorities. His relationships with women were intense, stormy, and brief—until he met one in Indiana who was a "born-again" Christian. She persuaded him to join their group. Some of the members were recovered alcoholics; he joined AA at their urging. For the 5 years immediately prior to follow-up, he remained abstinent and became a devoted member of his religious group. He moved to another city in the Midwest, worked steadily, earned an excellent livelihood as a salesman, and was planning to marry the woman who was instrumental in his recovery. Except for occasional mild "blues," he was asymptomatic. He also developed a number of hobbies, including the carving of wooden chess sets, from which he supplemented his income. His GAS score at follow-up was 73.

A Good Outcome in a Patient with Borderline Personality Disorder

A 25-year-old woman entered our unit at the urging of her parents. Her behavior had become chaotic and disruptive. Her illness had no discrete onset, as she seemed to have had serious behavioral problems throughout her life. As a child she was hyperactive, aggressive, and given to tantrums. At school or camp she would steal food and gorge on candy. Her tantrums grew more violent at menarche; scuffles with her parents took place in which each party hurt the other. Relationships with friends were stormy, and those with employers were chaotic. After quitting college in her third year, she worked but changed jobs frequently, often after outbursts of irritability. She became severely depressed at 20 following disappointment in a romantic relationship. In response, she made a suicide gesture with hypnotics. She began to binge on fattening foods, sometimes pocketing candy bars from the drugstore without paying for them. Her behavior became still more inappropriate at home, where she would alternate between appearing either unkempt or else vampishly attired. She also became obsessed with germs and took to bathing several times a day.

On the unit, the patient was at first irascible and overdramatic. Yet she was also tearful, depressed, and despondent about the future. Her response to her treatment, including antidepressants, was good, and by the end of her 10-month stay she had grown calmer and more mature. She resumed work, but now held a job in a responsible fashion for a number of years. On a few occasions she experienced mild bouts of depression; however, she continued to take her antidepressant medication. She married 2 years before follow-up contact and continued to work effectively at her job. Apart from premenstrual irritability, she was essentially well. Her GAS score at follow-up was 70.

A Good Outcome in a Dysthymic Borderline Patient

A young woman of 19 was helping to pay her way through college by working part-time in the university library. Both parents had died in a car accident when she was 10; she had then come under the care of a maternal aunt. Apart from this aunt and a cousin, she had no other living relatives. Her aunt developed congestive heart failure during the patient's freshman year (1962) and died 8 months later. The patient seemed unable to grieve (although she felt devastated) and quickly became depressed, withdrawn, and given to anxiety attacks and ruminations about suicide. Her cousin noticed that she failed to return home one evening and alerted the police, who found her wandering distractedly in the streets. They brought her to a nearby hospital, whose psychiatric crisis team then transferred her to our unit.

On arrival, the patient was depressed and showed psychomotor retardation, constriction of affect, and anhedonia. During her 19 months on the unit, her therapist met with her four times a week in 45-minute sessions and used no medications. Therapy concentrated on the key issues of (1) examining feelings related to loss and separation; (2) enhancing her capacity for pleasure; (3) working through the necessary mourning reaction over the deaths of her aunt and parents; and (4) building up ego resources preparatory to her function as a self-supporting adult. The unit's social and rehabilitative services played the primary role vis-à-vis the last-mentioned task. After a year and a half, she was re-enrolled at college, was doing part-time work again, and was ready to share an apartment with another convalescing patient.

Her course over the 23 years between discharge and follow-up was for the most part favorable. She completed college and found work as an editorial assistant in a publishing house. She married 4 years later and had two children; in the meantime, she rose to associate editorship in the same company. Her social life at follow-up was narrower than she would like. She was no longer fearful of losing friends as she once was (lest they "desert" her as her parents did), but remained rather shy and self-conscious and did not make friends easily. Occasionally she was overcome with feelings of loneliness and nostalgia, thinking about the desolation of her adolescent years. During such spells, she resumed therapy temporarily (on a less intense basis) and took a tricyclic antidepressant until her mood lifted. She never required rehospitalization. Besides her work and her family activities, she participated on a volunteer basis in a community charity organization. Her GAS score at follow-up was 71.

A Fair Outcome in a Patient with Borderline Personality Disorder

In 1966, a 24-year-old woman entered our unit following a severe suicide attempt with sedative drugs. She had been living with a roommate in New York City, where she was enrolled in graduate school. Her roommate, returning from a weekend trip a day earlier than planned, discovered the patient in a coma and summoned an ambulance. The patient's family consisted of her father (an executive in a large chemical corporation), her mother, and an older brother. Tensions between her parents had mounted to the point where her mother had recently made a suicide attempt, which in turn had sparked the patient's self-destructive act. Her father was a "weekend" alcoholic whose personality changed under the influence of alcohol from sanctimonious and unemotional to abusive and seductive. Her brother took the brunt of the abusiveness. Toward the patient, the father had begun to make sexually suggestive remarks from the time she was 13; he also made a number of sexual advances (kissing and hugging in a sexual manner, perhaps more), the frequency and full extent of which were never made clear. After one such confrontation when she was 15, she ran away, lived by her wits for several weeks, had several sexual encounters with strangers, and then reluctantly returned home. She could not bring herself to reveal to her mother what had been happening, but did plead with her mother to "go away somewhere" and take her and her brother. Throughout her college and postcollege years the patient grew increasingly dependent on her mother; she dated very little, despite many offers, because of her mistrustfulness toward men.

When the patient was first on the unit, the staff became aware of her night terrors and frequent nightmares (involving male attackers, large animals about to pounce, etc.). These, she reported, went back to early childhood, suggesting that her father had engaged in some form of abuse for many more years than she was able either to remember or to divulge.

Besides psychotherapy, she received occasional low doses of a neuroleptic when she became anxious after having had a particularly disturbing nightmare. She left the hospital after a year, no longer pursuing graduate school, but supporting herself instead as an administrative assistant. At follow-up she lived alone and rarely visited her family, waiting instead for her mother to visit her. She had a few friends, avoided the company of men, saw a therapist on a once-weekly basis, and continued to feel generally apprehensive (anxiolytics offered some relief). She still had recurrent (though less frequent) nightmares and was evasive even with her therapist about the events of her early life. Her GAS score at follow-up was 58.

A Fair Outcome in a Dysthymic Borderline Patient

A 22-year-old college senior was experiencing severe anxiety that began to encroach on his academic performance. He characterized his mental state as one of "existential angst," having to do mostly with uncertainty about the purpose of life in general and his own life in particular. He became detached and withdrawn, stopped seeing his girlfriend, broke off contact with most of his male friends, and started abusing marijuana. He also became depressed, and as his depression deepened he began to "self-medicate" with small amounts of alcohol or amphetamines. After graduation in 1968, his symptoms interfered with his looking for work (his degree was in engineering). He felt lost and hopeless about the future. In this context he developed insomnia, weight loss, and suicidal feelings. When he cut his wrist in a half-hearted suicide gesture, his mother insisted he enter the hospital. She had remarried the year before he came to our unit. An only child, the patient had lost his father when he was 7; his mother's remarriage made him feel there was no one left who was entirely "there" for him.

The patient responded favorably to tricyclic antidepressants. Though highly motivated for expressive psychotherapy, an alliance never developed between him and his therapist. Upon leaving the unit, he supported himself with a series of free-lance assignments. He found solace in Buddhism and eventually converted to that faith (he had been raised as a Methodist). He met a woman, also a fellow-convert, and began a long relationship with her. When this broke up about 5 years after his discharge, he made another suicide gesture. This led to his only subsequent hospitalization. The therapist at this hospital was more to his liking, and the patient continued to see him on an ambulatory basis. In recent years, he found steady work in an engineering firm, but felt at follow-up that he would "rather be doing something else." He lived alone, had a few friends and a few outside interests, and continued to derive satisfaction and a sense of belonging from his religious affiliation. Though often "down and discouraged," he had not been seriously depressed in the 12 years prior to follow-up; he no longer saw a therapist or took medication. His GAS score at follow-up was 60.

Marginal Adjustment in a Patient with Borderline Personality Disorder

The index admission of this 18-year-old woman was her second psychiatric hospitalization. She had come to the unit a year earlier (1963), remanded by the court as a person in need of supervision. She had become truant, rebellious, and sexually promiscuous since age 14, when her mother had left her in the care of an aunt. Her parents had divorced when she was 4; her mother was inconsistent as a caretaker, and for most of the years that followed she lived with her grandparents. All members of her immediate family were alcoholic. The patient herself drank to excess episodically after age 16. Shortly before her admission to PI, she mutilated her arms on two occasions with a razor, making only superficial cuts. These were acts of desperation, done in hopes of rescuing herself from the home of her punitive aunt.

On the unit, the patient was sullen, defiant, labile, and bored; at times, however, she was also depressed and preoccupied with thoughts of suicide. A fear of being pregnant intensified these symptoms. She was in fact pregnant but, despite her ambivalence, chose to raise the child. This she did, with the help of her mother and grandparents. Over the course of the 23 years till follow-up, she worked briefly at secretarial jobs but was fired repeatedly because of her willfullness. She had never abused drugs or alcohol since release from the index (which was also the last) hospitalization. She had few friends and led a constricted life, supported mostly by public assistance. Her suicidal feelings recurred after her daughter grew up and left home, but she was mistrustful of doctors and refused to seek help. Her GAS score at follow-up was 40.

CHAPTER TWELVE

Disorders Presenting with Psychosis

DIFFICULTIES IN DIAGNOSING THE PSYCHOTIC DISORDERS

Although the reliability of diagnosis is generally greater when one is dealing with psychotic disorders than with personality disorders, even the most sophisticated of the current structured diagnostic instruments do not yield perfect reliability or perfect discrimination between conditions that are conceptually similar. The possibility for confusion becomes even greater as we attempt to compare results between countries and between eras. Considerations of this sort affect whether we cleave to a narrow or to a broad definition of "schizophrenia," and whether we picture the prognosis in schizophrenia as uniformly poor or as quite variable.

In a comprehensive paper based on long-term follow-up studies, Angst (1986b) has attempted to clarify these issues, especially as they touch on differences between taxonomic customs between Europe and America. The tendency in Europe, as Angst point out, is to base the diagnosis of "schizophrenia" on symptoms; the label is therefore reserved for patients exhibiting a clear psychosis, not merely certain prepsychotic signs. The relevant symptoms are an amalgam of those outlined by E. Bleuler (1911), Kraepelin (1913), and Schneider (1959). More importantly, "The length of the previous psychiatric history or age of onset are not taken into account" (Angst, 1986b, p. 3). As a result, some cases of psychosis where depressive or manic symptoms occur in one phase or another of an otherwise nosologically schizophrenia-like disorder receive the "schizophrenia" label. Since affective psychoses have as a rule a better prognosis than, say, insidious-onset schizophrenia, studies that include a certain proportion of the former under the "schizophrenia" label, will cast "schizophrenia" in a more optimistic light than would other studies where such cases were rigorously excluded. Recovery may in fact occur in about a quarter of supposedly "schizophrenic" patients, where reliance is on initial symptoms only. Yet initial symptoms are what diagnosis, in the strict sense of the word, is all about. The currently popular solution to this dilemma in the United States is to employ a strict definition of "schizophrenia" emphasizing not only deficit or "negative" symptoms, but also chronicity of course. About this loading of the prognostic dice, Angst says the following:

> M. Bleuler (1972) stresses the fact that it doesn't make sense to include course into the definition and then use it again as a validator. Results based on selection of schizophrenics by the previous course are considered self-fulfilling prophecy, for instance, if we apply the 6-month criterion [i.e., in DSM-III] for defining schizophrenia. (1986b, p. 19)

Long-term follow-up studies of schizophrenia as defined by initial symptoms have made it clear for over half a century that cases presenting with affective symptoms, referential ideation, and confusion are much more likely to lead, years later, to complete recovery or to social recovery with minor residual symptoms; pronounced schizoid temperament has consistently been associated with a bad prognosis (Langfeldt, 1937). Langfeldt (1937, 1956) referred to some of the cases with depressive trends or mental cloudiness at outbreak of the illness, which had a better outlook than the more certain cases, as "doubtful" schizophrenia. Many of his "doubtful" cases we would call "atypical psychosis" (cf. Tsuang, Dempsey, & Rauscher, 1976) or "schizoaffective psychosis" (SA). Holmboe and Astrup (1957), in this connection, spoke of "reactive" psychoses and also of "typical" (schizophrenic) symptoms. The latter included more than we now include under the rubric of "negative signs" (or Huber's [1983] *Basissymptome*)—that is, not only passivity, but "primary delusions, religious megalomania, catatonic hebephrenic symptoms, haptic hallucinations and delusions of high descent" (Holmboe & Astrup, 1957, p. 58). These authors were at pains to point out that although reactive psychoses without typical symptoms rarely ended up with schizophrenic deterioration, not all patients showing the typical symptoms at the outset went on to a deteriorating course. In a similar way, Achté (1961) noted that recovery was rare (p. 232).

The narrow definitions tend to redefine "schizophrenia," as Angst mentions, so as to move psychotic patients with affective symptoms purely into the affective camp. Insistence upon 6 months or more of symptoms as an inclusion criterion reinforces this tendency and also selects out a subgroup of "schizophrenics" whose long-term outcome is almost uniformly bleak. Meanwhile, as Angst emphasizes, some psychiatrically ill relatives of narrowly defined schizophrenics have SA with either depressed or manic symptoms but without the chronic disability of the "index" cases. Scharfetter and Nüsperli (1980) noted that 4% of close relatives of schizophrenics had affective psychoses. The implication is that, to some extent at least, the distinction between schizophrenia and SA is arbitrary and based on symptoms, whereas from a genetic standpoint they may be linked.

Despite the diagnostic confusion and disagreement about prognosis alluded to in these remarks, some assertions enjoy wide acceptance. Patients with typical schizophrenia, for example, may recover in a minority of cases; only a few cases of schizophreniform illness (SF) turn into chronic schizophrenia (Angst, 1986b, p. 7). Also, whereas clinical symptoms present at admission to a hospital by themselves have little predictive power vis-à-vis outcome, those at discharge do— since the latter already reflect something about the *course* of illness (Angst, 1986b, p. 18). Apathy and other negative signs at time of discharge augur a chronic course. Premorbid adjustment is also a better predictor than admission symptomatology alone. Altogether, as Angst concludes, "follow up studies have not, so far, contributed to the classification of schizophrenia to a useful degree" (p. 21). The same argument holds for SA disorders as well.

Because of these unanswered questions in the realm of schizophrenia, we must endure a certain measure of arbitrariness in the definitions employed in the present study. I chose the DSM-III definition of schizophrenia (SZ) when rediagnosing the original records (almost all of which bore the rubber stamp "pseudoneurotic schizophrenia"). Given the patient population of the PI-500, this meant that the division I made, in relation to the 163 patients whose records justified a diagnosis of either SZ or SA, put 99 in the SZ group and 64 in the SA group. The differences between my results and those of Ciompi and Müller (1976), M. Bleuler (1972), and others, and the similarity to those of McGlashan (1984b), are primarily a function of definitional differences; they have little to do with whose definitional criteria were "better" or whose patients were "sicker." There is no assurance that, were the "real" schizophrenia to declare itself in the near future thanks to some external laboratory test, there would be more homogeneity than we are now seeing, with respect either to initial symptoms or to long-term outcome.

To illustrate the interrelationships among the various arbitrary diagnostic subgroups within the realm of psychotic disorders in the PI-500, I have drawn a Venn diagram (Figure 12.1) showing their regions of overlap and disjunction. In the actual assignment of individual cases to the different categories, I did not use "Bleulerian schizophrenia" or "substance-induced psychosis." I include those circles in the diagram for purposes of comparison with the other taxonomies under discussion. The small overlap between substance-induced psychosis and SA reflects the rare instance where follow-up of a presumably SA patient revealed a mistake in the initial diagnosis: One man, for example, should have received the diagnosis "alcohol-related paranoid psychosis" on admission (see Chapter Fifteen). The original literature on SF preceded the era of hallucinogen abuse (1962–present); the originators of the term would have assigned many of my SF patients to the compartment for substance-induced psychoses. Cases with typical affective and typical schizophrenic symptoms in about equal measure cannot be convincingly assigned to SA or to manic–depressive psychosis (MDP) and would occupy an intermediate zone— namely, the overlap region between these two conditions. In the diagram, SA

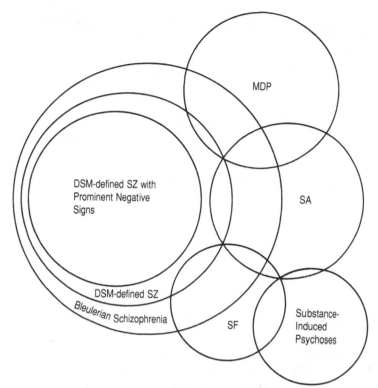

FIGURE 12.1.   Interrelationships among the psychotic disorders.

does not overlap negative-sign SZ at all, though actually one of the original SA (and one of the SF) patients emerged at follow-up as having chronic SZ.

The remainder of this chapter discusses outcomes for the PI-500 patients in the SZ, SA, and MDP groups.

THE SCHIZOPHRENIC PATIENTS

The life trajectories of the 99 schizophrenic patients within the PI-500 for the most part inspire pessimism. Only partially was this a function of the illness itself. Changing diagnostic standards also helped shape the resulting curve of outcome distribution. Also affecting the results heavily were the prevailing treatment philosophy when our schizophrenic patients were first becoming symptomatic, and the inadequate network of institutions and services then available for implementing this philosophy.

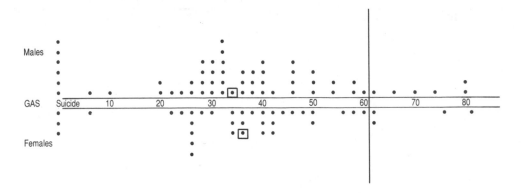

FIGURE 12.2.   Distribution of follow-up GAS scores in schizophrenic patients. Dots within boxes denote median scores.

Average Global Assessment Scale Scores

About five-sixths of the schizophrenic patients had Follow-up Global Assessment Scale (GAS) scores less than 60. As Figure 12.2 shows, the great majority were either "incapacitated" or "marginal" in their adjustment. These two categories accounted for 75% of the patients. A small, and roughly equal, proportion were either "fair" or dead from suicide. Outcome patterns for the two sexes were almost identical. The "good" and "recovered" categories were also roughly equal in size and represented even more exceptional outcomes.

The mean GAS scores for the male and female schizophrenics were essentially the same.

The findings in the present study concerning global outcome are closely compatible with those of McGlashan (1984b, 1986b) in his reports on the Chestnut Lodge follow-up study. The methodologically elegant Chestnut Lodge study is the current standard by which other outcome studies of schizophrenia—of patients in our culture and of similar socioeconomic status—are to be measured. The heterogeneity of results in other contemporary schizophrenia outcome studies around the world would seem to be more a function of variables such as social class, interval length, stage of life at last contact, and the like than of diagnosis (which is now fairly standardized). Definitional matters also come into play, as in the 5-year outcome study of Prudo and Blum (1987) from London. Their mention of "49% good symptomatic outcome" relates to the grouping together of 19% with "no residual psychotic symptoms/no further major episodes" plus another 30% with "less than a year in total episodes and some residual symptoms." In my schema, the latter would probably have follow-up GAS scores of 51–60 ("fair") or lower; my impression of about 10% "good" outcomes (GAS scores > 60) is perhaps not so strikingly different from Prudo and Blum's 19% "asymptomatic."

Other Points Concerning Life Course and Outcome

In general, schizophrenic patients who showed extremes of awkwardness or of bizarre behavior had poorer outcomes at follow-up than did those whose illness seemed confined to the realm of ideation. Although severe psychosis at the outset did not predict an unfavorable outcome, unfavorable outcomes were the rule where severity of thought disturbance was accompanied by marked and long-standing characterological peculiarity. Two schizophrenic patients with equally bizarre delusions upon entry to the hospital—one of whom had had friends throughout adolescence, the other not—would have outcomes more reflective of their relative abilities to connect up with others than of their thought processes at the height of their illness. One of the schizophrenic men, for example, had the delusion that germs were crawling out of his penis. A schizophrenic woman was convinced she was Satan's mistress, the embodiment of evil, to do penance for which she felt constrained to eat garbage out of refuse pails. The first patient had been friendless and eventually committed suicide, whereas the second had always had a number of friends. At follow-up, 18 years after discharge, she had long ago given up her self-denigratory delusions; she was working, married, and only moderately symptomatic (GAS score = 55).

Presence versus Absence of Paranoia

No symptom or trait *taken by itself* has great predictive power over the long term in schizophrenic patients. Paranoid patients may do less well at the time of release from the hospital, partly because, as Ritzler (1981) mentions, they "are not easy to engage in the process of treatment. Either suspicious, guarded, untrusting and hostile, or exceedingly grandiose and aloof, they are not well disposed to following treatment regimens [or] cooperating in psychotherapy" (p. 710). Allen, Tarnoff, Kearns, and Coyne (1986) did not find appreciable differences in status between paranoid and nonparanoid schizophrenics at discharge after long-term hospitalization. Unevenness in the old records made it difficult for me to divide the PI-500 schizophrenics methodically into categories, although some paranoid patients clearly did well eventually and others did not. A small proportion of the PI-500 schizophrenics were violent (two men committed manslaughter; another was gunned down while committing a crime). When I singled out patients with pronounced paranoid qualities during their hospitalization, and contrasted their outcomes with those of the schizophrenic patients with no striking paranoid features, I could establish two rosters containing 80 of the 96 traced schizophrenics. The remainder had a few or else fleeting paranoid features that defied neat categorization. Table 12.1 shows the results in the two nearly equal groups. The proportions in each group with follow-up GAS scores > 60 were not significantly different. The suicides tended

TABLE 12.1. PI-500 Paranoid versus Nonparanoid Schizophrenic Patients ($n = 80$):
Follow-Up GAS Scores

GAS score	Paranoid		Nonparanoid	
	Males	Females	Males	Females
>70	2	0	0	1
61–70	1	0	2	2
51–60	2	1	4	2
31–50	10	3	10	8
1–30	10	3	4	7
Suicide	3	3	2	0
Total	28	10	22	20
Average for patients who did not commit suicide	33.1	25.5	41.6	38.6
Average for males and females together	31.1		40.1	

Note. 16 traced schizophrenics were omitted because clinical data did not permit meaningful division into either of these two subgroups.

to cluster in the paranoid group; the average outcome GAS score for the nonparanoid patients of either sex was somewhat higher than that of the paranoid patients. Schizophrenic patients in general tend to communicate less with potential helpers about suicidal feelings than do depressed patients (Allebeck, Varla, & Wistedt, 1985); schizophrenic patients who are paranoid may be even more secretive in this respect.

Negative versus Positive Symptoms

Within the past few years, researchers have begun to look at outcome in schizophrenia from the perspective of "negative" versus "positive" symptoms (Andreasen & Olson, 1982; Crow, 1980; Lindenmayer, Kay, & Friedman, 1986; Opler, Kay, & Rosado, 1984; Strauss, Carpenter, & Bartko, 1974). Kulhara and Chadda (1987) have drawn attention to similarities between chronic schizophrenic and chronically depressed patients in relation to negative symptoms, noting that alogia, poor eye contact, inappropriate affect, and blocking are more (but not perfectly) specific for schizophrenia. Liddle (1987) found a correlation between psychomotor poverty and later impaired personal relationships, as well as a link between inappropriate affect and impersistence at work. For a detailed review of the subject, with comments on the probable familial nature of negative symptoms, the reader should consult the article by Pogue-Geile and Zubin (1988). For convenience, I reprint here a list by Kay,

Opler, and Fiszbein (1986, p. 443) of the more prominent symptoms in these categories. (To Kay et al.'s "negative syndrome," I would add "anhedonia.")

Positive syndrome
  Delusions
  Conceptual disorganisation
  Hallucinatory behaviour
  Excitement
  Grandiosity
  Suspiciousness
  Hostility
Negative syndrome
  Blunted affect
  Emotional withdrawal
  Poor rapport
  Passive–apathetic social withdrawal
  Difficulty in abstract thinking
  Lack of spontaneity and flow of conversation
  Stereotyped thinking

One should keep in mind that the condition we glibly call "schizophrenia," as though it were unitary, is more in the nature of a heterogeneous collection of symptom constellations, emphasizing one or another "nervous" traits. These traits (nervousness, shyness, nonconformity, etc.), in their milder forms, shade into the general population. Past a certain threshold of intensity, they stimulate a clinician to apply a term like "schizotypal personality" or "borderline schizophrenia" or "nuclear schizophrenia" (Claridge, 1987). Prominent "negative signs" are especially likely to trigger the diagnosis of (full-blown, DSM-III) SZ.

As Kay et al. (1986) mention, the "negative symptoms" overlap considerably with the "defect state" as described in the earlier European literature (Kraepelin, 1913). Huber (1983) continues to draw attention to the significance of the defect symptoms, under the heading of "basic" symptoms. The productive or "positive" features (especially delusions and hallucinations) have now become more important as diagnostic indicators (Feighner et al., 1972). Yet the negative signs often betoken a chronic course (Munk-Jørgensen & Mortensen, 1989; Pogue-Geile & Harrow, 1984), unless one is studying young patients with acute SZ (Lindenmayer et al., 1986), in which case the "negative symptoms" are associated with depression and a more favorable outcome.

The picture is complicated by the fact that the positive–negative dichotomy, though useful heuristically, does not divide actual patient samples so neatly: Some schizophrenic patients show both in abundance. Positive symptoms do not always predict better overall prognosis, since they are also associated with a more *stormy* course in certain patients, and with more frequent hospitalizations (Kay et al., 1986). Premorbid adjustment tends to be poorer in

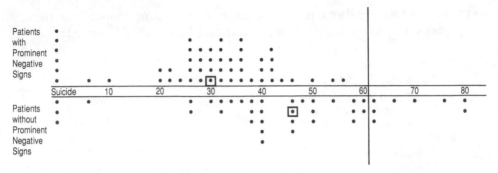

FIGURE 12.3. Presence or absence of prominent negative signs in schizophrenic patients: Follow-up GAS scores. Dots within boxes denote median scores.

those with the negative syndromes (Andreasen & Olsen, 1982), which are also more common in males (Huber, Gross, Schüttler, & Linz, 1980; Pogue-Geile & Harrow, 1984) and are associated in some schizophrenics with enlarged ventricles on computerized axial tomography (CAT) scans (Johnstone, Crow, Frith, Husband, & Kreel, 1976). Even in chronic schizophrenics, the negative features are apparently not irreversible, though Johnstone, Owens, Frith, and Crow (1986) found that they proved more durable than certain positive symptoms such as anxiety and depression (p. 62). In regard to CAT scan studies, Pearlson, Garbacz, Moberg, Ahn, and DePaulo (1985) felt they could identify a special subgroup of schizophrenics with (1) marked ventricular enlargements, (2) pronounced negative signs, and (3) early onset of illness.

I have attempted to review the records of the PI schizophrenics with respect to negative versus positive symptoms. In the absence of methodical ratings made at the time of admission, I have had to "make do" with the unevenness in the quality of the records, with memory, and with the recollections of my colleagues. I subdivided the traced schizophrenic patients into (1) a group with the prominent negative symptoms in Kay et al.'s (1986) list, with or without concomitant positive symptoms; and (2) the remainder group, without prominent negative symptoms. Almost without exception, the schizophrenic patients were on a regimen of neuroleptic medication, which may have caused some blunting of affect (Rifkin, Quitkin, & Klein, 1975). I had no way of controlling for drug effects in my assessment.

The follow-up GAS scores of the 52 traced schizophrenic patients with prominent negative symptoms were rather homogeneous: Half the scores ranged from 30 to 49, and none exceeded 55. The mean scores, 31 for the males and 34 for the females, were below those of the remaining schizophrenics, $\chi^2 = 13.8$ with Yates's correction, $df = 1$, $p < .01$. Figure 12.3 illustrates these findings.

More than half the traced schizophrenic patients exhibited the "negative syndrome" (52 of 96, or 54%); of those who did, only 2 had ever married, whereas 9 of the 42 remaining patients had married. The negative syndrome was also associated with a poorer work history. In the PI-500, the proportion of males with prominent negative symptoms did not exceed that of the females.

The PI-500 schizophrenics—most of them urban, middle- to upper-middle-class, brighter than average, and in their 20s at the time of index hospitalization—were not a representative group. At follow-up, in their late 30s to early 50s, they did not seem to be showing the kind of improvement or mellowing that Bridge, Cannon, and Wyatt (1978) noted in a sample of schizophrenics once they passed the age of 55, or that Harding and colleagues (Harding, Brooks, Ashikaga, Strauss, & Breier, 1987; Harding & Strauss, 1985) reported in the mostly rural, lower-middle-class patients of their Vermont study. Nevertheless, the negative syndrome, especially when found in combination with other factors conducing to a poor outcome, will probably emerge as an important predictor of chronicity and marginal adaptation. Huber et al. (1980) made this point in connection with their longitudinal study, adding that maladaptive, *non*syntonic premorbid personality (especially of the schizoid type), if present in the clinical picture alongside the "basic symptoms," was particularly likely to be correlated at follow-up with chronically poor adjustment.

The defects underlying the positive symptoms may be quite different from those responsible for anhedonia and affect-blunting. In the lives of schizophrenic patients, the two categories of symptoms often appear to strike a certain balance—one in which the delusions and hallucinations play a "defensive" role, much as Freud (1911) hypothesized in the Schreber case, and as Beck (1959) suggested in connection with persecutory delusions ("a man who has the whole F.B.I. chasing him must be a very important person").

In some of the PI-500 schizophrenic patients, the defect responsible for the eccentric mode of thought appeared to coexist with the negative syndrome throughout the life course; if anything, it may have aggravated the negative syndrome by driving the patients in on themselves. One of our male schizophrenic patients, for example, had a flat trajectory: His GAS score of 30 at follow-up was equally valid 19 years earlier, when he first became known to us. A highly intelligent man, he had a painful awareness of his own illness, referring spontaneously to the "defensive" uses his psychosis had acquired: "I go back into delusions as an escapism thing . . . it's idiotic, but I do it." But autistic thought and neologistic speech (positive symptoms) had been noticeable features of his condition for so long as to enforce his social withdrawal (a "negative" symptom) by causing others to turn away from his "weirdness." Whereas the better-functioning paranoid schizophrenic patients spoke with perfect coherence about their unrealistic convictions (thus appearing to the world as more "paranoid" than "schizophrenic," and to those who agreed with them as not ill at all), this man betrayed the peculiarity of thought in every sentence. As he told me in describing his lifelong isolation, ". . . it's a person-transparency thing. People can see through me to what is inside. [It's] a passive cathexis—something from inside that is leaking—like, a latent homosexual thing.''

Like many of the still-dysfunctional schizophrenics, the patient described above was never suicidal. This was true in the PI-500 of half the schizophrenics, whether male or female. Being isolated and out of work, not having a mate, having to rely on public assistance—shortcomings that one might naively suppose would inspire suicidal thoughts in many persons (especially those raised in comfortable circumstances)—served as the triggers of suicidal behavior only in a small fraction of the schizophrenic patients who were still living alone and in reduced circumstances. In the chapter on suicide (see Chapter Four), I mention some of the factors that may have contributed to the nine suicides among the PI-500 schizophrenics. Several who died really needed years-long sanctuary, but were compelled to live in what were for them unstable and unsafe surroundings. The lack of sanctuary was itself the reflection of professional overoptimism about the efficacy of analytic psychotherapy and of the neuroleptics to normalize the lives of schizophrenic patients. With this came the program of deinstitutionalization. This policy led to the closing or refurbishing of some inadequate facilities. But on the negative side, overzealous deinstitutionalization impeded the development of more integrated and more humane networks of structured settings that many schizophrenic patients still require, often for several decades, when their illness is more active. In the 1980s, models for the treatment of schizophrenics began to emphasize rehabilitation and a graduated series of structured settings from full-scale hospital to sheltered apartments and workshops. These facilities were not consistently available to the schizophrenic patients of the PI-500, some of whom lived instead as homeless people; others, as wards of the community, were shunted back and forth between the main hospital and meager ''single-room occupancy'' dwellings.

The lives—and deaths—of these schizophrenic patients make it clear that we cannot really speak of the natural history of their condition in the abstract, but only in relation to the types of treatment they received (or failed to receive) during the follow-up interval. Yet, in the absence of carefully controlled studies of various treatment modalities, we cannot make categorical statements about the efficacy of the various treatments. The excellent study of Gunderson et al. (1984)—which compared two treatment approaches in schizophrenic patients, with randomization to one or the other modality—represents an important step in clarifying questions about efficacy.

Counterintuitive Results

As in all the diagnostic groups, there were many counterintuitive results among the schizophrenics (see also Chapter Fifteen). The following vignette concerns a patient whom the hospital staff felt would do well, but whose adjustment at follow-up was marginal.

A woman of 20 entered our unit because of auditory hallucinations, delusions of shifting content, and inability to complete her studies. The unit personnel found her particularly likeable. A combination of shyness, compliance, attractiveness, and solicitousness of others made her a "model" patient. Upon discharge, she returned to her studies, still encountering considerable difficulty, and remained for a time with her therapist from the unit. But a few months later she went to Texas, ostensibly to be near some of her relatives. We had no word of her during the next 16 years, apart from a request for some information. She wrote our hospital 10 years ago, using what appeared to be her married name, which I will call (pseudonymously) "Delabrière." Only a few Delabrières existed in the phone directories of Texas and the neighboring states. Surely one of them must be the husband or one of his relatives. But no one had ever heard of an "Emilie Delabrière" who had come into the family in recent years.

Eventually I traced this patient through the chain of therapists involved with her care. The current therapist informed me that she had been living for the past 7 or 8 years in a rurally situated religious community dedicated to the care of emotionally handicapped persons. There she received bed and board and performed light duties. She took maintenance-level neuroleptics under the guidance of the therapist. Her life was stable; she fit in well with the other members of the community. Because of her social anxiety, she seldom left the grounds. Her thought disorder was now encapsulated, manifesting itself as an atypical erotomanic delusion. Although she had not had male companions in many years, she fancied herself married—to an imaginary Mr. Delabrière, whose namesakes in the Southwest I had stumbled onto during my original tracing efforts.

The patient in the vignette above was doing reasonably well in a less pressured environment. Those who had worked with her over the years came intuitively to this realization and advised her to seek out a community that would offer her a simpler and more predictable life, in a setting that would meet her spiritual and physical needs. Many of the schizophrenic patients of the PI-500 benefited from similar recommendations or else gravitated toward similar environments on their own. We sometimes concluded on behalf of patients still on the unit that they would do better in a less competitive atmosphere, and arranged a transfer to a hospital or other facility that provided a more appropriate setting. We occasionally did so with reluctance, as though such a move represented "giving up" on the patient. In retrospect, if we had made similar recommendations less haphazardly and with greater conviction, we would have helped a greater percentage of our schizophrenic patients. Such was the *Zeitgeist* in the '60s and '70s that we aimed too high. And even in cases where our aim was more accurate, we could find few programs and few places that had the ideal characteristics. A propos that *Zeitgeist,* I can also recall situations where the hospital personnel already understood the need for a less competitive setting, but could not convince the parents to scale down their hopes that their children would one day fulfill their expectations. This was particularly true with highly successful families of schizophrenic children who had very high IQs. Suggestions about sheltered settings and the like were repugnant to these families. I have the impression that a few of the schizophrenic patients who committed suicide were caught in this kind of disharmony between parental expectation and their own capabilities.

Changes in Diagnostic Standards

Confounding any comments we might wish to make about outcome in schizophrenia is the matter of changing diagnostic standards. Vaillant (1963) noted some years ago that the frequency of relatives with affective psychoses was much higher in families of fully remitting schizophrenics than in the families of schizophrenics who, at long-term follow-up, proved to have an unfavorable course. Contemporary diagnostic standards would probably require us to place quotation marks around the "schizophrenics with affective heredity," calling them "manic–depressives originally misdiagnosed as schizophrenic." Similarly, the Swiss outcome studies of Ciompi and Müller (1976) and M. Bleuler (1972) are hard to compare with recent American studies, since the broader criteria of E. Bleuler (1911) may contain a greater proportion of "false positives" (particularly of MDPs) than would be true of samples selected by the narrower criteria now in use here. In part, schizophrenia now appears to have an unfavorable outlook because of our current, more Kraepelinian view that favorable cases may not have been examples of the real thing. Between this and our emphasis throughout the era of the PI-500 on "cure" (which we could not effect) rather than on trying to minimize social disability (which we could have facilitated), it is small wonder that the outcome results in the PI-500 schizophrenics appear as unfavorable as they do (cf. Vaillant, 1978).

THE SCHIZOAFFECTIVE PATIENTS

Notes on the Diagnosis; Results of Other Studies

The schizoaffective patients in the PI-500 showed a wide range of outcomes at long-term follow-up. In this, they resembled the patients with MDP. As noted in the chapter on outcome patterns (see Chapter Thirteen), patients in either of these groups were almost as numerous at the extremes of outcome as in the middle; that is, there were nearly as many suicides or recovered patients as there were patients with "fair" and "good" outcomes. This was particularly true of the female schizoaffective patients, who were distributed almost equally within each outcome compartment (see Chapter Three).

Schizoaffectives form a diagnostically controversial group. The diagnosis of "schizoaffective disorder" was reluctantly accorded a berth in DSM-III "for those instances where the clinician is unable to make a differential diagnosis with any degree of certainty between *affective disorder* . . . and schizophrenia." All authors who accept the term (van Praag & Nijo, 1984; Winokur, 1974) or who prefer a somewhat different label for a fundamentally similar clinical picture (e.g., Tsuang et al.'s [1976] "atypical psychosis"), draw attention to the acute onset, usually with life stress precipitants. "Schizoaffective" patients are also notorious for appearing under one clinical guise this year and under a different one the next, exhibiting what has been called "occasion variance." Manic signs may be uppermost during one crisis, cognitive aberrations during another crisis, and depressive symptoms in the one following. Others show an unvarying clinical picture.

van Praag and Nijo (1984, p. 14) found that schizoaffectives made better overall adjustments at a 4- to 7-year follow-up than schizophrenics, both occupationally and psychopathologically (i.e., the schizoaffectives were ulti- mately less symptomatic). These authors noted that schizoaffectives with mood-congruent delusions—melancholic, manic, "ecstatic"—did better than those with mood-incongruent delusions, the latter resembling classic schizo- phrenics more closely in both symptom picture and outcome. Those with mood-congruent delusions, conversely, resembled the classic manic–depressives more closely in their life course. Angst (1986a) drew similar conclusions from his large follow-up study of 173 depressive and 215 bipolar patients: Full remissions were more likely in those with congruent delusions. The latter were twice as commonly noted as the more schizophrenia-like incongruent delusions. Angst felt it was meaningful to reclassify those with incongruent delusions as schizoaffective. About the *incidence* of psychogenic provocation, van Praag and Nijo commented only that this factor was "virtually the same" (1984, p. 17) across all the diagnostic groups of their study.

In their follow-up study over a much longer period (30–40 years), Tsuang and Dempsey (1979) reported combined outcomes (averaging marital, residen- tial, occupational, and psychiatric statuses) for their schizoaffectives ($n = 85$) that were intermediate between the worse outcomes of the schizophrenics and the generally better outcomes of the manic–depressives. Opjørdsmoen (1989) registered a similar impression. Elsewhere, Tsuang et al. (1976) mentioned that an outcome considered significantly improved was seldom associated with schizophrenia (8%), much more often associated with the schizoaffective or "atypical" psychosis (44%), and still more often noted among manic– depressives (58%). The features that characterize "atypical" psychosis are outlined in Table 12.2. A patient who meets Feighner criteria for schizophrenia, but who also shows six or seven of the attributes of "atypical psychosis," is then reclassified in this way.

Angst, Scharfetter, and Stassen (1983), meantime, argue for the preserva- tion of the schizoaffective concept, having noted the frequency of depressive and

TABLE 12.2. Features Found in Association with "Atypical" Psychosis

Feature	Schizophrenia	"Atypical" psychosis
Age of onset	Under 25	30 or older
Marital status	Single	Married
Premorbid adjustment	Poor	Good
Self-reproach	Absent	Present
Auditory hallucinations	Present	Absent
Precipitating factors	Absent	Present
Educational level reached	Lower	Higher
Gender	Male (more likely)	Female (more likely)
Persecutory delusions	Present	Absent
Motoric symptoms	Present	Absent
Recovery from previous episodes	No	Yes

Note. From Tsuang, M. T. (1986) Atypical psychosis. Grand Rounds, New York Hospital, Westchester Division, March 21. Reprinted by permission of Dr. Tsuang.

manic symptoms among schizophrenic patients (p. 259). Using a cluster-analytic approach, these authors believe that the data supported a *continuum* concept "of psychopathological subgroups with a lot of overlap, which may also differ to a certain extent in other respects such as course, genetics and response to treatment" (p. 259). I have expressed similar views in a previous publication (Stone, 1980a).

Van Eerdewegh et al. (1987) studied a large group ($n = 621$) of affectively ill patients in the National Institute of Mental Health collaborative project. Using a "manic" dimension and a "schizophrenic" dimension, they divided the patients into four main groups: unipolar (387), bipolar (159), schizounipolar (30), and schizobipolar (45). The last two groups constituted the schizoaffectives. On average, the schizoaffectives spent more time in hospital, and had more numerous hospitalizations before the index admission, than did the MDP (unipolar and bipolar) patients. This was especially true of the schizobipolar ("schizomanic") patients.

Global Results

The outcome of the PI-500 schizoaffectives can be grouped according to the categories mentioned in Table 12.3, where, for didactic purposes, the suicides have been classified along with those whose follow-up GAS score was between 1 and 30 as "incapacitated." We can condense the groupings further into "incapacitated," "little or no improvement," and "significantly improved" (GAS scores > 60), a schema that divides the schizoaffective patients roughly

TABLE 12.3. Outcome in Traced PI-500 Schizoaffective Patients (*n* = 61)

Outcome category	Males (*n* = 21)	Females (*n* = 40)	Combined	
			n	%
Incapacitated	5	14	19	31
Suicide	5	9	14	23
GAS score = 1–30	0	5	5	8
Marginal (GAS score = 31–50)	7	9	16	26
Fair (GAS score = 51–60)	0	5	5	8
Good (GAS score = 61–70)	4	7	11	10
Recovered (GAS score > 70)	5	5	10	17

into thirds. The average GAS score of the still-alive schizoaffectives was 55, placing them below the borderlines and schizophreniform patients, at the same level as the PI-500 manic–depressives and above the level of the schizophrenics. But, as noted in Figure 3.1 (see Chapter Three), the median score in the SA patients was 46 (in contrast to 54 for the MDP patients), owing to the larger proportion of suicides among the SA group.

Because the schizoaffective patients numbered only 64 in the PI-500, further compartmentalization creates groups that make statistical analysis risky because of their small size. From Table 12.3, for example, it appears as though the male patients exhibited bimodality: 12 did very poorly, none were in the "fair" range, and 9 did well. But this could be sample artifact. The well-functioning group did not differ appreciably in symptomatology when first hospitalized from those who did poorly. Six males had "schizobipolar" characteristics on admission; of the five of these patients traced, one committed suicide, two had marginal functioning at follow-up, two were recovered. (In Angst's [1988] experience, schizoaffective patients with bipolar episodes tend to do better than those with exclusively unipolar episodes—an observation based on much larger numbers of follow-up schizoaffective patients.) Males were more apt to be "schizomanic" than the females (6 of 20 males as opposed to 2 of 41 females), $\chi^2 = 6.94$, $p < .05$ with Yates's correction.

The female schizoaffectives, who were more evenly divided over the outcome spectrum at follow-up, also showed no sharp differences in symptoms between those who did best and those who committed suicide. The suicides and the still-alive incapacitated patients did, however, tend to have more schizoid personalities and to have remained delusional throughout their stay on the unit. Perhaps the greater shyness of the poorest-functioning SA patients is an example of the point made long ago by Chase and Silverman (1941) in connection with schizophrenics: "[E]xtravert temperament and adequate pre-psychotic life-adjustment offer a more favorable outlook, in contrast to introversion and inadequacy" (p. 363).

Background Factors

The schizoaffective patients in the PI-500, besides showing heterogeneity of initial clinical picture and of outcome, also seemed heterogeneous as to the patterns of contributing genetic and environmental factors. Strong evidence of genetic factors, for example, was discernible only in 12.5% of the original schizoaffectives, if we use as a criterion the presence of functional psychosis in a parent (seven patients had one such parent; in an eighth, both parents were ill). Five of the affected parents (4%) were manic–depressive; four schizophrenic (3.3%). In a small number of families, we found not full-blown psychosis but merely one or another of the Kraepelinian "temperaments" (irritable, depressive, manic) in one of the parents.

In the majority of the remaining schizoaffective patients, onset of illness had usually followed some traumatic event, such as the breakup of a romantic relationship or the death of a parent. Given the frequency of antecedent losses across all diagnostic groups in the PI-500, this was not a striking finding. What does warrant our attention, however, is the incest rate among the female schizoaffectives, which at 27% was the highest for any diagnostic subgroup in the study. Since only one of the incest victims had a parent with psychotic illness (a schizophrenic mother), we may be dealing with subgroups where genetic liability is not much intermixed with the more severe forms of psychogenic trauma, and vice versa. Physical abuse by a parent played only a minor role in the schizoaffectives as a group (three instances), though this brutality played a major role in the families where it occurred. One schizoaffective woman suffered both sexual and physical molestation at the hands of her father. We cannot readily assess the impact of abuse upon suicide in the PI-500 schizoaffectives, given that the suicide rates in the entire group and in the incest subgroup were both 22%.

Some of the schizoaffectives had been so severely traumatized, and their illness followed so closely upon the heels of a major incident (incest, beating), that we can make a convincing claim that their acute illness was a *phenocopy* of the hereditary/familial schizoaffective psychosis. Instead of exhibiting a latent condition made manifest (by some life event, such as the early death of a parent), these patients may have come into the world *not* especially vulnerable genetically, only to succumb to a condition in every way mimicking a mixed psychosis—a condition set in motion purely by the same extremes of sexual/physical abuse that, under other circumstances, give rise to the syndrome of multiple personality. Here we may legitimately speak of a "*posttraumatic* psychosis," akin to the "posttraumatic neurosis" except in severity. Certainly, reality-testing may give way under the impact of severe trauma; "multiple personality" is not the only resulting syndrome. I had occasion recently to interview a young woman who had been molested sexually by a male relative. In addition, her mother, an adherent of a charismatic religious sect, had abused her daughter in various ways under the pretext of purifying her body against the blandishments of Satan: She would lock her daughter in a closet without food so that the girl would have inside her as little "dirt" as possible. She would then "cleanse" her further by scrubbing her vulva with steel wool. Later the young woman made a suicide gesture and was brought to a hospital. There she revealed the fantasy that the woman who did these things was not her "real" mother at all, since her "real" mother, a kindly lady always dressed in white gowns, lived "somewhere in a faraway city." At times she spoke as though this was indeed merely a fantasy (diagnosticians then considered her "borderline"). But at other times, the fantasy hardened into conviction, and in this delusory state, the same diagnosticians considered her "schizoaffective."

Another, scarcely less poignant, example occurred in the PI-500. One of the nominally schizoaffective patients was a woman of 17 whose parents had divorced when she was 11. She had lived subsequently with her mother, or else with her grandmother, until economic circumstances made either arrangement difficult. At 17 she went to stay with her father—a successful businessman with a history of alcohol abuse. Within a short time he molested her; she then cut her wrists in a suicide gesture and was hospitalized. Upon admission, she was so incoherent and evasive that for several months the staff members were unable to piece together her story. She struck strange postures, laughed and cried by turns, and sometimes heard voices taunting her about the incest. Throughout her 5-month stay, she remained uncommunicative and tearful, eventually eloping from the unit and returning to live with another relative. Fourteen years later, I learned that her posttraumatic psychosis (as I now characterize her condition) had lifted shortly after she resumed life at the safer of the homes available to her. She remained coherently rational ever since, although she eschewed the company of her father. A year after she left the hospital, she was well enough to resume schoolwork and enter college, where she eventually completed training in elementary school education. At follow-up, she was employed and engaged to be married.

Though 2 of the 10 SA female incest victims have committed suicide and another 2 were leading marginal lives at follow-up, 4 (including the last-mentioned patient) were doing well. As with the borderline females, incest seems to have made a number of them ill who might not have otherwise succumbed, but apparently it did not preclude eventual recovery (especially where the initial traumatization was not too severe or involved a brother rather than a father).

THE MANIC–DEPRESSIVE PATIENTS

The manic–depressive patients described here are the 39 for whom chart review, in accordance with DSM-III criteria, justified a diagnosis of MDP. This number does *not* include the borderline patients who subsequently became manic–depressive (see Chapter Five). Of the 38 traced patients, 25 were bipolar;

4 had bipolar II illness; 8 were unipolar; and 1 was psychotically depressed on admission, with mild depressions (not requiring hospitalization) subsequently.

Suicide

Three of the four suicides were in unipolar patients; the other, in a bipolar patient. The numbers of patients in the various subgroups are too small to lend themselves to generalizations. These suicides (three of which occurred 1, 12, and 15 years after the index hospitalization, plus a fourth while the patient was in the hospital) do raise several questions: Is there a higher incidence in one versus another diagnostic group? Do suicides in MDP cluster during certain age periods? The present study cannot shed light on these questions, but several studies with large numbers of MDP patients have been completed; these either provide partial answers or else highlight current controversy.

Weeke and Vaeth (1986), for example, looked at mortality after 7 years in 2,168 manic–depressives (19% were bipolar) and noted that bipolars had a higher rate of deaths by causes other than suicide, but had a likelihood of suicide similar to that of the unipolars. The authors took into account the 5% of unipolars who, in their series, later showed bipolarity. Mortality rates were equal for the two genders and did not show dependence on age at first admission. Perris (1966) and Dunner, Gershon, and Goodwin (1976) reported a higher risk of suicide in bipolar patients; Angst, Felder, and Frey (1979), in their 14-year follow-up, found a higher suicide risk (10%) in unipolars compared with bipolars (3%).

In a more recent study, based on 37 suicides out of 212 deaths, Angst and Stassen (1986) reported a tendency toward *earlier* age of onset in these unipolar and bipolar patients who did eventually commit suicide. In contrast to Guze and Robins (1970) and Tsuang (1978), both of whom stated that suicides tended to occur within 10 years or so of index hospitalization, Angst and Stassen found that the suicide risk in MDP remained roughly the same in each phase of life, after the illness had declared itself. In comparison to the manic–depressives who had died of natural causes or causes other than suicide, the suicide group showed shorter cycle lengths between recurrences and spent a greater proportion of their life ill (30%) than did those who did not commit suicide (19%). As Angst and Stassen (1986, p. 160) point out, controlled studies of either psychotherapy or somatotherapy in MDP usually concentrate on samples of 100 or less, followed over brief time periods. They fail to explain how it is that the suicide rate has remained in the 10% (for bipolars) to 15% (for unipolars) range, despite the supposedly improved treatment approaches of the past generation. Actually, the pharmotherapy now available may, as these authors mention, diminish the suicide rate to some degree, to the extent that the drugs may reduce the intensity of symptoms and the frequency of relapse. This would argue for long-term prophylaxis rather than reliance on medication only if and when symptoms return.

Life Events and Life Trajectory

The role of life events in MDP is another area of controversy. The illness, especially its manic phases, appears to follow an internal rhythm related to central nervous system (CNS) neurotransmitter activity fluctuations that are relatively independent of external stresses. Yet not all investigators subscribe to this view. Ambelas (1987) compared 50 manics in their first episode with manics experiencing a relapse. Life events (e.g., death in the family, loss of job) had occurred in two-thirds of the first-episode manics, but only in a fifth of those with a second or third episode. This apparent susceptibility was independent of gender in Ambelas's experience, though Dunner, Patrick, and Fieve (1979) found that life events were more likely to trigger a manic episode in males. Ambelas felt that younger patients more often showed the life event–mania sequence and speculated that perhaps these events might advance the clock by as much as 20 years in some cases. The birth of a child sometimes acted as a precipitant in fathers, not just in mothers. Ambelas's finding is similar to that of Marneros, Rohde, Deister, Fimmers, and Jüremann (1988), who found that in schizoaffective patients life events more often precipitated a first than a subsequent outbreak of illness. In the present series, a life event had ushered in the psychosis in half the MDP patients, including half (13 of 25) of the bipolars.

Whereas Kraepelin (1921) spoke of a *restitutio ad integrum* as characteristic of MDP, we now recognize that many manic–depressives have serious underlying personality disorders (including borderline personality disorder [BPD]) and lifelong problems in social or occupational adjustment. Lithium brings about this long-lasting "restitution" in some bipolar patients, but not in all. These differences in life trajectory were discernible even within the small subgroups of the present study. At least five of the bipolar patients had been asymptomatic and essentially normal, usually on maintenance lithium, from the time of leaving the unit to that of follow-up. Another patient, incorrectly diagnosed as "schizophrenic" on review, was bipolar in retrospect—and had been well for many years, including the 13 years immediately prior to follow-up, when he stopped taking his lithium. One man had been asymptomatic on lithium for 25 years, but was working below his potential, deriving most of his financial support from his wife's family. Seven of the bipolars and one of the bipolar II patients had been chronically ill and dysfunctional since leaving PI, with many relapses and rehospitalizations. Some had negativistic personalities and were noncompliant about their medications, keeping their condition in a more active state than it would presumably otherwise be. These same personality attributes militated against the formation of a therapeutic alliance as well (some became "help-rejecting paranoid" persons), which also diminished their chances of a smooth life course. Several of the manic–depressive patients were quite the opposite—compliant and highly motivated to maintain a therapeutic relationship—and these qualities apparently helped to sustain them over difficult times. This was true even with some of the bipolar and predominantly manic patients, despite the common tendency of manics to exhibit denial of illness, grandiosity, insensitivity to emotional nuances, and inconsistency about the maintenance of contact with a therapist.

This raises, as a corollary, another important question, especially in relation to the bipolar patients. When a therapeutic relationship appears to ward off suicide in a manic–depressive, does this speak to the efficacy of the therapy per se? Or does the phenomenon reflect the increased likelihood that the patients who cling to life, who have the least anhedonia, and so on, will reach out to a therapist as a way of creating a stronger buffer against the urge to commit suicide, whereas certain other patients who are more anhedonic, more inclined to "give up," will fight shy of help and kill themselves no matter what? I felt that such distinctions were relevant to the MDP group in the PI-500 (as well as to several BPD patients who became unipolar). Three unipolar suicides in this series, for example—two female MDP patients and a BPD-turned-unipolar male—seemed destined not to form a therapeutic alliance with anyone, owing to adverse personality factors that long antedated their psychosis. Sometimes the personality abnormality was itself a product of the underlying illness and took the form of lifelong irritability and hostility, of a sort that demolished relationships with everyone (family members, potential friends, therapists). Thus we cannot always say that a good therapeutic relationship would have "saved" certain affectively ill patients, since this ignores pre-existing personality factors that might have rendered this impossible. The same paradox, where "the rich get richer . . . ," holds true among alcoholic patients: Some have favorable personality attributes that allow them to "click" with Alcoholics Anonymous (AA) and thus get even better, while others who are angry with the world, contemptuous of AA, and so on, continue to drink until their habit kills them.

Early life events may also have an impact on the course of MDP. Hällström (1987), in his study of women with major depression, noted an increased frequency of corporal punishment during childhoods, of poor relations with mothers, and of generally unhappy childhoods, compared with the experiences of a control group. Parental brutality was too uncommon in the manic–depressive patients of the present series (see Chapter Seven) to permit any generalizations. One adolescent male committed suicide as a direct result of his father's "soul murder." The other patient who experienced severe abuse made an excellent adjustment, as did one whose mother was abusive only on one or two occasions.

In McGlashan's Chestnut Lodge series unipolar depressed patients had long-term outcomes that were similar on most variables studied to those of the BPD patients (McGlashan, 1986a). Average Health–Sickness Rating Scale scores were 60 for the unipolars ($n = 44$ traced) and 64 for the borderlines ($n = 81$). Percentage ever married, work quality and level, hospital time, and continued treatment time after discharge were also similar. In the present series there were only eight unipolar patients, two of whom were well at follow-up, three of whom were "fair," and three of whom committed suicide. Even if combined with the two patients admitted for a psychotic depression, they constitute too small a group for comparison with McGlashan's unipolars.

Half the manic–depressive patients were rehospitalized at least once during the follow-up interval. The median follow-up GAS score of those who *never* required rehospitalization was 65: this was 20 points higher than the median figure for the ever-rehospitalized group.

Parental Disorders

Of the 76 biological parents, 7 had an affective psychosis (3 were bipolar); all 7 were among the parents of a bipolar I or II patient. Another 11 parents had milder conditions within the affective spectrum (e.g., cyclothymia, major depressive disorder). In the PI-500, there was no significant difference between MDP patients with negative family histories and those with ill parent(s), in relation either to percentage well at follow-up or to the presence of psychotic symptoms at index hospitalization.

With respect to psychotic symptoms, Winokur, Dennert, and Angst (1986) mentioned that a significant portion of unipolar and bipolar patients exhibit such symptoms at one time or another. From a genetic standpoint, Winokur et al. felt that the tendency toward psychotic symptoms did not seem to behave as an independent variable. Delusional depression, for example, did not breed true in families and may have been related instead to certain as yet undetermined nonfamilial, nongenetic factors.

Alcoholism, which Kraepelin (1921) found as a common accompaniment of MDP, was surprisingly rare among the parents of the MDP patients in this series (only 1 of 76 biological parents). Only three of the patients became alcoholic. This may relate to the high proportion (71%) of patients from Jewish backgrounds in the MDP group, during an era when alcoholism rates among Jews in this country were still quite low. The overrepresentation of Jewish patients among the manic–depressives (27 of 38), compared with the schizophrenics (43 of 99), was significant, $\chi^2 = 7.8$, $p < .01$. A number of investigators in recent years have challenged the notion that alcoholism may in some cases be a phenotype of MDP, concluding that the mood disorder and nonaffective concomitants, such as alcoholism, reflect *independent* genetic transmission (Grove et al., 1987). Grove et al. feel that the co-occurrence of these factors in a patient is more likely to be the result of extrafamilial factors, or of familial factors related to the nonaffective conditions.

The relationship between plasma catecholamines and psychotic versus nonpsychotic depression before and after dexamethasone challege has been the subject of several recent studies (Rothschild et al., 1987; Schatzberg et al., 1987). The era of the PI-500 ended before such studies could be carried out routinely. Future follow-up studies of manic–depressive patients might benefit by incorporation of key biochemical determinations into their design, in the event that prognostic significance may attach to some of the results (e.g., high suicidality/aggressivity with low CNS serotonin; greater tendency to psychotic depressions in those with particularly low postdexamethasone plasma norepinephrine; etc.).

Summary

In summary, nearly half the manic–depressive patients, whether bipolar or unipolar, had had a benign course at follow-up. Four committed suicide; the remainder showed residual symptoms and had a stormier course, characterized by repeated episodes and rehospitalizations. Like the schizoaffective patients, their course and outcome as a group showed more variability (and less predictability) in course and outcome than the schizophrenic patients, whose follow-up GAS scores clustered in the marginal range, or than the dysthymic borderlines, the majority of whom recovered.

Outcome Patterns

LIFE TRAJECTORIES IN PREVIOUS STUDIES

In a follow-up study where several hundred patients were traced by one investigator, even the most precise data necessarily reflect the functioning of each patient at the moment of the interview. What is important, nonetheless, is not so much the level of that momentary functioning, but the precise shape of the life course from birth through the period of index hospitalization to the follow-up time many years later. Harding and Strauss (1985) have pointed this out in their chapter on the course of schizophrenics whom they followed for several decades. To prepare a life chart that accurately portrays the year-by-year state of such key variables as work, social and intimate life, and general emotional health requires periodic assessments at brief intervals—something quite beyond the scope of a lone investigator using a retrospective technic. To be sure, a handful of the patients or their relatives in the present study were so candid and so precise in their recollection of details concerning the past 10 or 20 years that a life chart could be constructed. Such life charts are rudimentary and sketchy, compared to those made by investigators moving along the life trajectory in lockstep with the patients—yet they are not without value.

Life trajectories have been presented in a variety of ways by epidemiologists of mental illness. M. Bleuler (1972), for example, illustrates the natural histories of schizophrenic patients he followed by means of diagrams where the peaks represent poor functioning and the valleys indicate good functioning or freedom from symptoms. Thus, the overall clinical picture of a certain "Klara E.," who suffered from late-onset paranoid schizophrenia, was charted as shown in Figure 13.1. This woman had functioned well until age 49, had then remained severely incapacitated until almost 60, and had later recuperated to the point of showing only minor symptoms and disability for the last 7 years of her life. Many other patterns were discernible among the 208 schizophrenics in M. Bleuler's large series.

Ciompi and Müller (1976) used a similar method in their book on the long-term follow-up of schizophrenia patients. These authors, having traced the

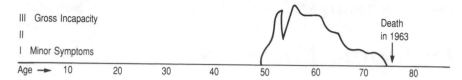

FIGURE 13.1. Overall clinical picture of "Klara E." Adapted from Bleuler, M. (1972) *Die Schizophrenen Geistessörungen* (p. 294). Stuttgart: Thieme Verlag. Adapted by permission.

life course of several hundred patients, grouped the various trajectories into a smaller number of schemata based on M. Bleuler's typology. The schemata that emerged from their investigations permitted still further generalizations into simple, wave-shaped, and atypical forms (p. 73). The diagrams shown in Figure 13.2 are representative. Ciompi and Müller's book (1976, p. 14 ff.) also contains a most useful and exhaustive review of the major long-term (ranging from 5- to 56-year) follow-up studies of schizophrenics, from Rennie's in 1939 through Huber's study in 1973.

Huber and his colleagues in Bonn (Gross & Huber, 1973; Huber, Gross, Schüttler, & Linz, 1980) discerned over six dozen patterns in the 502 schizophrenics they followed for an average of 21 years. These patterns could be compartmentalized into 12 main categories, a figure only somewhat greater than the 8 types generated by Ciompi and Müller's observations. The latter, identifying onset as either acute or chronic, course as either wave-like or simple, and end state as either mild-to-recovered or moderately-to-severely-impaired, created eight (2 × 2 × 2) possibilities.

Harding and Strauss (1985) relied upon more complex methods of representation. Whereas their Swiss and German predecessors utilized diagrams of global functioning, the authors of the Vermont study analyzed functioning using five-tiered flow charts—one each for work, social support, residence, medications, and mental health, respectively. As with M. Bleuler's diagrams, peaks and valleys indicate "good," "problematic," or "poor" functioning in any given area.

Léon (1989), in a 10-year follow-up study of 101 schizophrenic patients in Colombia, South America, could discern some nine patterns of life course. The most common were the "episodic recurrent," the "continuous stationary," and the "continuous, severe." These were associated with poor outcome. Patients with a more favorable life course tended to exhibit the "single episode" or the "episodic, occasional" course. The latter two accounted for 21% of the sample.

Much more long-term follow-up work has been done in the domain of schizophrenia than in that of borderline conditions. Few have thus far attempted to work out life trajectories or even posthospitalization life courses of borderline patients, apart from McGlashan (1985). In his Chestnut Lodge study, McGlashan noted several typical patterns among the 81 patients with DSM-III-defined borderline personality disorder (BPD). One such pattern was characterized by a relatively long period of poor functioning (5–10 years, usually during a patient's 20s or early 30s) followed by gradual (at times, more rapid) recovery. In some borderlines followed into their late 40s to early 50s, however, there was a loss of support system (often enough owing to divorce or breakup of a sexual partnership), with a subsequent downturn in functioning after the patients had maintained rather good functioning for several years. Borderline patients seemed more than ordinarily vulnerable to this kind of "midlife crisis" because of their tendency to remain rather demanding and irascible, heightening the likelihood of alienating a spouse or intimate companion.

Using patients with DSM-III-defined schizophrenia (SZ) and unipolar depression as comparison groups, McGlashan found that, while two-thirds of the schizophrenics were either continuously incapacitated or marginally adjusted at follow-up, and only rarely well or recovered, the DSM-III-defined borderlines

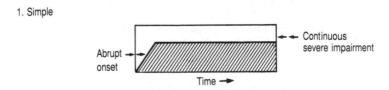

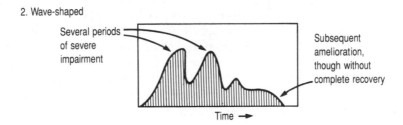

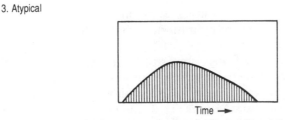

FIGURE 13.2. Ciompi and Müller's three main types of life trajectories. Adapted from Ciompi, L., and Müller, C. (1976) *Lebensweg und Alter der Schizophrenen* (p. 73). Berlin: Springer-Verlag. Adapted by permission.

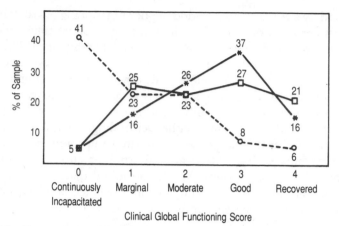

FIGURE 13.3. Frequencies of global functioning scores since discharge for BPD (asterisks; *n* = 81), schizophrenic (circles; *n* = 163), and unipolar depressive (squares; *n* = 44) groups. From McGlashan, T. H. (1986a) The Chestnut Lodge follow-up study: III. Long-term outcome of borderline personalities. *Arch. Gen. Psychiatry 43:* 20–30. Reprinted by permission.

were doing poorly (incapacitated or marginal) only in a fifth of the cases. Half the borderlines were considered "good" or "recovered" in their adjustment. The distribution in global outcomes among the unipolars more nearly resembled that of the borderlines. These observations are illustrated in Figure 13.3, reprinted from McGlashan's 1986a report.

Using the same 5-point scale (from 0 = "continuously incapacitated" to 4 = "recovered"), McGlashan provided another chart plotting the global outcome score in the borderlines according to their average ages at each of several 5-year follow-up intervals. As noted in Figure 13.4, the borderlines were usually struggling through their late 20s and early 30s, during which life phase they were only moderately well (working more than half the time, a few friends, a small amount of time in structured settings, some asymptomatic periods); they finally gained higher ground during their late 30s and early 40s. Some slipped back later on, as alluded to above, through subsequent failure of support systems (especially in the realm of close relationships), such that the group average at age 57 descended to the 2.4 level.

In biological systems of any large size, one expects normal gaussian distribution with respect to key variables: Roughly two-thirds of the individuals should demonstrate "average" readings, a sixth should surpass these averages, and a sixth should fall back. Figure 13.3 shows that the average global functioning score in McGlashan's 81 borderlines was 2.48, corresponding to an outcome between "moderately impaired" and "good." Because the *typical* outcome of the borderlines was "good," however, the curve is bowed to the right: The modal point overlies the score 3.0. When portrayed according to this

5-point schema, the schizophrenics' outcomes do not even describe a bell curve, skewed or otherwise: Their average score was 1.2, but the *peak* of the curve was at the extreme left (41% with scores of 0).

As we compare the results in the Chestnut Lodge patients with those in the PI-500, we should keep in mind that the Chestnut Lodge patients were on average 5 years older than the PI-500 patients, and were contacted at intervals averaging 5 years longer beyond discharge (21.5 vs. 16.5). The PI-500 patients are now mostly in their late 30s and 40s; many of the Chestnut Lodge patients are already in their 50s. Also, the outcomes for the PI-500 patients are recorded as Global Assessment Scale (GAS) scores—specifically, as the latest or most typical GAS level. The distributions of the GAS scores within all diagnostic subgroups of the present series do describe "bell curves," varying in flatness or lopsidedness with respect to their modal points.

The flattening of the bell curve is particularly noticeable when plotting outcome in patients with manic–depressive psychosis (MDP) and schizoaffective psychosis (SA). In the extreme example, a straight line overlying a parallel to the abscissa (graded according to outcome level) would indicate that an equal number of patients fell into each of the compartments. A symmetrical but gentle curve, as in Figure 13.5, should correspond to a situation where there were *nearly* as many patients at the extremes as in the central regions. This is what a number of investigators have observed in follow-up studies of bipolar and schizoaffective patients. Outcomes in these two groups are similar, as one may note in Table 13.1, reprinted from Angst, Felder, and Lohmeyer (1980). Here, the two extreme interpretations of this curve are as follows: (1) All bipolar patients have a checkered life trajectory, spending some time "well," some time "incapacitated," but the bulk of their life "fair"; or (2) bipolar patients are

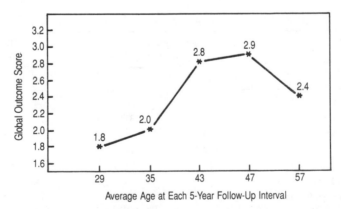

FIGURE 13.4. Global outcome score by follow-up age (in years) and interval, BPD group. From McGlashan, T. H. (1986a) The Chestnut Lodge follow-up study: III. Long-term outcome of borderline personalities. *Arch. Gen. Psychiatry 43:* 20–30. Reprinted by permission.

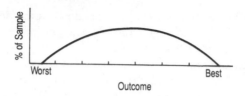

FIGURE 13.5. Bell curve illustrating the type of outcome distribution often found in studies of manic–depressive and schizoaffective patients.

probably divisible into two small groups who are always either "well" or "ill" and a large group whose function is always "fair."

Later, in discussing the patterns that emerged as the present follow-up study progressed, we shall have a chance to look once again at the question: How much and how well can we predict, given some knowledge of *group* outcome, concerning the life trajectory of the patients who made up that group?

Meanwhile, we must address briefly another issue raised by the disparity between Huber and the Swiss investigators (Angst and Ciompi) over the *number* of outcome patterns one might expect the data to reveal. Huber spoke of 73 types (Gross & Huber, 1973); Ciompi, of 8 (Ciompi & Müller, 1976). Huber later regrouped his 73 into 12 broader patterns. In part, the seemingly correct number is probably a function of our brains' internal "wiring." We are more adept at recognizing different patterns (e.g., similar vs. different faces) than at recalling their precise number and the separate name for each. Large numbers of named patterns tend to collapse into smaller, more manageable numbers of broader categories. There may be some meaningful criteria that justify Huber's elaboration of 73 "patterns" of life trajectory. From a *practical* standpoint, nevertheless, Angst, Ciompi, and Huber himself worked with a dozen or less.

TABLE 13.1. Degree of Remission in Two Patient Groups

	Schizoaffective disorders		Bipolar disorders	
	n	%	*n*	%
Full remission	40	26.7	34	35.8
Partial remission	52	37.7	26	27.4
Chronic course	3	2.0	—	—
Ongoing episode	22	14.7	12	12.6
Death during episode	17	11.3	7	7.4
Suicide during episode	5	3.3	3	3.2
Organic brain syndrome	9	6.0	13	13.7
Unknown	2	1.3	—	—
Total	150		95	

Note. From Angst, J., Felder, W., and Lohmeyer, B. (1980) Course of schizoaffective psychoses: Results of a follow-up study. *Schizophr. Bull.* 6: 579–585. Reprinted by permission.

LIFE TRAJECTORY METHODOLOGY IN THE PRESENT STUDY

By definition, mental *illness* is the opposite of "wellness" and implies some deviation downward from the level of social and occupational functioning of average people, or from any other arbitrary level one finds useful. In the GAS, the decile 61–70 corresponds to "some mild symptoms . . . generally functioning pretty well . . . most untrained persons would not consider [the patient] sick." A GAS score of 61 provides a useful cutoff point between "ill" and "well." Plotting the GAS scores over frequent intervals permits one to assess the amount of time spent below this minimal level of good function, throughout the life course up till the moment of (latest) follow-up. This exercise corresponds to the meteorologist's method for measuring "degree days" during winter—that is, the cumulative number of degrees, day by day, by which the temperature outside is less than comfortable room temperature (68°). If, for example, the average temperature on January 1 was 40°, on January 2 was 45°, and on January 3 was 37°, that would add up to 82 "degree days" for the 3 days. In retrospective long-term studies such as the present one, information is too skimpy to allow measure of "degree days"; we will have to be satisfied with a grosser measure of "degree years." In Figure 13.6, I have illustrated this notion, using the life trajectories of three borderline patients followed at fairly frequent intervals (every year in Case 2; every 5–6 years in Cases 1 and 3) over 22 years or longer. The GAS levels are plotted; those portions of the life curve spent *below* a GAS score of 61 are shaded. The first patient (Case 1) had a rocky course for the first 10 years but did well more recently. Still subject to spells of depression and somewhat bitter about the past at her latest follow-up, she functioned in the mid-60 GAS range after her late 30s. Cumulatively, she showed 148 "degree years" over a 23-year span (i.e., 6.4 per year). This would correspond to an average GAS score of 53.6 since she left PI. This number happens not to reflect her typical functioning, since she was consistently worse during the first decade and consistently better afterwards.

The patient in Case 2, agoraphobic and self-mutilative initially, left the hospital only mildly phobic. She was able to work when her younger child turned 4 and functioned as a clinically recovered person until her late 30s and early 40s, when she divorced and later remarried to an unstable man. There was considerable marital strife in the new marriage, pushing her into the area of "degree days" for the first time in 20 years. In "degree years," she showed 209 above 60 and 20 below for a total of −189 (− 8.6 per year), corresponding to an average GAS score of 68.6 over the whole span.

The patient in Case 3, a borderline who has become manic–depressive, almost never worked after discharge, was living a constricted life with her second husband at latest follow-up, and was on medication consistently the whole 24 years. Her "degree years" totaled 348, 14.5 GAS points per year below "good" functioning; this corresponds to an average GAS score of 45.5, which, given the straightness of her life trajectory, was actually her usual level.

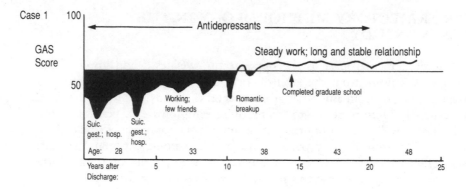

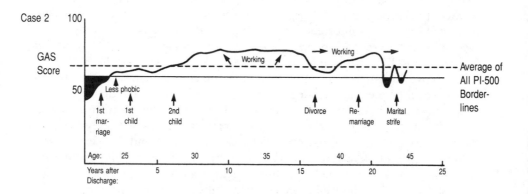

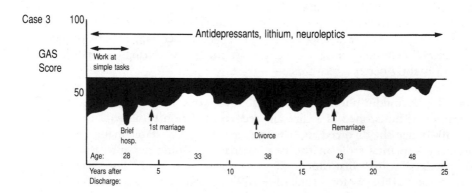

FIGURE 13.6. Life trajectories of three PI-500 borderline patients, plotted according to GAS scores at fairly frequent follow-up intervals. Portions of each trajectory below a GAS score of 61 (''degree years'') are shaded.

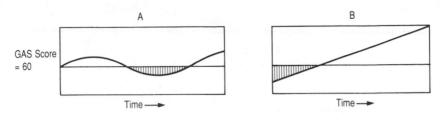

FIGURE 13.7. Two different types of life trajectories with roughly equivalent "degree years."

Life trajectories that are equivalent in "degree years" are not necessarily experienced in the same way. From the patient's standpoint, it is much better to have logged a number of difficult years in the beginning and to have become well lately than to have had ups and downs of about equal duration year in and year out. Of the trajectories in Figure 13.7, for example, B is clearly preferable. By the same token, conditions usually associated with a trajectory of Type B will often be regarded as prognostically better than will those associated with Type A. I have paid special attention, therefore, to patient variables that augured well for eventual recovery, in contrast to variables that predicted a more oscillating course.

In the material that follows, I hope to demonstrate some of the outcome patterns discernible within the PI-500. Examination of the patterns predominating in any given diagnostic subgroup may then enhance our predictive powers concerning similar patients encountered currently, and may shed some light on the root causes behind the "favorite" trajectories of certain subgroups. Why, for example, should there be waviness in one group, linearity in another, and irregularity in the life course of still another group?

As an aid to this exercise, I have developed my own catalog of patterns—not as ambitious as Huber's 73, nor yet as simple as Ciompi's 8. I have relied on Ciompi's schema, however, adapting it in a way I felt would better highlight the natural history of the PI-500 series (containing, as it did, three times as many borderlines as schizophrenics). I generated the 15 patterns by collapsing the outcome levels at follow-up into three: "good" (GAS scores > 61), "fair" (GAS scores = 51–60), and "poor" (GAS scores < 51, including suicides). These three levels, multiplied by five basic trajectories (gradual incline, steep incline, undular, linear, and atypical), yield 15 patterns. They are illustrated in Figure 13.8, where the words "slow," "quick," "wavy," "linear," and "atypical" are used to denote the different trajectories.

Armed with this schema, I could then match up the life course of each traced patient with one of the first four trajectories, failing which the pattern was called "atypical." Since seven out of eight patients are still alive, I could not speak so much of "end result" as of *latest* level at the time the patient was traced. Only for a few patients was I able to prepare a life chart as dense with details of work, social life, and treatment as the ones prepared by Harding and Strauss

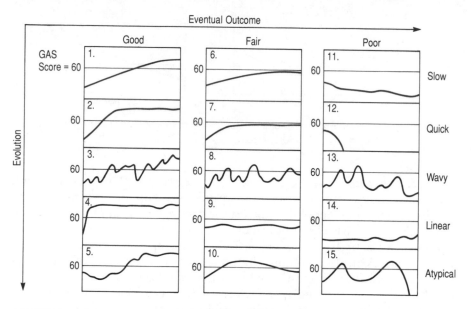

FIGURE 13.8. Some common life trajectories in formerly hospitalized patients of the PI-500.

(1985). Those were the patients my colleagues and I had followed ever since discharge or had continued to contact over the years with exchanges of letters. But most of the follow-ups were retrospective and at the mercy of the generosity (or taciturnity) of the respondents.

OUTCOME PATTERNS IN THE BORDERLINE DOMAIN

I was able to reconstruct the overall trajectory of the life course during the follow-up years in all but 19 of the traced borderline patients. Two-thirds of the patients had "good" outcomes; a sixth had "fair" and a sixth "poor" outcomes. The predominant patterns among the good-outcome patients were those of "quick" recovery (40%) and "slow" or "atypical" recovery (20% each). These ratios were approximately the same for those with BPD as for the dysthymics and other borderlines. No predominant patterns emerged among the patients with a less favorable life course. Of interest was the finding that a quarter of the worst-functioning BPD patients showed a "wavy" course, consistent with the fluctuating moods of the bipolar illness many went on to develop in the posthospital years. Another quarter (10 of 38) of the BPD patients with poor outcomes committed suicide shortly after leaving the hospital, and thus showed the "quick" (in this case, quickly downhill) pattern.

The "atypical" trajectory was usually the expression of 5–10 years of substance abuse and chaotic life, followed by abstention and rapid recovery. In other cases, the initial dip reflected severe depression with recurrent suicidal gestures and occasional rehospitalizations, until a higher and stable plateau was reached sometime in the fourth decade of life. Four of the BPD females showed a life course otherwise compatible with trajectory 1 in Figure 13.8 (slow recovery), except that the linearity was interrupted in midcourse by a sudden downturn (often, a romantic breakup with a suicide gesture and rehospitalization) and subsequent resumption of the gradual uphill trend. The resulting shape was as shown in the top half of Figure 13.9. Several others held high ground for many years until a divorce or breakup in their mid-30s led to a modest downturn; however, they remained within the region of recovery, as shown in the bottom half of Figure 13.9.

OUTCOME PATTERNS IN PATIENTS PRESENTING WITH PSYCHOSIS

The Schizophrenic Patients

Table 13.2 summarizes the distribution of outcome patterns I noted among the schizophrenic patients. The predominant pattern among these patients was a "linear" trajectory. Three out of five schizophrenics exhibited this pattern,

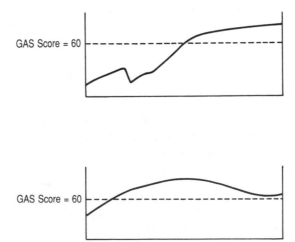

FIGURE 13.9. Two variations on trajectory 1 in Figure 13.8, exhibited by female BPD patients in the PI-500.

TABLE 13.2. Outcome Patterns in the Schizophrenic Patients (*n* Traced = 96): Number in Each Subtype

	Follow-up status		
Pattern of change	Good	Fair	Poor
Slow	4	2	5
Quick	4	0	4
Wavy	0	2	6
Linear	0	0	59
Atypical	1	0	1

Note. Uncertain, 8; untraced, 4.

remaining over the years at about the same functional level ("poor") as when they left the unit.

The few who showed "quick" recovery included the fée counterculture woman who later married a protective husband (see "Attractiveness," Chapter Eight); the woman who sought psychosurgery for what was probably a severe obsessive–compulsive/erotomanic disorder rather than true schizophrenia (see "Lobotomy," Appendix B); and a man who was killed in a car accident when returning home for Thanksgiving. He had gone to graduate school right after leaving the unit, had worked full-time, and was engaged to be married. A fourth patient also completed graduate school shortly after leaving the hospital and worked in the computer field ever since. He lived alone at follow-up but had a fairly wide circle of friends.

The recovered patient with the "atypical" course was the one mentioned in "Religious Cults" (Appendix B), who checked in with his psychiatrist whenever he noticed himself getting preoccupied with cabalistic mysticism. He showed the ladle-shaped pattern that was common among the borderline patients.

Eight of the schizophrenic patients had a "wavy" trajectory (two with a "fair" and six with a "poor" outcome), characterized usually by multiple brief rehospitalizations followed by longer periods of somewhat better functioning. One young woman left the unit, completed college, made a suicide attempt, spent a few months in another treatment facility, met and lived with a boyfriend in a shabby area where she was twice raped, and at follow-up was living with another friend in a less run-down neighborhood. She was seldom able to work and continued to receive support from her family. One of the males went through a similar succession of up and downs until the final down of his suicide. Another male had a course typical of certain schizoaffectives, which alternated between lows—generated by depressive episodes, suicide attempts, and rehospitalizations (four in 18 years)—and better phases, in which he worked, took courses, and (briefly) married. Figure 13.10 sketches his life course since 1972.

Of the four schizophrenics showing "slow" but steady improvement, one was a man who took various odd jobs when first discharged and required two week-long rehospitalizations during the year he left the unit, but who then was able to complete on-the-job training in a computer-related company. At latest follow-up, he had held a good position there for over 10 years, and had also developed a steady relationship with a woman he planned to marry. Initially he was preoccupied with fears that his coworkers were making invidious comments about him or that his boss disliked him, but these fears grew much less intense over the years—partly through therapy, partly through the realization (now that he was a respected employee of many years' standing) that the environment could not have been as malign as he had imagined or he would not still be on the payroll.

The usual life trajectory among the schizophrenic patients of this study was, in contrast to the one described above, quite flat, or else one of no more than gentle fluctuations—unvarying marginal functioning with an occasional downturn and rehospitalization. One such patient left our unit and lived for the 16 years from discharge to follow-up with her immediate family or relatives. She had many of the "negative" signs (see Chapter Twelve), but was quite fearful in the presence of strangers. Although rehospitalized only once (briefly) because of delusions that returned during a time when her medications needed readjustment, she was never able to work or to maintain a friendship. If she skipped her medication for a few days, her family noticed the return of bizarre thoughts.

The Other Diagnostic Groups

Briefly, among the *schizoaffective* patients, a "linear" course with "poor" outcome was the most common (15 examples); this pattern was followed by "quick" change for the worse (8, including many of those who committed suicide in hospital or within a few years after discharge) or "slow" recovery (8). Recovery via an "atypical" pattern was also common (6).

Two patterns accounted for half the outcomes among the *manic–depressives:*

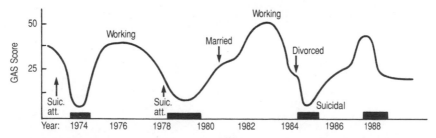

FIGURE 13.10.   Life course since 1972 of a schizophrenic patient in the PI-500. Black bars indicate periods of rehospitalization.

an "atypical" course with eventual "good" outcome, and a "wavy" course with "poor" (usually marginal) outcome.

The *schizophreniform* (SF) patients were most apt to show one of two patterns: a "good" result via "slow" recovery, or an "atypical" course. The latter, as with many of the borderlines, represented several years after hospitalization of continuing substance abuse, followed by abstinence and rapid recovery.

CHAPTER FOURTEEN

Effects of Therapist and Type of Therapy

A study of the natural history of psychiatric patients will not usually be able to shed much light on the relative efficacy of various forms of treatment. This is all the more true of retrospective studies, especially when the variable we are weighing happens to be subtle, such as contrasting forms of psychotherapy. Long-term follow-up is even more handicapped in this regard, owing to the large number of intervening events during the 10- to 20-year interim and to the difficulty in reconstructing the typical nature of the therapeutic process at the time. Was the psychotherapy consistently transference-oriented? Did the interventions shift from supportive to expressive at a certain point? Was the supportive therapy analytically informed and intensive (e.g., three or four sessions a week lasting 45 minutes each) or very matter-of-fact and nonintensive (e.g., one or two sessions a week lasting 20 or 30 minutes each)? Even if we have enough data at hand to address these questions adequately, we still need to be concerned about the issue of matched populations (are the "comparison groups" truly comparable?).

THERAPIST EFFECTS

With respect to the PI-500, I did not think it possible to assign the patients in a consistent manner to dichotomous groups, such as "exploratory therapy, working consistently with the transference" versus "supportive therapy with no allusions to the transference." Because the therapists were trainees, however, I was able to classify them, using the reports by the unit's administrators and supervisors, into a few broad categories of general competence. We rated the therapists according to a number of qualities, including integrity, maturity, empathic capacity, psychological aptitude, cooperativeness with the ancillary staff, decisiveness, grasp of the relevant literature, general grasp of clinical situations, professional demeanor, candor, and emotional "warmth." We could agree most readily on the least effective therapists, some of whom showed commendable integrity and good general knowledge but little ability to understand psychodynamics or the symbolic overtones of their patients' comments. A few therapists were actually mendacious, unprofessional, or exploitative. We could agree less readily on the "best" therapists, since we could not be certain that the qualities the supervisors most admired were the ones that made them the most effective therapists with their patients. One man we considered "average," for example, was not average in the recollection of his patients: All I contacted at follow-up remembered him fondly and felt that he had been largely responsible for their recovery. In their eyes, he was certainly a "best" therapist.

I sought, at all events, to compare the outcomes of patients who had worked with a "best" therapist to the outcomes of those whose therapists had been the least competent. Because of the long stay on our unit, some patients worked with several therapists, especially if they entered the unit near the time of the academic rotation of residents. In developing two lists—patients with a "best" and patients with a "worst" therapist—I omitted any who had worked with one of each. Any differences that might emerge would still have little to do with the efficacy of exploratory therapy, analytically informed supportive therapy, purely reassuring/re-educative supportive therapy, or any other therapeutic approach. All the therapists aimed, as far as their abilities allowed, toward at least a supportive technic bolstered by analytic insights on their part regarding where the patient was "at" from moment to moment. Beyond that, each therapist tried to work directly with the transference–countertransference field, focusing mostly on the here-and-now; there was less emphasis on the distant past. Differences in results, if any, would therefore reflect not so much technic as the general competence and "humanness" of the therapists.

Among the schizophrenic (SZ) patients, the outcomes in the two groups showed little variation and were not significantly different. The severity of the underlying condition seemed to be the overriding factor determining outcome.

Among the larger group of borderlines, the patients with the "best" therapists were more likely to appear in the good-to-recovered category (GAS scores > 60) at follow-up (47 of 63, or 75%); only about half (17 of 32, or 53%) of the patients with a "worst" therapist reached this level. Figure 14.1 shows the distribution. However, the average follow-up GAS score was only slightly higher in those with a "best" than in those with a "worst" therapist (69 vs. 63). This is a narrower difference than the one I reported earlier (Stone, 1987), at a time when I had not yet traced a few borderlines (with a "best" therapist) whose outcomes happened to be in the marginal range. The median scores were nearly the same as the average scores.

The presence of marked antisocial features—enough, for example, to justify a second diagnosis of antisocial personality (ASP) by DSM criteria—would presumably militate against the efficacy of the conventional psychotherapies. Having many such patients in a sample would tend to create a bias against the

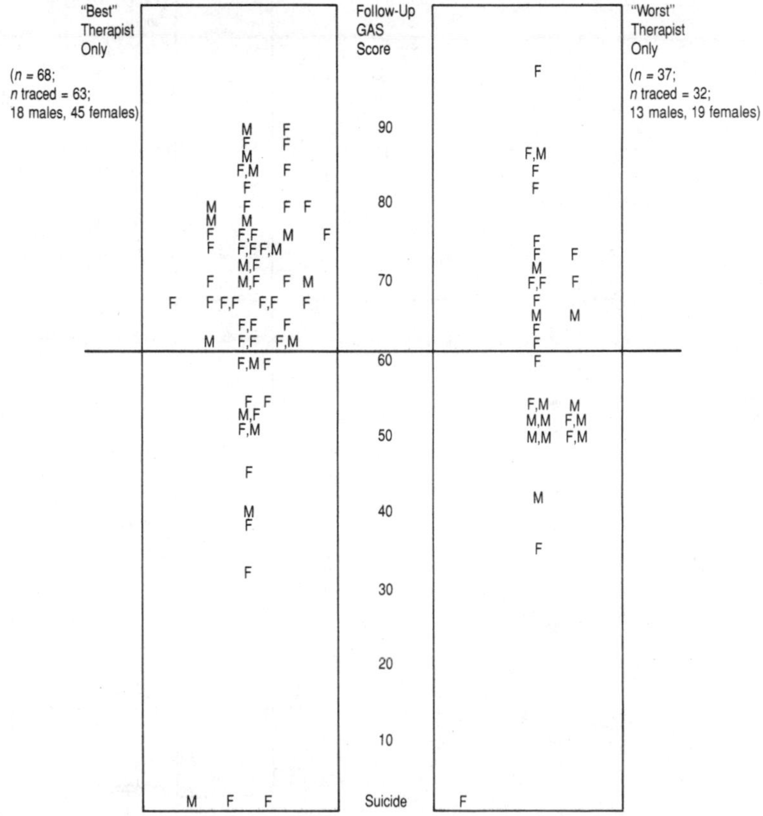

"Best" Therapist Only	Follow-Up GAS Score	"Worst" Therapist Only
(*n* = 68; *n* traced = 63; 18 males, 45 females)		(*n* = 37; *n* traced = 32; 13 males, 19 females)

```
"Best"                          Follow-Up                  "Worst"
Therapist                       GAS                        Therapist
Only                            Score                      Only

(n = 68;                                      F            (n = 37;
n traced = 63;                                             n traced = 32;
18 males, 45 females)                                      13 males, 19 females)

                   M     F        90
                   F     F
                   M                          F,M
                 F,M     F                    F
                   F                          F
              M    F    F F       80
              M    M
              F   F,F    M    F
              F   F,F,F,M                      F
                 M,F                           F      F
              F  M,F    F  M      70           M
          F   F F,F  F,F   F                 F,F      F
                                              F
                 F,F    F                      M      M
              M  F,F   F,M                     F
                 F,M F             60          F

                 F    F
                M,F                           F,M     M
                F,M               50          M,M    F,M
                                              M,M    F,M

                 F

                 M                40          M
                 F

                 F                                   F
                                  30

                                  20

                                  10

          M   F   F           Suicide    F
```

FIGURE 14.1. Effects of having a "best" versus a "worst" therapist among the borderline patients.

revelation of a therapist/therapy effect, if such an effect were present. The males were more likely to exhibit antisocial features than the females; the borderline males assigned to a "worst" therapist were more often antisocial (7 of 13) than were those assigned to a "best" therapist (2 of 18). Since we made the assignments randomly (with very rare exceptions), I do not know how to account for this difference other than as a chance phenomenon.

Subtracting the antisocial patients from the reckoning yielded "best"- and "worst"-therapist groups of female borderlines with identical average GAS scores at follow-up (68). Their partitioning into two broad compartments (GAS scores ≤ 60, GAS scores > 60) was now nearly equal: 76% (34 of 45) of those with a "best" therapist had scores above 60; 68% (13 of 19) of those with a "worst" therapist had such scores. Significant differences were found only in the male borderlines (without antisocial personality). As Figure 14.2 illustrates, the average GAS score in males of this group with a "best" therapist was 71 (rounded off); in males with a "worst" therapist, it was 52. By partitions, 13 of

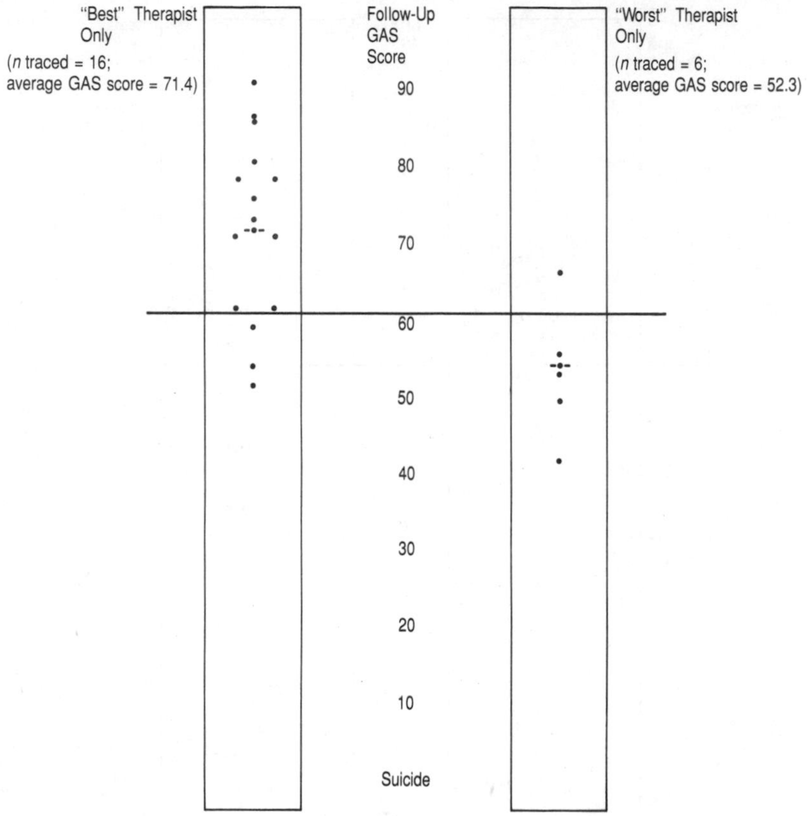

"Best" Therapist Only		Follow-Up GAS Score		"Worst" Therapist Only
(*n* traced = 16; average GAS score = 71.4)		90		(*n* traced = 6; average GAS score = 52.3)
		80		
		70		
		60		
		50		
		40		
		30		
		20		
		10		
		Suicide		

FIGURE 14.2. Effects of having a "best" versus a "worst" therapist among male borderlines without ASP. The dot with lines on either side indicates the median case in each group.

16 with a "best" therapist had GAS scores > 60, as against 1 of 6 in the "worst"-therapist group ($p < .001$, Fisher's exact test). Here we may be in the realm of statistically significant differences of clinically not very meaningful phenomena, whereas some differences may have existed in the clinical material (e.g., superlative therapists may indeed have had better success than mediocre therapists) that the present study cannot demonstrate.

One can begin to appreciate how problematical tests of therapeutic efficacy are—the more so when one takes into consideration the fact that most comparison studies, even randomized studies, concentrate on two or more therapeutic approaches, and must *assume* equal efficacy of the therapists. Ethical constraints would militate against a design utilizing "worst" therapists on purpose as a "control group" for excellent therapists, in the study of one form of psychotherapy. We gather impressions about the impact of "best" versus "worst" therapists only from necessarily imprecise naturalistic studies. The more scientifically correct a research design in the study of psychotherapy is, the less similarity it has to treatment as it is "in nature." Question and method tend to pass each other by. Time creates another problem: Follow-ups at *brief* intervals are probably better indices of possible benefits from a particular therapeutic technic. Life has less opportunity to introduce extraneous variables into a short as opposed to a long interval. But short-term follow-up of borderlines fails to capture their potential for ultimate clinical improvement (as we and several other groups of investigators have noted), and thus also yields a distorted picture.

Quite apart from their ability (or lack of it) to understand symbolism, form a therapeutic alliance, and so on, certain therapists have (1) keener clinical judgment regarding suicidality and (2) greater vigor in taking the steps necessary to thwart a suicide attempt than do some of their colleagues. But this, too, is hard to measure. Suicide is a rare event; therapists do not compete with one another using cloned sets of suicidal patients to see who loses the fewest patients. In examining the list of suicides in the PI-500, I can see two instances in which greater clinical perspicacity would have saved the day. The *day*. Not necessarily the year, let alone the remaining lifespan that (actuarially, at least) awaited those patients. One was the friendless borderline woman mentioned in Chapter Four, both of whose parents had recently committed suicide. The other was a schizophrenic man whose therapist had apparently overlooked some fairly striking clues of suicidal intent. Both patients killed themselves while on brief passes from the unit.

The suicide rate is already high in the PI-500 borderlines (see Chapter Four). How much of this is accounted for by therapist effect? I am uncertain. But I believe that therapist insouciance and misjudgment account for only a small portion; the rest has to do with severity of illness and with systemic effects, such as the inability of the mental health facilities at that time to provide adequate haven for our patients' most vulnerable years.

The other factors also contribute to the obfuscation of the therapist's role. Ours was a hospitalized population. We simply cannot disentangle the effects of the one-to-one therapy from those of the interactions with the nursing staff and other supportive personnel. Pharmacotherapy (which almost every patient received in some form), group therapy, family therapy, and (in selected cases) behavior therapy played their part alongside the dyadic psychotherapy. Some patients expressed special gratitude toward a particular therapist, but in reality the gratitude might better have been expressed toward the "collective"—the entire personnel and its *esprit de corps*—in which the "primary therapists" (as they are now known in hospital circles) were sometimes the dominant and curative force, sometimes a subsidiary element whose effects were much less noticeable.

EFFECTS OF TYPE OF THERAPY: EXPRESSIVE VERSUS SUPPORTIVE

Through long-term follow-up of the PI-500, I sought primarily to answer questions about the natural history of patients hospitalized for various emotional disorders. I was interested, at the same time, in studying the efficacy of different forms of psychotherapy in these categories of patients—most especially, of psychoanalytically oriented psychotherapy. The latter is also known under several other overlapping though not entirely synonymous terms (e.g., "expressive therapy," "exploratory therapy," "dynamic therapy," and "insight-oriented therapy"). Whether measure of its efficacy is amenable to scientific methodology is an open question.

Randomization of the newly admitted patients into two groups—one to receive expressive therapy, one to receive supportive therapy—would have been most useful. In 1970, we carried out a pilot study relying on this technic. We were able to include only a dozen patients in each group. The admitting staff of the unit accepted for randomization only those patients aged 19 or over who appeared to be amenable to expressive therapy. The expressive therapy was to focus on interpretive work, clarifications, and dream analysis. The supportive therapy was not to exceed 50 minutes per week (usually as five 10-minute sessions, or else a 20-minute session plus two or three brief meetings), whereas the format for the expressive therapy was three 45-minute sessions per week.

One serious flaw in the research design consisted in our utilizing the same therapists ("PGY-3" residents) for both groups. They were not at all enthusiastic about supportive therapy and may well have transmitted to the patients receiving this therapy their impression of its being second-best. Looking at outcomes 20 years later, we may actually find an advantage to this flawed design if, and only if, the old "supportive" group did as well as the "expressive" group. Such a result would incline us toward the belief that the specific form of the psychotherapy did not make much difference, since everyone did well—even those with whom their therapists had spent little time. If the supportive group had significantly *worse* outcomes, we could always criticize the design, claiming that supportive treatment carried out by those who were really skilled at it and enthusiastic about it would have yielded a result comparable to that achieved by the more intensive therapy. If *optimal* expressive therapy, using therapists more seasoned than our second-year resident trainees, clearly outperformed optimal supportive therapy in a large group of borderline patients, we could at last claim superiority for the expressive mode—only to have to wonder, nevertheless, whether some other technic would have been superior to both. Expressive therapy might be good, in other words, but not necessarily the treatment of choice.

And who is to say, regarding the few "failures" in the expressive group, whether the cases were somehow "hopeless" (thus not reflecting any shortcoming of the treatment chosen) or whether they had been merely mismatched—capable of getting well if they had been offered, 20 years ago, some *other* form of therapy? The reader can already begin to grasp the elusiveness of the questions raised here: Even if we were evaluating the results of an ideally constructed psychotherapy study, we would be left 10 or 20 years later in the position of someone examining a cat's cradle through a cracked lens. I will mention here just one objection to any assertion we might make, based on a randomized technic: What if patients' *knowing* they are participating in such a study casts a pall over the whole process (especially if they regard their assigned treatment modality as the "off-brand")? The patients in our small pilot study raised such objections when assigned to the supportive group, since some of their dormitory mates were getting hours of therapy, while they got only minutes. A better design would be a naturalistic one: Therapists at a large psychiatric facility would treat some borderlines on a unit wholly devoted to expressive therapy; others would treat a matched population of borderlines on another unit devoted to supportive therapy. The allocation might depend, not on randomization and signed consent forms, but on which patients had this or that type of insurance coverage. Here the two modalities could eventually be compared without the hospital's tipping its hand to the patients that they were a part of a research protocol.

Leaving the hypothetical to one side for the moment, we may ask whether the experience with the PI-500 sheds any light on the vexatious questions about the efficacy of therapy. Here, I think, the answer is a qualified "yes."

The pilot study, containing only half a dozen borderlines in each category, yielded nothing of statistical significance, though it did give rise to a few interesting anecdotes. Although there were some borderlines with a fair outcome and others who ultimately recovered in both the expressive and supportive groups, two of the former supportive-group patients expressed to me their consternation at having received such brief and perfunctory treatment while at the hospital. They had heard that PI was a bastion of analytic excellence; why, then, had they been given short shrift? I reminded them of their agreement to accept whichever of the alternative therapies was dictated by the randomization, sympathizing with them at the same time over their irritation. One of them was not content until he finally had a long course of expressive therapy at another hospital a few years later. I am prepared to believe that had we offered him this experience at PI, he might have become emotionally strong enough to have stabilized without the subsequent hospitalization. I am in no way prepared to convince the reader of this, knowing that to do so would require either (1) personal acquaintance with the patient or (2) a book of prodigious length.

Considering that the format of 5 or 10 minutes a day was really a caricature of supportive therapy, we can make a more convincing case that sometimes expressive therapy was *not* necessary: Several of the supportive-group borderlines in the pilot study had excellent outcomes at follow-up, though they received no more than this skimpy "curbside" treatment at PI and *no* therapy in the years that followed. Presumably, had expressive therapy been an indispensable ingredient of their eventual recovery, its absence ought to have consigned them to a mediocre outcome or worse. With the borderline man alluded to just above, this seemed to be the case. But it was not so with many others. Indeed, as I inspect the outcome registry, I note as many phenomenal recoveries (typical GAS score > 90) in borderlines who eloped, having had a therapist of less than average skill, and who never re-entered therapy, as in borderlines who were gifted at making psychological connections and who remained with the same excellent therapist for many years. If one uses a GAS score of 80 as a cutoff point, 50 of the PI-500 borderlines (31 females, 19 males) achieved outcome scores in this range.

What was the role of expressive therapy in the successful outcomes of these 50 borderlines? Here I can only offer some impressionistic comments. At least 10 were highly insightful, motivated, and able to work well with transference themes and with dreams. Expressive therapy appeared to facilitate not only recovery from the original symptoms, but their maturation to levels of integration they had never attained before. Several permanently outgrew the "suicide game," by which I refer to their tendency, characteristic of their life before and during (the early phase of) hospitalization, to manipulate others by threats of suicide. One man overcame his corrosive jealousy: Obsessed before his hospitalization with the image of his fiancée making love to another man, he had several times assaulted her without provocation. In the course of his treatment, he overcame this symptom. At follow-up, he had remained well for the past 24 years, both at work and in the sphere of intimate relations. (This man is also discussed in "Pathological Jealousy," Appendix A.) A young woman of 17 did well in the expressive mode, though she became mired after several months in an eroticized transference she could not get past. An impasse of this sort was a common problem with the adolescent borderline women and their male therapists. Treatment in the case just mentioned shifted to a supportive mode, and eventually she made a splendid recovery.

Expressive therapy proved altogether too difficult for a number of the PI-500 borderlines. A few succumbed to what was in effect an iatrogenic psychosis. Changes in the personal lives of the resident/therapists occasionally precipitated these reactions, especially marriage or the birth of a child. The news of such events traveled fast within the tight community of the PI-500. That one or another patient was reacting strongly to the event was obvious to everyone; less obvious were answers to the questions of which patients were capable of tackling the attendant emotions within the context of expressive therapy, and which patients were too fragile for such exploration. The superior clinical judgment of a more experienced analyst might have made these distinctions more readily, one could argue, and might thus have prevented the regressive (at times, catastrophic) reactions these events unleashed. Be this as it may, expressive therapy, under the circumstances prevailing on our unit, proved overwhelming to a number of the patients.

One borderline woman of 20, for example, became acutely anxious before her therapist's forthcoming wedding. She dreamed of being ripped apart by *little green monsters*. The obvious interpretation about her extreme envy did not calm her. She eloped and picked up a bellicose man at a bar, who beat her up; further interpretations about the acting out were also unavailing. The relationship with her therapist was never restored afterwards to its proper cooperative level. She left the hospital a while later, discontinued the work with her therapist after a few months, and left for another part of the country. At follow-up over 20 years later, despite this unpromising beginning, she had done unusually well, thanks in part to periodic stretches of supportive therapy with a different therapist (see also Chapter Fifteen).

At least four of the borderlines with the best outcomes suffered these paradoxical reactions to expressive therapy. The contributory factors are not all of a piece: One patient had been an incest victim and was unable to tolerate in the intense therapy the forced reliving of her father's exploitation; another, who had not been an incest victim, ended up in a sexual relationship with her therapist; a third had a rather insensitive therapist, eventually eloped, and did well on her own; the last became suicidal under the impact of transference interpretations she was unable to handle. I am not sure what generalizations one can make concerning which borderlines should *not* be given a trial of expressive therapy. The intolerant group at PI happened all to be fragile women with male therapists—in some cases, overzealous ones. Borderline patients who have been incest victims, who have been attacked repeatedly by a parent, who have lost one or both parents through suicide, or who are for whatever reasons inordinately fragile and clinging should inspire in us a certain hesitation concerning the advisability of expressive therapy, at least in the early phases of treatment. Some (but not all) will become amenable to a more insight-oriented approach after a suitably long "induction period" of supportive therapy. Many will get well without ever making the transition to expressive therapy.

The warning note I have introduced here is partly anachronistic: Therapists of the 1960s were apt to rely upon analytic methods for borderline patients in a less discriminating fashion than is true today. In the PI-500, the patient who raised the most vehement objections to expressive therapy was a borderline woman, both of whose parents had manic–depressive psychosis (MDP); she had been in a classical analysis with a prominent analyst before she came to out unit. With supportive therapy and appropriate medications, she eventually recovered. I believe most clinicians today, in treating a borderline patient with these vulnerabilities, would have selected the latter regimen to begin with.

Waldinger (1987) has made a valuable contribution to our understanding of expressive therapy and its role vis-à-vis borderline patients. Among tactics and approaches that the clinicians participating in this study felt were valuable, Waldinger mentions stability of the treatment framework; increased activity of the therapist (compared to the technic with a neurotic analysand); tolerance of the patient's hostility, rendering the self-destructive tendencies no longer gratifying; and an ability to help the patient translate actions into their corresponding verbal equivalents. Waldinger makes the point (1987, p. 273) that there are many nonoverlapping subpopulations of "borderlines"—some clinging, some more paranoid, some highly impulsive, others less so, and so on. Certain clinicians advocating one particular approach (1) may have a personality optimally suited to one special category of borderlines, and (2) may gradually acquire a caseload through appropriate referrals of similar patients. The position taken concerning such issues as early use of the negative transference versus avoidance of such focus may in large part be the outward manifestation, an epiphenomenon, of a clinician's particular skills and preferences. All clinicians are in a way correct regarding the recommendations they make about technic. But even the most astute and experienced clinicians must struggle against the tendency to immure themselves within a solipsistic world that cannot easily be generalized, to the much larger and more variegated domain of *all* borderline patients. Our literature is handicapped by the need for great care in preserving confidentiality. Except in supervision, we cannot communicate the minute details about our patients that alone would enable us to determine whether the borderlines treated successfully by Adler, Bryce Boyer, Chessick, Giovacchini, Gunderson, Kernberg, Masterson, Rinsley, Searles, and Volkan (all with their own methods) closely resemble our own borderlines or not. In any case, as Waldinger emphasizes, the *actual* technics of various well-known clinicians are probably much more similar—in the mixture and in the timing of various supportive and expressive interventions—than their writings would lead one to suspect.

How wide is the applicability of expressive therapy within the large domain of borderline patients? Here, I believe, inspection of the PI-500 and their outcomes provides some useful estimates (though little in the way of definitive answers). What I would like to propose, in tackling this question, is a response based half on observation, half on a thought experiment. We may begin by looking at the PI-500 in its entirety: 550 patients, mostly selected, for whom expressive therapy was to be the mainstay of their therapeutic regimen. They cannot all be considered ideal candidates for this modality, especially in the light of contemporary practice. We would do little injustice to the realities of this population if we eliminated from the roster patients who exhibited a clear-cut and nontransitory psychosis. A small number of the PI-500 schizophrenics were amenable to expressive therapy—specifically, two of the male patients who improved via "integration" rather than by "sealing over"(McGlashan, Levy, & Carpenter, 1975) and whose outcomes at follow-up were in the good-to-recovered category. For didactic purposes, we may place the clearly psychotic patients to one side and narrow our domain from 550 to the 299 borderlines plus the 7 who functioned at the "neurotic" level.

Suppose now, focusing on the borderlines only, that we trim our roster further by excluding the alcoholic and other seriously addicted patients, whose amenability to expressive therapy was questionable at best, and whose needs would have been served by the appropriate "Anonymous" groups plus supportive therapy. Patients with ASP are notoriously resistant to the interventions of expressive therapy. Patients with anorexia nervosa and/or bulimia nervosa severe enough to warrant residential treatment are seldom ideal candidates for this approach, primarily because of their strong tendency to denial of illness; in addition, their body image distortions often have a tenacity

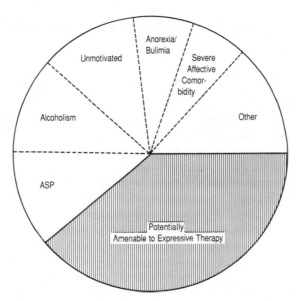

FIGURE 14.3. Distribution of the 299 PI-500 borderlines with respect to expressive therapy. The total number of "potentially amenable" patients was 132.

reminiscent of delusion. Hilde Bruch, it is true, advocated an analytically oriented therapy and claimed good success (Bruch, 1978). But she was writing in an era when the behavior modification technics currently employed had not as yet been developed. Her claims of cure appear to have been unrealistic. A few of the eating-disordered patients did seem to respond well to exploration of their dynamics, but I suggest that we trim the roster of this group as well.

In a similar vein, we may subtract those borderlines with serious affective comorbidity—of the sort inspiring the more biologically oriented consultants to speak of them as affectively disordered patients with borderline features, while others speak of borderline patients with affective features. A number of patients were simply unmotivated and signed out after 3 or 4 months. Finally, we may reduce the ranks by excluding the extremely hyperactive, the intractable agoraphobics, those with severe paranoid or "inadequate" personalities, and those traumatized so severely by shattering early loss or by parental abuse (sexual or physical) as to render exploration too painful. With this process completed, we are left with some 132 presumably amenable borderlines who had no glaring reason not to improve with expressive therapy.

Figure 14.3 shows the result of this narrowing process, and gives the approximate size of the nonamenable compartments. Many patients had more than one attribute arguing against the utility of an analytically oriented approach (e.g., alcoholism plus ASP), such that the compartments would actually overlap to varying degrees.

The next step in the refinement of these impressions is to review outcomes in the 132 potentially amenable borderlines. Some clearly did not benefit from expressive therapy, in the sense that they (1) eloped from the hospital a few months after their arrival and never re-entered therapy even on an ambulatory basis; (2) had a marginal life in the intervening years; or (3) probably could have been helped by this form of treatment if they had been in better hands, but happened to have bad experiences with their hospital therapists. This group numbered 30 (10 males, 20 females). If we assume for the moment that the remainder all did well, we could claim that 102 of the original borderline patients appeared to have had good experiences with expressive therapy. We would not be entitled to claim a causal connection; at the most, we could say that expressive therapy was indeed instrumental in helping these patients, though we would be left wondering whether another method (e.g., purely supportive therapy) might have done as well. The *maximum* level of benefit for expressive therapy with this group of hospitalized borderlines is thus in the range of 33%.

As for the *minimum* level of benefit, I can identify 42 patients (12 males, 30 females) for whom the claim of benefit via expressive therapy appears quite reasonable. These patients usually remained for many years with the same therapist; worked well with transference issues, dreams, and the like; and had excellent and lasting recoveries. The minimum level of benefit would therefore be in the range of 14%. The same caveat applies: Some or all these patients might have done as well with alternative methods; the natural-history approach does not permit us to decide this question. Giving expressive therapy the benefit of the doubt—as a method that *was* helpful to these patients, even though we cannot show that no other therapy would have led to similar results—we arrive at the elimination process illustrated in Figure 14.4.

Several ambiguities surround the borderlines, numbering 60, who fell between these extremes. Expressive therapy was *probably* useful for 30 (10 males, 20 females), though their outcomes were less impressive ("good" as opposed to "clinically recovered"). Here we cannot resolve the question: Did they fail to reach higher levels of adaptation because they were intrinsically more vulnerable or poorer in personality assets than were the recovered patients? If so, then expressive therapy may have helped them get as far as they did, and perhaps no other modality could have done better. Or did expressive therapy fail to promote the gain (into the "recovered" range) that an alternative method might have effected?

For the remaining patients, I do not have enough evidence to permit comment on the role of psychotherapy; 5 patients remain untraced.

To summarize, my experience with the PI-500 suggests that expressive psychotherapy—with its focus on confrontation concerning paradoxical attitudes, on transference, and on interpretation (of dream material, of the here-and-now, and to a lesser extent of the patient's historic past)—is effective with somewhere between one-seventh and one-third of a carefully selected

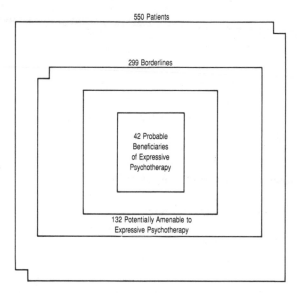

FIGURE 14.4. Elimination process to establish number of patients for whom expressive therapy was probably beneficial.

group of hospitalized borderline patients. To be conservative, I should add that many such borderlines do as well with other, largely supportive forms of therapy and that a small number, though suicidal and self-destructive when admitted, make equally dramatic gains after nothing more than a period of sanctuary in the safe environment of the hospital. Even the "expressive therapy" offered at PI, though supervised by experienced psychoanalysts, was seldom purely expressive. The nature of the patients' serious symptoms, especially in the early phases, demanded supportive measures. The therapists, not yet finished with their training, lacked the skills necessary to maintain a more "expressive" atmosphere during certain tense moments, when seasoned therapists might still have preserved a more neutral tone. One might better speak of the *balance* between dynamic/interpretive/*expressive* interventions and reassuring/exhortatory/educative/*supportive* interventions, acknowledging that few of the PI-500 patients received a predominantly expressive treatment (until they left the hospital.

In the absence of convincing evidence that expressive therapy was the *sine qua non* of recovery in these hospitalized borderline patients (i.e., supportive/ intensive therapy twice or thrice weekly might have yielded the same good results in *any* of the patients), we should view expressive therapy as *one of several competing and about equally effective modalities* that should be chosen, *not* because expressive therapy is (1) superior or (2) alone capable of promoting recovery, but because this form of therapy happens to be congenial to the training of certain psychotherapists and to the culture and personality of certain borderline patients. The curative element is probably the soothing and growth-promoting relationship that successful therapists are able to foster over time with their borderline patients (Giovacchini, 1982). Expressive therapy becomes one of several "languages" in which this healing dialogue can be carried out. I am prepared to believe that the dynamic/interpretive aspects of expressive therapy may have more specific value for a subgroup of ambulatory borderline patients, who eventually rise to adaptive heights they might not have reached with supportive therapy.

This issue lies outside the scope of this follow-up study, though Wallerstein (1986) addresses the controversy in his admirable monograph on the Menninger study (which included predominantly ambulatory patients). He too was led to conclude that although expressive therapy was useful in a portion of the 42 patients he followed, supportive therapy was often as effective and tended to be underrated by the therapists. With hospitalized borderline patients, made fragile either by constitutional factors or by the abuse of caretakers (or both), our role as therapists is to catalyze the natural restorative forces within our patients, so that they may at last resume their positions on the path toward maturation and self-development. More often than we are accustomed to acknowledge, this facilitation stems from our adequacy as surrogate parents rather than from our cleverness as interpreters.

CHAPTER FIFTEEN

Counterintuitive Results

The most recent follow-ups of the PI-500—in effect, the latest chapters in the story of their natural histories—are filled with counterintuitive results. Happily, more patients of whom we expected the worst did well than vice versa, especially among the borderlines. The schizophrenic (SZ) patients, it is true, have generally done worse than we anticipated, particularly those with prominent "negative signs" or those who clearly met the now more stringent diagnostic criteria. But, here, our optimism was seldom as keen as our pessimism was gloomy on behalf of certain drug-abusing, chaotic borderline patients.

One can divide the unexpected successes into several categories, reflecting the main reasons for the original pessimistic forecast. These are as follows: (1) the wildly impulsive, (2) the intensely suicidal, (3) the antisocial, (4) the seriously addicted, and (5) the grossly psychotic. This list is reminiscent of the four dimensions associated with treatment difficulty in hospitalized patients that Allen, Colson, and their colleagues at the Menninger Clinic outlined (Allen, Colson, et al., 1986; Colson et al., 1986)—namely, (1) withdrawn psychoticism, (2) character pathology, (3) violence–agitation, and (4) suicidal–depressed behavior. A number of our patients fell into more than one of the five categories; a few fell into none. (An example of the latter was a highly narcissistic and grandiose borderline patient contemptuous of the hospital's efforts and seemingly unmotivated for any real change.)

Conversely, those who had unexpected grim or tragic outcomes included a few patients in each diagnostic category who were unusually intelligent, attractive, or likeable, or else who entered the unit with relatively mild symptoms and only a brief history of dysfunction.

I cannot be precise in enumerating all of the patients with counterintuitive outcomes, since my selections were of necessity somewhat impressionistic. I relied mostly upon the prognostic comments appended to each admission note by the therapist. Where these were perfunctory or at odds with firm recollections of my own, I relied upon memory. I cannot relate all their stories for several reasons. For one thing, the detailed biographies of these three dozen patients would double the length of this book; also, in some cases, the details themselves are so unusual as to defy adumbration while still safeguarding confidentiality.

BORDERLINE PATIENTS

Unexpected Success in "Poor-Prognosis" Borderlines

At least 21 borderlines belonged to this category. Seven had abused alcohol or drugs severely and shown marked antisocial characteristics; of these, two were incest victims, had been "runaways" before coming to PI, and had eloped a few months later from our unit. Two had been delinquents on probation. Two, through chronic lying, had defeated their therapists' attempts to achieve a therapeutic alliance. Four had made serious suicide attempts; another four were wildly impulsive, including two female adolescents who had given out-of-wedlock children up for adoption, were chronically truant, and came from fragmented and unsupportive families. I have sketched the life course of several of these patients elsewhere: the man with episodic dyscontrol and temporal lobe epilepsy (see Appendix A); the woman with pseudologia fantastica (see Appendix A); the alcoholic woman rescued by Alcoholics Anonymous (AA) after having "disappeared" for many years (see "Missing Persons, Vagrants, and the Homeless," Appendix B); and one of the men who barely survived a near-death experience stemming from a narcotics overdose (see "Almost-Suicides," Chapter Four). Arguably the best outcome was that of a shy and isolated young man admitted after a brief psychotic episode precipitated by LSD. The drug activated dormant fears of being homosexual, unleashed murderous fantasies about his parents, and mobilized self-destructive impulses, the most flamboyant of which led him to a (luckily unsuccessful) attempt at autocastration. Nineteen years later, this man had become a "pillar of his community"—a prosperous and socially minded businessman, equally effective and gratified in his roles as husband and father.

Several of the female patients, markedly ambivalent about motherhood, had developed an uncanny knack for picking men with dissimilar tastes, dissimilar backgrounds, and dissimilar habits—until they reached an age where the whole question of motherhood became moot. One such woman, self-centered and embittered to the point of alienating staff and fellow-patients alike during her 2 years on the unit, carried on one affair after another with men who abused her physically. Mostly they were drifters and ne'er-do-wells from the end of the socioeconomic spectrum opposite to that of her wealthy parents. She had little sense of direction in life and still less capacity for work, yet she demanded to be taken seriously about her "art." At the time we knew her, this consisted largely of formless splatters on canvas, all red—rather as though a Jackson Pollack had confined himself to one color. Her social habits seemed sure to condemn her to a life of isolation. She would knock on the doors of friends, unannounced, at midnight and stand amazed that they did not welcome her with open arms. A year after she left the hospital, having enrolled aimlessly in this course and that at a junior college, she left for another part of the country.

Since this patient had been only modestly self-mutilative and suicidal while in hospital, I expected to find her alive, but still languishing in her directionless existence. She was more than alive: Twenty years later, she had somehow become the proprietress of a commercial art establishment and had married (at age 40) a suitable and devoted man; both partners were content to forgo parenthood. Her success was more than could be attributed to her attractiveness (which was considerable) or to her talent (which obviously surpassed our original estimates). Somewhere during her late 20s, she had acquired self-discipline and a capacity for hard work. One is reminded of Kolb's list (1982, p. 221) personality assets whose presence helps offset the effects of the many pathological traits we are so much better at enumerating in our patients. Kolb's list is so useful that it warrants repetition; hence I give it below (with one addition, that of "charm").

A. Related primarily to the external world
  1. Courage
  2. Curiosity
  3. Flexibility
B. Primarily task-directed; also related to constancy in relationships
  1. Commitment
  2. Perseverance
  3. Responsibility
C. Primarily related to personal relationships
  1. Humor
  2. Empathy
  3. Trust
  4. Charm

Usually, these qualities, if they are destined to emerge in a particular person, have already manifested themselves before the age at which most of the PI-500 patients were hospitalized. As for the patient in the vignette above, the "late onset" of her perseverance and self-discipline was thus as counterintuitive as her overall recovery.

The "natural advantages" discussed elsewhere (see Chapter Ten) figured importantly in the unexpected successes of certain borderline patients: Those who were likeable, attractive, or talented were especially likely to overcome their original handicaps. But some of the borderlines with a counterintuitive recovery lacked even these qualities—most noticeably, three delinquent male adolescents remanded to us by the courts, and two males heavily involved with polydrug abuse. These patients seemed, during their days at PI, to have nothing going for them. None of these five showed signs of recuperation when they left the unit; all had a "ladle-shaped" life trajectory (see Chapter Thirteen), spending 5 or 10 years close to skid row before shaking the drug habit and recovering.

The quality of family life is surely another important variable. Leff and Vaughn (1980) and others have recently drawn attention to the ill effects, especially upon schizophrenics, of families high in "expressed emotion"; usually this refers to parents who are hypercritical, volatile, and noisy. Their children, even if temperamentally calm and dispositionally obedient, may nevertheless be jarred into all manner of nervous or destructive behavior. Here we are dealing, in words of one syllable, with "good kids from bad homes." The opposite situation—irritable, abusive children born to placid, sensitive parents—also occurs (see Spungen, 1983). Prognostically, we might expect that "good kids from bad homes" would eventually make much better adjustments, once liberated from the traumatizing environment, than their opposite numbers. Of the 21 borderlines with unexpectedly successful outcomes, at least 8 came from deplorable homes, yet were apparently of good character all along, underneath rather a thick carapace of defiance and rebelliousness. Their hidden goodness was, one might say, begging to be uncorked and released by some protective person or by some favorable life situation. For many of the PI-500, the hospital and its caring personnel provided just these catalysts. But with the aforementioned "delinquents" we could, at the time, neither see nor actualize their good qualities.

In several instances what was counterintuitive was not so much the unexpectedly favorable result, but rather the way in which the patient achieved this result. One man, who exhibited borderline functioning (but did not have DSM-III borderline personality disorder [BPD]), had been severely agoraphobic for many years both before and after his 14-month stay on our unit. Ill since adolescence, he led a marginal existence for some 20 years after he left the hospital, getting by on disability payments and some help from his family. He had been in conventional psychotherapy, much of it analytically oriented, for 30 years. Finally, in his mid-40s, he tried (at the recommendation of a friend) a marathon week of "primal scream" therapy. For the first time in his life, he felt in touch with his emotions and was no longer so afraid of the world. From the end of that week to the time of follow-up (6 years later), he was largely asymptomatic. In addition, he expanded his circle of friends greatly and made a splendid success in business. This vignette constitutes a scientifically unassailable argument for the efficacy of psychotherapy in a particular case—but no one, least of all within the confines of traditional psychiatry, would have predicted the variety of psychotherapy that would finally have unleashed this man's potential for a gratifying life.

Unexpected Failure in "Good-Prognosis" Borderlines

Some of the borderline patients considered to have a good prognosis at admission were still rather ill, compared with an ambulatory population. Ours was, after all, a hospitalized series. This subgroup consisted either of patients with comparatively minor symptoms, less than serious suicide gestures, and the like, or else of patients whose relatively serious initial symptoms were counterbalanced by unusual degrees of talent, attractiveness, intelligence, or appeal. Of the several dozen such patients, most vindicated our estimations and were therefore not "counterintuitive" examples. Where the outcome is poor in the face of many natural advantages, one suspects high genetic loading for mental illness or an abysmal environment, or both.

The three borderlines whose life course most egregiously fell short of expectation were all uncommonly attractive women. One was artistically talented and extremely intelligent. Another came from a prominent family, was rather self-effacing, and elicited great sympathy from the unit personnel because of her agreeable personality. The third came from a family even our staff considered "warm and supportive"—no small compliment if one reflects that, in an era when to invoke constitutional factors was still taboo, we generally blamed the parents for everything. But the first two women were incest victims, having been forced into sexual relations by older male relatives. The third was, and remained, severely agoraphobic. She also evolved along the lines of recurrent depressive illness and probably began with adverse constitutional factors predisposing her to manic–depressive psychosis (MDP). The two incest victims, despite their many engaging qualities, were notably lacking in two of the positive traits Kolb (1982) mentioned as fostering good personal relationships: They had neither trust nor humor. The molestation had destroyed their trust; their mistrustfulness had undone every effort they had made over the years to establish an intimate partnership. As Henriette Klein once mentioned (1980), "where there is no trust, there is no love"; this means, not that the mistrustful are incapable of falling in love, but rather that they eventually extinguish love and demolish relationships through jealous taunts, carping criticism, or possessiveness. The third woman demonstrates a particularly malignant aspect of agoraphobia—namely, the fact that wholesale avoidance of the external world disrupts the feedback mechanism normally permitting one to experience the innocuousness of once-dreaded situations. Like a collapsing star, the patient's world soon closes in on itself until the "black hole" stage is reached: The patient becomes, for all intents and purposes, invisible to the world outside.

Counterintuitive results showed up, as I have mentioned, in all diagnostic groups. Although each patient with a surprising outcome is worthy of study, for sake of brevity I confine my examples from these other categories to the next largest group—the schizophrenic patients.

SCHIZOPHRENIC PATIENTS

Unexpected Success in "Poor-Prognosis" Schizophrenics

A few of the schizophrenic patients who were still diagnosed as such after reclassification by DSM criteria were, at latest follow-up, clinically "recovered" or even well with minor symptoms. In two or three instances, the improvement has been so durable that the patients would have appeared to any new consultant as having "schizotypal personality" (STP), frank psychosis having long disappeared. Some might wish to challenge the original diagnosis. In one case, however, the diagnosis rested on a most solid foundation: The patient progressed from "childhood autism," with social isolation and hallucinations, to eccentric behavior and bizarre magical thinking throughout adolescence. He refused to play with other children, daydreamed constantly, exhibited thought-blocking, and had strange religious/philosophical preoccupations and delusory ideas concerning his teachers and classmates. His magical thinking was replete with veiled erotic symbolism: He was terrified of parochial school lest, in case of fire, the nuns could not find the keys hidden deep in the folds of their skirts; he walked stoop-shouldered lest the (imaginary) cockatoo perched on his shoulder fall off. He was able to make a few friends, however, and had several brief infatuations, Quixote-like, with inaccessible girls. An excellent student, he attended college for a while, but dropped out because of hallucinations of people ridiculing him. He spent a year and a half at PI in a string of crises and eventually eloped a few weeks before his therapist was due to leave the unit. He had none of the "natural advantages" I refer to elsewhere (see Chapter Ten); his intelligence was average for the patients in the series. His father, who died during the patient's adolescence, had been a stern disciplinarian, not without a jovial side; his mother was nurturing, though moralistic. They, too, seemed "average."

Far from making the "average" adjustment for the schizophrenic patients of the PI-500, however, this patient's life trajectory carried him, 24 years later (at age 50), to the second highest level achieved by his diagnostic counterparts. He married, converted his once bizarre philosophizing into conventional and supportive religious interests, and made a successful career in the business world. At the time of follow-up, he had worked in the same company for 23 years and had never been rehospitalized. His hobby of writing short stories sustained him during the few "ups and downs" of the immediate posthospital period. He had not required medications or therapy for 20 years. It would be of the greatest importance to understand the factors that contributed to this impressive and lasting recovery, achieved in a schizophrenic patient who scarcely relied upon our profession for help at any point.

Another of the patients in this diagnostic group who did unexpectedly well was one whose original illness, as his therapist described it in great detail in the old records, seemed of an unmistakably schizophrenic stamp. Besides auditory hallucinations and persecutory delusions of a sexual nature, the patient also exhibited bizarre and extremely "regressed," primitive behavior throughout much of the early part of his lengthy stay at PI. Several members of his immediate family appeared also to suffer chronic schizophrenic illnesses, for which they spent long periods in hospitals on several occasions. The patient had aspirations to be an artist, which no one among the staff took very seriously—partly because he had dropped out of college and had never completed any major goals; partly because he seemed so disorganized.

The patient responded to neuroleptics, improved gradually, and by the time of his discharge was speaking in a somewhat pressured way about his artistic ambitions. His therapist characterized the latter as grandiose. These new features—pressured speech and grandiosity—intensified to the point that his therapist, working with him now as an outpatient, began to see him as having bipolar MDP. Lithium then led to a total clinical recovery. After several years, the patient secretly discontinued taking the lithium to see whether he would remain well without it. He then went to a different part of the country, married, and realized his artistic strivings to the point of becoming a respected and self-supporting portrait painter. At follow-up, he still saw a therapist with some regularity, but had been continuously well and on no medications at all for 14 years. He spoke with great candor about his illness and with profound gratitude toward the hospital and his old therapist. Of the 240 original patients with a psychotic disorder on admission, he was one of three with a follow-up Global Assessment Scale (GAS) score of 90 or above.

In retrospect, this man exemplifies the point made by Vaillant (1963) concerning certain good-prognosis "schizophrenics" who, in the light of long-term follow-up, most likely had MDP to begin with. Another point the case illustrates concerns the poor predictive power of hallucinations and delusions as compared with the "negative signs" of schizophrenia (see Chapter Twelve). The evidence has been with us a long time: E. Bleuler (1911) described, among the "schizophrenic" patients he knew of, eventual recovery in a hebephrenic professor, in the jurist Schreber, and in the composer Schumann (p. 210)! Contemporary biographies of Schreber and Schumann point to affective, not to schizophrenic, psychoses (Niederland, 1984; Ostwald, 1985). One could also add Freud's "Wolf Man" (see Gardiner, 1971), earlier considered "schizophrenic," but in all likelihood a manic–depressive with a strong family history of MDP.

One patient who was originally diagnosed as "schizophrenic" and whose life course was unexpectedly good was, in retrospect, neither schizophrenic nor manic–depressive. Yet the nature of her breakdown, which occurred in the transition from home to college, satisfied DSM criteria for schizophrenia. She showed predominantly the "positive signs," having exhibited persecutory delusions for 11 months before coming to our unit. She never abused drugs. As a child, she once experienced febrile convulsions. Family life was tempestuous; discipline was stern. The parents portrayed men to their two daughters as predatory, and sex as repugnant. The patient became inhibited, perfectionistic, and preoccupied with cleanliness—traits whose appropriateness were challenged in the liberated atmosphere of her college dormitory. She made no real progress while on our unit; was too shy to "open up" with her therapist; and 5 months later, in response to a crisis in the family, eloped and returned home. Her symptoms promptly abated, and within a few years she re-enrolled in college and went on to graduate school. At follow-up 24 years later, she had a managerial position in a large corporation and maintained an active social life (GAS score = 81). She had never been ill or required psychiatric care since she left the unit. In retrospect, her original illness was really in the nature of a schizophreniform disorder (SF) (or "acute schizophrenic reaction")—which, as defined in DSM, is not supposed to exceed 6 months in duration. The time criterion cannot, however, be taken as an absolute and is not a proper *diagnostic* sign in any case, since it is a reflection of the course and not of the symptoms. Since there was no way of knowing she was not a "typical" schizophrenic when she left the hospital, we assumed that she would show persistent impairment in some areas, as did the majority of those whose original records supported a diagnosis of schizophrenia.

Unexpectedly Poor Outcome in a "Good-Prognosis" Schizophrenic

A 20-year-old woman of half French-Canadian, half Native American background became ill when her parents separated, during her sophomore year at the Sorbonne in Paris. When she got the news, she became withdrawn, suspicious, and referential, and heard voices urging her to kill herself. She tried to jump from a bridge spanning the Seine but was restrained by passers-by, and later by the police who brought her to a hospital. For a time, she was delusional about wires that she imagined were buried within her body to administer painful shocks. Another set of voices told her she was "no good." She was no longer suicidal when she arrived on our unit, but she showed blunting of affect. Unusually attractive and polite, she became a favorite of staff and patients alike. Neuroleptic medication led to rapid clearing of symptoms. Her high intelligence seemed to augur well for resumption of studies and eventually for a successful career.

After a year on the unit, she left to enroll at a local college and to live in a halfway house. At this time, she was on maintenance doses of thioridazine. A few months later she re-entered the unit, having become suicidal again, though she had been doing well in her coursework and at a part-time job. She responded to increased doses of thioridazine, and was able to leave the unit 3 weeks later. The remainder of her course is described in Chapter Twelve: This is the patient who at latest follow-up was living in a rural religious community, able to perform light duties in exchange for bed and board. As her life has unfolded, it becomes clear that the balance between fragility and personality assets, though we could not sense it at the outset, was tilted toward the side of fragility.

CHAPTER SIXTEEN

Afterword

The remarks that follow represent in part a summary of the findings, in part a commentary upon those findings. The summary is not complete, but rather focuses on the unusual or surprising. Most of my remarks relate to the borderline and to the schizophrenic (SZ) patients, who together made up about three-quarters of the PI-500.

THE BORDERLINE PATIENTS: GENERAL OBSERVATIONS

1. Given enough time, about two out of three hospitalized patients with borderline personality disorder (BPD) will get better, if we define "better" as a Global Assessment Scale (GAS) rating > 60 that is valid throughout most of the past few years up to the time of (long-term) follow-up contact. The measure of "enough time" can be only approximate. Borderline patients often begin to improve as they enter their 30s. This may relate to a developmental "mellowing" that occurs in most people as they pass the stormier stages of adolescence and early adult life. If this were the only factor, borderline patients of 19 or 20 might have to wait 10 years to reap the advantages of this maturational process. For some patients, however, adequacy of the treatment program (which itself spans several years) may play a large role. In this case, improvement might begin to take place 6 or 7 years after the initial crisis, whether that crisis occurs at age 20 or at age 25. The majority of hospitalized BPD patients remain dysfunctional for the first few years after hospitalization in a way that makes them indistinguishable, on average, from a similar group of SZ patients (cf. Carpenter & Gunderson, 1977; Modestin & Villiger, 1989).

2. The timetable of potential recovery in borderline patients depends in part upon the presence or absence of substance abuse (alcohol abuse, drug abuse, or both). Patients who never abused substances tended to show an accelerated pattern of improvement. Patients who did abuse substances but who eventually recovered did so only when they brought their drug or alcohol misuse

under control. In some cases of alcoholism, the patients were at greater risk of suicide, fatal or crippling accidents, and the like—some of which could have been reduced, if their treatment had dwelled more emphatically on this issue (see Rich, Fowler, Fogarty, & Young, 1988).

3. The suicide risk in any sample of patients with BPD will depend upon such factors as the average age of the sample and the prevalence within the sample of patients with major affective disorder (MAD) comorbidity and of patients who abuse alcohol or drugs. Those in their early 20s are passing through a decade of high suicide-proneness in our culture (greater in males than in females). The 9% suicide rate in the PI-500, as contrasted with the 3% rate in McGlashan's Chestnut Lodge series, may reflect the fact that the average age of the PI-500 was 5 years below that of McGlashan's patients. Of the 17 BPD suicides, 15 occurred within 6 years of their stay on the unit. Suicide risk in those with BPD × MAD, especially if they go on to develop unipolar or bipolar illness, may not diminish as the patients pass beyond age 30 (see Angst & Stassen, 1986). The higher the proportion of such patients in any BPD sample, the greater may be the likelihood of a continuing loss, over the years of a long-term follow-up, through suicide.

In any large series of BPD patients, some suicides will have the quality of inevitability, either because of the severity of underlying depressive illness or because of the severity of traumatic factors in the early environment. (Chapter Four contains several examples of such suicides in the PI-500, including one case of mother–son incest.)

Clinicians who utilize both the phenomenological criteria of DSM or of Gunderson and the psychostructural criteria of Kernberg in determining which patients are borderline may find that the eventual suicides occur chiefly in the ranks of the DSM or Gunderson BPD patients, and much less often among the borderline personality organization (BPO) (but non-BPD) patients. The dysthymic (D) borderlines (those with BPO × MAD but no BPD) of the PI-500, a group resembling Grinker's Type IV borderlines, thus far contain no suicides. Alcoholism was also low (6%) in this group.

4. Contrary to common psychiatric opinion in the past, patients with antisocial personality (ASP), though they may appear blasé and impervious to guilt, do under certain circumstances commit suicide. Their suicide rate is considerable (see Rich, Ricketts, Fowler, & Young 1988). Those who commit suicide do so not out of remorse but out of a sense of being cornered. Persons with ASP are prone to alcoholism and other substance abuse. In the present study, the suicide rate was especially high among the BPD × ASP patients who abused any substances; it was zero in BPD × ASP patients who did not abuse substances.

5. Borderline patients who either commit suicide or remain dysfunctional at long-term follow-up are likely to have been victims of parental physical abuse, transgenerational (especially parent–child) incest, or other negative factors. In some instances, early loss of a parent sets in motion an unfortunate sequence of events whose cumulative effect is to make someone "borderline" who might

not otherwise have become so, or else to render the life trajectory unfavorable where it might otherwise have been favorable. One example of this snowball effect may begin with death of a mother during a daughter's adolescence, followed by a father's incestuous advances and then by the girl's running away and engaging in drug abuse, promiscuity, and suicidal behavior. Another example may begin with death of a father and remarriage by the mother to a man to whom her son cannot adjust, followed by the son's abusing drugs, joining an antisocial gang, and so on.

Borderline patients with an unfavorable life course whose early life has been devoid of traumatic factors or serious loss are apt to show evidence of constitutional handicaps, whether in the form of genetic liability for affective illness, attention deficit disorder, childhood hyperactivity, and the like, or in the form of constitutional abnormalities resulting in partial complex seizures or other "organic" disturbances. Adolescent males with BPD are especially likely to manifest this kind of "organic" substrate.

In general, poor outcomes in *male* borderlines are associated with antisociality, alcohol abuse, and elopement from the hospital; poor outcomes in females are linked with a strong history of suicidal gestures or attempts (see McGlashan, 1988).

6. Unexpectedly good outcome in certain borderline patients may be a function of positive "soft signs" whose long-term effects are to outweigh the more easily recognized negative "hard signs." Likeableness (and the absence of marked hostility or mendacity), candor, perseverance, talent, attractiveness, and the like may win out eventually over traumatic factors (if they are not too severe), florid symptoms at the height of the illness, and so on (see Aldrich, 1986). Personality attributes that elicit positive responses from therapists and other mental health professionals with whom the patient comes in contact enhance the likelihood of a good therapeutic alliance and of a favorable outcome. The same attributes enhance the likelihood of establishing a harmonious sexual partnership or other close bond, which in turn exerts a supportive and stabilizing effect. As they approach their 40s, many borderline patients—perhaps three out of four—lose the tempestuous qualities that once identified them as cases of BPD. But they often remain brittle, such that unanticipated losses in midlife (e.g., sudden death of a spouse) may reawaken part or all of the old borderline symptomatology (e.g., becoming frantic when alone, making suicide gestures). Borderline patients with irritable and disagreeable personalities tend to have an unfavorable life course, partly because they alienate those upon whom they depend, push spouses to divorce who might otherwise have remained with them, or the like.

THE SCHIZOPHRENIC PATIENTS: GENERAL OBSERVATIONS

1. The tighter a definition of "schizophrenia" one uses, and the greater the role that "negative signs" play in the clinical picture, the worse are a

patient's chances for recovery. Global functioning at nearly any moment within the course of a 10- to 25-year follow-up will, if the patients resemble the PI-500 schizophrenics, most likely be in the marginal range.

2. If many of the schizophrenic patients in this series had made significant gains by the time of follow-up contact (most are in their 40s at this writing), we would not, owing to the lack of a research design, have known how to explain the improvement. Treatment was multimodal. Most patients received analytically oriented ("expressive," "exploratory") psychotherapy, pharmacotherapy, group and family therapy, and the like. In the *absence* of improvement, we cannot claim that any of these modalities—including the psychotherapy—was especially helpful. The original treatment philosophy of the unit, which held that one lengthy hospitalization (emphasizing analytically oriented psychotherapy) would prove definitive in helping young schizophrenics recover, constituted a hope that the final results did not justify.

3. In the present series, the schizophrenic patients who committed suicide tended *not* to abuse alcohol (1 out of 9), whereas the borderline (BPD) patients who committed suicide *did* tend to abuse alcohol (7 out of 17). This difference by itself is not significant ($p > .05$), though it would become so ($p < .01$) if one were to add the schizoaffective suicides (14, with *no* alcoholics). Hopelessness figures importantly in the mind-set of most suicides, but in the PI-500 the schizophrenic and schizoaffective patients seemed to have felt hopeless about different issues than were weighing on their borderline counterparts. Among the borderlines, the loss of a key relationship was usually primary. Among the schizophrenic (and, to a lesser extent, the schizoaffective) patients, the key issue seemed to be despair over ever being able to achieve any of the most mundane life goals, let alone the lofty ambitions their parents had entertained for them during the days of their childhood—before their handicap had begun to manifest itself.

OBSERVATIONS ON PSYCHOTHERAPY WITHIN LONG-TERM HOSPITALIZATION

Evolving Views on the Needs of Schizophrenics

Neuroleptic drugs, beginning with chlorpromazine, have been in use in the treatment of schizophrenia for about 35 years. Reasonably effective in alleviating the "positive signs" of the condition (the delusions and hallucinations), these drugs seemed to offer great hope of restoring schizophrenic patients to normality. The need for prolonged hospitalization grew less urgent over time, and by the mid-1960s, the bleak facilities that once housed schizophrenic patients in such large numbers began to shut down. "Deinstitutionalization," as this process came to be known, and relocation of the patients to their homes or to less dehumanizing settings within the community were the watchwords of the day. Those who worked in the mental health community spoke of "percentage of time out of hospital" as a measure of the program's success.

We have begun to learn more recently that improvement as gauged by a lower percentage of time in a hospital does not always coincide with improvement in the quality of life for schizophrenic patients. And sometimes the alternative settings were as dehumanizing as the old ones. One "missing man" of the PI-500, who turned out also to be a homeless man (see Appendix B), had given up the bleak four walls of the institution for the still bleaker four tires of the car under which he slept, in cold and warm weather alike, in a local parking lot. Another of our schizophrenic patients killed a homeless man in a random act of violence. Still another killed himself after his therapist died—the only one with whom he had felt rapport among the many he encountered in his brief career as a "revolving-door" patient.

Our schizophrenic patients had not begun as "no-hopers." They came from supportive families. They had attended, and some had completed, college. There was realistic hope that they could have led a satisfactory (though not full) life in a sheltered setting, where they could have been content, productive, and relatively symptom-free. This hope was all too often extinguished by the unrealistic hope of the mental health community that, with pharmacotherapy and intensive psychotherapy, they could be "all" better. Sometimes the personnel of our unit did recommend to the parents of a schizophrenic patient that they place less reliance on a "cure" through psychotherapy and accept the idea of transfer to a less demanding treatment setting. Usually this meant residing in a therapeutic community in a rural setting or living and working at Fountain House in New York City, rather than re-enrolling in college or resuming a fast-paced job in the city. But the parents were often full of unrealistic hopes, too, and would not accept these less glittering alternatives. Had they known that the "half loaf" of dignity but little wordly success was the *whole* loaf for most of their schizophrenic children, I believe they would have lowered their expectations in this more realistic way. But in the 1960s and 1970s, we were not as yet convinced that the whole loaf was beyond reach.

We could not speak with authority to the parents or to the patients themselves, because to do so would have required the long-term follow-up results that were not to become available for another 10 or 15 years. Worse still, the kinds of therapeutic environments that could have provided these patients with dignity, pleasure, and a sense of usefulness were scarcely available at that time in the United States. The long-term supportive/rehabilitative model that I now feel is appropriate to the care of schizophrenic patients is already operational in many countries. In Switzerland, Ciompi (in Bern) and Angst and Scharfetter (in Zürich) direct outstanding programs, where the patients have the opportunity for as long as necessary to acquire high-level skills under the tutelage of excellent craftsmen. The Fountain House branch in Lahore, Pakistan, under the direction of M. Rashid Chowdery, is a supervised community where some 120 schizophrenic patients live, work, and maintain themselves. In their 25-year follow-up of schizophrenics in Japan, Ogawa et al. (1987) found that drug therapy, though it diminished the number of patients with severe defects, did not increase the proportion who recovered, whereas intensive aftercare did. They refer to their treatment model as *seikatsu-rinsho* ("procedure for the development of living skills"), a model in every way similar to the humanistic rehabilitative model at last coming into vogue in our country.

Some centers here in the United States now have all the elements in place: hospital, day hospital, halfway house, sheltered apartments, superior crafts program, and recreational facilities. Among the best are the Menninger Clinic in Topeka, Kansas, and the Chestnut Lodge Hospital in Rockville, Maryland. At these centers, as at their counterparts in Switzerland and elsewhere, not only are all these mechanical elements in place, but the human element is present in its finest form. In these centers one finds therapeutic personnel, across all disciplines and within all ranks, who create for their SZ patients an environment of dignity, patience, compassion, and respect. Ideally, schizophrenic patients need to have humane environments of this kind available to them for years at a time—if necessary, for life.

Part of the reason for the dismal outcome of the schizophrenic patients in the present study lies in the scarcity of sheltered and non-time-limited therapeutic settings in the United States. All too often we have poured chemicals into such patients at the outbreak of acute symptoms, have quashed those symptoms just in time for their insurance benefits to expire, and have then left the patients to their own devices. A particular "prognosis" is not so much inherent in the schizophrenic illness itself as it is the expression of a dynamic equilibrium between the condition and its treatment. Granted, the condition is not an easy one; our symptom-oriented treatment has been, nevertheless, an egregious failure.

As Vaillant (1978) wrote in his essay on the prognosis and course of schizophrenia, "We are as capable of making schizophrenia worse as we are of ameliorating it" (p. 23). Vaillant's summarizing remarks are as appropriate today as they were over 10 years ago:

> If we shield the [schizophrenic] patient from too-intrusive families or hospital treatment; if we offer hospitals that provide shelter and community rehabilitation rather than involuntary incarceration . . . ; if we learn to use group membership to support and not to threaten; then, although we may not increase cures, we can minimize social disability. (p. 23)

Benefits of Hospitalization to Borderline Patients

Compared with the schizophrenic patients, the borderline patients in the PI-500 were for the most part more capable of utilizing the long-term hospitalization either as a springboard to self-sufficiency or at least as a major step in this direction. Few required rehospitalization. For most of the borderline patients, especially in the dysthymic and "other BPO" groups, the index hospitalization often appeared to be definitive, in the sense that it lifted the patients from serious dysfunction to a level of autonomy. Unfortunately, it is not possible to determine in a naturalistic study whether and when the lengthy index hospitalization actually spared a patient the necessity of additional hospitalization later on. In a number of instances, the long hospitalization served as a bridge between home and either college or full-time work. The gain was one of psychological independence, and sometimes of financial independence as well. For some of the patients, an 8- to 18-month hospital stay was unnecessary—as in the case of the adolescent who eloped in order to return to his own high school. For most of the borderline patients, a stay of 9 months to a year seemed about right; this enabled them not only to get over their initial symptoms, but to accomplish a major piece of work in the area of tolerating being alone and, more importantly, of conquering the tendency to handle stressful situations via self-destructive acts.

General Discussion

The present study sheds less light than I had hoped it might on the topic of long-term hospitalization. As mentioned in the preceding chapter, proof of failure is much easier to determine than proof of success. This would remain true even with a randomized research design: The longer the follow-up, the more tenuous the connection between outcome and treatment.

Currently, psychiatry has turned away from long-term intensive psychotherapy of patients in residential treatment. The reasons for this have more to do with economics and changing orientation (toward the more biological therapies) than with compelling scientific evidence. Given the chronic self-destructiveness of some patients and the chronic psychoticism of others, there will always be a need for centers that can offer long-term care. Such centers, including the long-term unit at PI, provide sanctuary; act as containers for destructive impulses and barriers against destructive influences from the outside; and serve as a catalyst for growth, sometimes even as a molder of character. Among the PI-500, a number of wayward youths (adolescents who were in need of supervision) and delinquent adolescents remanded by the courts made excellent recoveries after their downhill spiral was checked by long-term hospitalization.

Many chronically suicidal borderline patients were able to make use of their year or year and a half on the unit to reach higher adaptive ground; they never resorted to self-destructive behavior throughout the years of follow-up. Patients who had suffered betrayal within the family (whether in the form of abuse, humiliation, or incest) and who showed the kinds of personality deformation that result from such environments were able in many instances to use the long-term unit as a "corrective emotional experience" (Alpert, 1954, 1959). The necessary deprogramming (in relation to a destructive home) and reprogramming (the gradual learning that at least some people are nurturing and trustworthy) is not something that can be compressed into a 30- or even a 90-day hospitalization.

But what is the place of psychotherapy within a long-term hospitalization? Here, I believe, the present study is informative. The patients of the PI-500 all had serious problems in the areas of identity formation, work, and intimacy. These were, in effect, "requirements" for admission to the unit. Some form of supportive psychotherapy was therefore appropriate for all. Depending upon the particularities of each case, this therapy might include elements of suggestion, reassurance, problem-solving, group pressure, re-education, and so on. With the majority of the schizophrenic patients, rehabilitation plus supportive psychotherapy constituted an optimal program. The difficult question concerns expressive (analytically oriented) psychotherapy for the borderline patients. The question requires consideration of several interrelated issues: amenability, applicability, efficacy, and necessity. A borderline patient might, for example, be amenable to expressive psychotherapy, yet this modality might not be applicable if the patient were in the midst of a mild crisis and needed only brief supportive treatment. The reverse would be true in a borderline patient who was chronically suicidal but not at all psychologically minded. If the patient were both self-destructive *and* psychologically minded, expressive therapy might appear effective (I say "appear" rather than "be," because proof is so hard to establish). The most demanding task—demonstrating that certain borderline patients could have recovered in no other way—is well beyond the powers of the present study and may remain elusive for many years to come. In my own view, I think that a number of such borderline patients exist (more among the ambulatory than among the hospitalized), and that some were included in the PI-500. But this is an article of faith. I feel more convinced, though this too is an article of faith, that what was particularly helpful for many of the borderline patients was the lengthy hospitalization itself, with all its interacting components, including the frequent sessions in whatever form they took.

This last assertion—about lengthy versus brief hospitalization—gives rise to a testable hypothesis. One could match appropriately selected borderline patients (those with high suicidality, high psychological aptitude, low antisociality) with respect to age, gender, socioeconomic status, and the like, and offer one group a "definitive" long-term hospitalization, while their matched "controls" received only brief (30 days or less) hospitalization(s). Follow-up at regular intervals over at least 10 years might yield an answer to the question about optimal length of stay. Ideally, one should make available to each patient in the long-term group one therapist and one team, consistently available over the entire time of inpatient care and preferably beyond.

How, then, is a long-term follow-up study informative about psychotherapy? Here, I believe, long-term follow-up, which Dr. Stanley Heller (1986) has aptly called the "psychiatrist's microscope," informs us largely in the negative. Expressive therapy cannot be the treatment of choice for schizophrenia, for example, given the generally poor outcome of the schizophrenic patients in the PI-500 and similar studies who received this form of therapy. By the same token, expressive therapy cannot be the treatment of choice throughout the whole domain of borderline patients, given the generally favorable outcome regardless of whether they had been in expressive therapy, mostly supportive therapy, or (as in a number of instances) in milieu therapy only, with no further therapy during the many years of follow-up.

Instead, we are left with a situation where the "right" kind of psychotherapy for borderline patients depends upon (1) the definition of "borderline" that is used; (2) a variety of patient factors (life events, diagnostic comorbidities, etc.); (3) therapist variables (relating not only to the personality of the therapist, but to the therapist's previous training, exposure to competing schools of thought, etc.); (4) the *Zeitgeist* and the respective cultures within which therapist and patient were raised; (5) family factors (supportive?, intrusive? obstructionistic?); and (6) economic factors.

All this means that the optimal therapy for a borderline patient remains in many particulars a highly subjective matter, not dissimilar to the complexities involved in choosing a friend or a mate. One usually decides on a case-by-case basis. Even with borderline patients who are highly motivated for expressive therapy and who present no obvious contraindications, the matter of "which therapist?" is often problematic. Borderline patients are highly sensitive to nuances of a therapist's style, to age, to gender, and to a host of other variables. For reasons of this kind, some of the PI therapists who showed enthusiasm, integrity, maturity, and emotional availability, but little skill at understanding the unconscious, did as well or better with their borderline patients than did some of their colleagues who understood symbolism well but who had less of those human qualities.

By demonstrating which subgroups of borderline patients responded poorly or not at all to expressive therapy, long-term follow-up performs a useful service in narrowing and in better defining the patient parameters within which this form of therapy would be effective (either exclusively or in conjunction with other treatment modalities). The present study suggests that borderline patients with dysthymic symptoms, high motivation, high psychological-mindedness, low degrees of intrafamilial trauma, and only a minimum of impulsivity may respond well to expressive therapy. Patients in whom these features are present alongside substance abuse, eating disorders, or other impulse disorders will usually require participation in a limit-setting group (Alcoholics Anonymous, Overeaters Anonymous, etc.) as well. Intensive supportive therapy with a skillful and enthusiastic therapist may, however, lead to equally good results in many cases.

The PI-500 results point in the direction of remarks by Robert Michels (1988)—namely, that an Axis I diagnosis usually makes a difference with respect to the treatment plan, whereas Axis II (i.e., personality disorder) diagnoses carry little prescriptive significance for a particular type of psychotherapy. All therapists require training and a workable theoretical model of mental function and dysfunction. Without these, they will seldom be effective as therapists. But the training and theoretical model need not be identical for all. As Michels (1988) has mentioned, therapists who are enthusiastic and who clearly convey their interest in understanding their patients will have the best results. They can also afford an occasional technical mistake, because their patients will continue to respect their sincerity and effort.

All this leaves me with the ironical conclusion that long-term follow-up helps to demonstrate in a (reasonably) scientific manner that one cannot define "optimal psychotherapy," for borderline patients especially, in a (rigorously) scientific manner. In place of determinism and proof, we are left with the messiness of humanism, educated guesses and faith. Psychotherapy, it would appear, is often useful in bringing about significant change; despite the scientific pretensions of those who advocate particular systems, however, the "ideal type" of therapy remains elusive and nonspecific. Jerome Frank (1988) has addressed this topic most eloquently: "The claim of most psychotherapists to be applied behavioral scientists is essentially a rhetorical device to enhance the credibility of their procedures . . . by invoking the prestige of Western science" (p. 290).

Psychotherapy is best viewed not as science but as art—specifically, the art of what Spillane (1987) has called the "noble rhetoric." Within the framework of this noble rhetoric, there exists an "ethical hierarchy of language and values, based on the principle of responsible autonomy" (p. 217). Psychotherapeutic practice requires attention to this hierarchy of values.

Patients who would respond well to a predominantly psychoanalytic psychotherapy are those who have an "internal locus of control" (Foon, 1987). Those with an external locus of control respond to more highly structured therapies, to approaches that emphasize limit-setting, and so forth. Borderline patients, especially those with BPD as defined by DSM, tend by definition to have external loci of control. Almost all need a structured therapy that includes limit-setting, whether or not they are also amenable to an expressive therapy. If an expressive therapy is used, it should probably stress an interpersonal approach. As Holmes (1988) points out, this interpersonal approach will aim not at carving out some "ultimate reality" concerning the patient's past, but at constructing a transferential matrix to which "the unconscious of both therapist and patient contribute" (p. 281).

DESIGN OF FUTURE FOLLOW-UP STUDIES

Long-term follow-up studies should have as a subsidiary goal the development of recommendations for improvements in the design of future follow-up studies. Because a high trace rate is essential to the success of any such study

(O'Connor & Daly, 1986; Sims, 1973), investigators should rely more upon a prospective than upon a retrospective design, whenever this is feasible. A prospective design makes it easier to keep in touch (every year or two, for example) with the former patients. Meticulous records (including names, maiden names, addresses, phone numbers, etc.) on all close relatives are also crucial to the success of the study. Analysis of the characteristics of patients who improve or do not improve will aid in the selection of treatment modalities most likely to benefit similar patients in the future. A natural-history study, such as the PI-500, helps establish the percentage of improvement in patients with various syndromes, life events, and so on. This in turn enhances the predictive powers of clinicians and permits better pathway analysis of different life scenarios and their usual outcome. We can, in other words, aspire to more scientific answers concerning who should receive what combination of therapeutic interventions. These efforts should increase our ability to tailor for each patient a treatment program that is more rational and effective. This is no small accomplishment. We should not be disheartened that the psychotherapeutic component of this treatment program will remain—though scientifically informed—at its core an art, a "noble rhetoric," unprogrammable, pragmatic, flexible. Psychotherapy will remain the "human" part of treatment, which, like good parenthood, we can recognize and emulate, but can never precisely measure.

Unusual Syndromes

Any sample as large as the PI-500 is bound to contain a small number of oddities, rarities, and unusual syndromes. Some of the conditions mentioned here are not so uncommon at certain centers specializing in such cases, but they were rare at PI. Eugene Bliss in Salt Lake City, for example, "collects" cases of multiple personality; similarly, cases of episodic dyscontrol get referred to Anthony Andrulonis's unit at the Institute of Living in Hartford. We saw few such patients at PI—partly because we felt they would not be readily amenable to expressive psychotherapy, partly because they are seldom encountered to begin with.

If the reader is looking for a definitive answer to a question such as "What becomes of patients with Munchausen syndrome?", this book will be disappointing. We had only one such patient. Nevertheless, even single-case reports are useful if enough similar ones can be culled from the literature. In hopes that the rarities reported below may be added to others accumulated elsewhere, and thus assist in delineating life course and outcome in such instances, I append the following vignettes.[1]

ASSASSINATION OF JOHN F. KENNEDY: DELUSIONS OF RESPONSIBILITY

Despite the pretensions of the Warren Commission, no one knows who killed President John F. Kennedy. It can be stated with authority, however, that everyone physically residing in New York City that day was innocent (at least of pulling the trigger). Nevertheless, from psychiatric emergency rooms throughout the city and, indeed, from all over the United States, reports came in of acutely psychotic persons claiming responsibility for Kennedy's death. Many of these men (they were usually men) were considered "paranoid schizophrenics." They were often in a state of anguish, guilt-ridden to the point of suicide—though one was often sensible of a certain grandiosity in these patients in supposing themselves the protagonists of the "crime of the century."

At PI we treated two *soi-disant* assassins, who were admitted to our unit a month or so after the event. Both were called "paranoid schizophrenics" at the time; only one

[1]The conditions described occurred before or during hospitalization.

would still be considered to have schizophrenia (SZ) by DSM criteria. At follow-up, the young man who was schizophrenic had never worked, had not been on speaking terms with his parents for some time after discharge from PI, and had lived in a sheltered residence near home for the past 22 years. By his parents' account, he sounded normal half the time; the other half, he was "in his own world"—though he was no longer preoccupied with guilt over Kennedy.

The other young man had what would now be viewed as an acute schizophreniform illness (SF). He had several close relatives with severe emotional disorders, but these were all depressive in nature. He quickly got over his delusion after coming to our unit, worked well (in the expressive mode) with his therapist, and was never been in therapy after discharge. At follow-up, he was extremely successful at his work (an executive post in the publishing industry) and had two small children. Economically, he had outstripped both his "normal" brothers and everyone else in his immediate family. He had also written a book.

CAPGRAS SYNDROME

A favorite diagnostic entity of psychiatric trainees, Capgras syndrome involves delusions of overinterpretation, described by Sérieux and Capgras in 1909 (see Capgras & Reboul-Lachaux, 1923; Guelfi, 1982). In these, the subject reasons falsely when confronted with an affect-laden stimulus, arriving through erroneous deductions at a false but personally significant conclusion. The most dramatic example concerns the conviction that someone to whom the subject is ordinarily quite close (e.g., the mother) is experienced as "not really" that person, but merely as a "double." There was a proliferation of such syndromes in the psychiatric literature of the last quarter of the 19th century—the age of "paranoification," when every minute variant of paranoia was regarded as a distinct condition. Usually, but not always, a Capgras case will emerge as a subtype of schizophrenia. The condition was rare at the turn of the century, and is rarer still now. Still, Signer (1987) found 212 cases to review from the English and French literature. The female-to-male ratio was 2:1, and about half also showed signs of affective disturbance.

The one case of Capgras syndrome among the PI-500 was that of a schizophrenic man in his early 20s. When first admitted, he sometimes insisted his mother was a "fake stand-in" wishing to trick him by her verisimilitude. In the 20 years between discharge and follow-up, he more often than not acknowledged the validity of his mother's claim (that she was in fact his mother), though his paranoia by no means disappeared. Instead, it took a different channel: He espoused a bizarre religion that he practiced alone (he never joined a cult; see Appendix B), one of whose rituals (if it could be called a ritual) was that he not bathe. When confronted by his parents about his hygiene, he would retort, "Years ago they didn't bathe!" He was referring to the 13th-century Albigensians in Provence, who, as Ladurie (1978) reminds us, "did not shave, or even wash, often" (p. 141). This is another example of erroneous reasoning of the sort that interested Capgras. This man has never worked, and in recent years, has never left the house, causing his parents considerable anxiety, now that they are nearing 70, as to what will become of him. It was with a poignant note of resignation that his mother told me, "On the one day I finally persuaded him to take a bath, there was no hot water."

In the example above, the family interaction throughout childhood had been (as far as we could reconstruct) benign; the constitutional factor was severe. Sometimes Capgras syndrome may develop in the reverse situation—where the environmental factor is malignant. A 20-year-old Australian woman who was making suicide gestures, for example, was hospitalized on a unit specializing in exploratory psychotherapy. She maintained the delusional belief that her mother was only a "double," her "real" mother being a "lady in white" who lived somewhere in the remote regions of her continent. In actuality, her mother was a religious fanatic given to scrubbing her daughter's vulva with steel wool before church to render her pure enough to attend the ceremonies. In this instance, the syndrome can best be understood as part of a posttraumatic stress disorder (PTSD), so severe as to mimic a schizoaffective psychosis (SA). At this writing, she is slowly beginning to recover, after 2½ years in the hospital and enforced separation from her parents.

Perhaps half of Capgras patients are schizophrenic; their outcome is determined more by their underlying psychosis than by the particularities of the case. The hospitalized woman described by O'Reilly and Malhotra (1987), for example, was delusional for years, turned many people into "doubles" (not just the members of her immediate family), and eventually stabbed to death another woman on her unit whom she believed (via projective identification) had wanted to harm her daughter.

DE CLÉRAMBAULT SYNDROME (EROTOMANIA)

The term "erotomania" has been used by the French for many years. Esquirol devoted considerable space to this variant of "monomania" in his 1838 textbook. Though most of his erotomanic patients (almost invariably women) were obsessed with passionate feelings toward a man (usually of higher social status or in a position of authority) who remained unaware of these emotions, or who did not even know the woman in question, some also suffered the delusion that the man secretly returned this love. Esquirol's first case occupied an intermediate position: The woman claimed that she could not have endured her anguish (caused by the "interference" of her parents and friends) were it not for the "power communicated to her" (somehow) by the object of her affection (1838, p. 36). De Clérambault (1942) concentrated upon the variant where the woman is convinced she is loved in secret by a man of high station (often a political figure, movie star, religious leader, etc.). Supposed proof of this love comes in the form of subtle signs and clever hints decipherable only by the erotomanic woman. The plasticity of the delusion is such that the woman can even deal with the "lover's" rebuff or indifference (should she actually confront him) on the grounds that "he needs to be discreet" or "he needs to test my devotion."

De Clérambault syndrome is considered rare; this passive variant (of being loved) is certainly less common than the active form (of deluded loving). The latter is often seen in the form of a "transference psychosis" during psychotherapeutic work with psychotic-level female patients. It has been shown recently (Ellis & Mellsop, 1985) that De Clérambault syndrome is not specific to any of the prototypic psychoses described in modern psychiatry: It can occur in manic–depressive psychosis (MDP) as well as in schizophrenia (Signer & Swinson, 1987).

In the PI-500, there were many instances of erotic transference psychoses. Clinically, these were, as would be expected, transitory and less malignant in the borderlines; they were more long-lasting and serious among the psychotic patients. Three schizophrenic women, for example, not only remained "in love" with their therapists, but continued to be preoccupied with them day and night for years afterwards, would write them steamy letters at frequent intervals, and would lie in wait for hours to catch a glimpse of them going to work or returning home (many years after leaving PI and the care of these psychiatrists). This intrusiveness was difficult to deal with: One patient made a near-fatal suicide attempt when her affections were "repulsed," another hung around the doctor's office, and so on. The only solution was of course judicious neglect, since a return letter (begging the patient not to write any more) or a phone call (urging the same) would only whet such a patient's appetite for further contact.

Only one case in the PI-500 actually fit De Clérambault's description: that of a newly married woman who was convinced that a teacher in one of her literature classes—of whom she was deeply enamored—was communicating his own love to her through the page assignments given to the class. Thus, if the first word of the first page of the reading material began with an "L," this stood for "love"; if the letter was an "R" (her last initial), this signaled that the paragraph contained sentiments mirroring his own affection for her; and so on and on.

This woman was not schizophrenic, though she was regarded so throughout her stay at PI; she exemplified instead a pure paranoid disorder, several other instances of which were to be noted among her close relatives. Her condition might also be regarded as a "delusional psychosis" (Jørgensen, 1986), though her outcome ultimately was better than the outcomes Jørgensen noted (1987) in his relatively short-term (2-year) study. The rest of her personality, outside the area of (as Esquirol would call it) monomania, was well intact. Her year of psychotherapy at PI made little dent in the solidity of her conviction. Twenty years later, however, the delusory ideas had faded, at first into obsessions and finally, into fond "memories." She completed graduate work in the humanities and, at follow-up, occupied a respected position in her field.

DYSLEXIA (STREPHOSYMBOLIA)

Intelligent and able to converse in Latin . . . [Charlemagne] never
could master reading, nor was he, in spite of having the best tutors,
ever able to write his name. —DeRosa (1988, p. 45)

Dyslexia may be a significant problem for about 12–15% of school-age children. The syndrome occurs preponderantly in males, perhaps at a ratio of 9:1. Reading disorder represents a final common pathway for a host of etiological factors. Neurological peculiarities may be relevant to some cases. Hynd and Cohen (1983), for example, mention a study pointing to a tendency in a dyslexic population for the right parieto-occipital region to be larger than the left—the reverse of the usual situation (p. 84). Sinistrals are more apt to show this pattern than dextrals, and are more prone to reading disorders. In other children, dyslexia occurs without discernible neurophysiological abnormality, and may be set in motion or aggravated by emotional disorders. Attention deficit disorders may be associated, at least transitorily, with some form of dyslexia. Some children at high risk for SZ are dyslexic; those at high risk for MDP, however, are not (Kestenbaum, 1982), and in fact often read earlier than usual and have a higher Verbal than Performance score on the Wechsler Intelligence Scale for Children (WISC).

One might suspect that a population of hospitalized patients such as made up the ranks of the PI-500 might show a modest overrepresentation of dyslexics, but this did not appear to be the case.

A borderline adolescent in the PI-500 exhibited one of the common manifestations of dyslexia—namely, left–right reversal of letters ("strephosymbolia"). This condition did not figure prominently in her illness, the main symptoms of which were premenstrual depression and irritability. There was no history of emotional disorders in her immediate family. Later she was noted to have a hypoglycemic tendency (see below). At follow-up 13 years later, she was asymptomatic, had a wide circle of friends, and was doing outstanding work at a professional school. Her reading was now fluent. A propos her old symptom, in recent years she developed a strong interest in a language with a right–left "reversal" (as a Westerner experiences it)—namely, Arabic.

DYSMORPHOPHOBIA

The unwieldy term "dysmorphophobia" connotes a delusional conviction of being ugly (Koupernik, 1982; Morselli, 1866) and has come to include the paradoxical situation in which a beautiful woman imagines herself misshapen or ugly (Hay, 1970). In an earlier report, I mentioned some of the unusual dynamics that may underlie these cases (Stone, 1985a). Some attractive women who have been incest victims, for example, develop a kind of defensive dysmorphophobia, as though harboring the illusion of being unattractive will somehow ensure that men will find them so also, and will therefore cease to molest them. In other instances, the condition serves to neutralize (in the eyes of the patient) the envy of, say, a less attractive sister. In a similar (and paradoxical) vein, a conviction of exterior "ugliness" may serve as a defense against the eruption into consciousness of a true ugliness of *character*. Dysmorphophobia may occur in women with pathological attachments to their fathers, providing a rationale for avoiding involvement with men their own age. Occasionally one will encounter males with similar preoccupations about being "ugly." Dysmorphophobia is not a true phobia in the sense of dreading something real, like snakes or bridges; it is rather an obsessive preoccupation that may vary in intensity from an overvalued idea (in a borderline person) to outright delusion. The latter is not specific to any particular psychosis. There were at least 10 dysmorphophobic patients in the PI-500; 7 were borderline, 2 schizophrenic, and 1 schizophreniform.

The fates of these 10 patients were diverse. Two young women committed suicide; the schizophreniform woman did very well academically, although she never made long-lasting relationships with men; the two schizophrenics (one of whom was male) did reasonably well. The schizophrenic woman had been sexually molested by a family member, and was later molested by a therapist. She showed something akin to a "multiple personality" (see below) at the hospital. The two patients who committed suicide came from unusually bleak environments (querulous, alcoholic parents, etc.); dysmorphophobia had been only a minor problem (see also Chapter Four).

Of the remaining five borderlines, one was not traced; at follow-up, the others were all either clinically well or recovered (Global Assessment Scale [GAS] scores of 65, 70, 72, and 90). In two, the chief contributory factor was not one of the paradoxical mechanisms mentioned above, but rather a hypercritical parent who perpetually undermined the daughter's self-confidence about her appearance. Both appeared to respond well to an expressive psychotherapy while at PI. Though most of the nine patients I traced were preoccupied with their faces, one was convinced (delusionally) that her breasts were disfigured.

The male borderline patient in this group remained overconcerned about his face for about 2–3 years after discharge, but at follow-up had, in the opinion of his parents, "become a different person—very outspoken, confident." He later completed a professional school, married, and had two children.

EPISODIC DYSCONTROL

Under the rubric of "episodic dyscontrol" is to be found an etiologically heterogeneous collection of disorders, often manifesting themselves in adolescence as some variety of "borderline" condition. Attention deficit disorder may be an accompanying feature, or else a learning disorder. Trauma, encephalitis, or epilepsy (including temporal lobe disorder) may have been in the background as a pre-existing or inciting factor. The symptoms of "minimal brain dysfunction" or of a limbic system disorder may be present. Usually, the patients are male, and show "aggressive and hyperactive behavior and academic difficulties during childhood, and antisocial acting out with drug/alcohol abuse during adolescence" (Andrulonis et al., 1982, p. 677).

Not all clinicians use Andrulonis et al.'s terminology, but all are familiar with the kinds of aggressive/impulsive syndromes they are referring to. On an inpatient unit with borderline adolescents, there are usually a few such patients at any given moment. Among the PI-500 there were very few such patients, simply because we instinctively felt, during the initial screening process, that patients with (what was later to be called) episodic dyscontrol are best approached by behavioral, limit-setting, and psychopharmacological means rather than by analytically oriented psychotherapy.

Several male adolescents with learning disorders, hyperactivity, and impulsive aggressivity are described elsewhere in this book. There were only three or four altogether; one eventually killed three people (see "Gradations of Antisociality," Chapter Six).

The one patient from the PI-500 who best exemplifies the episodic dyscontrol syndrome was a young man, aged 17 upon his admission, who had been subject to explosive outbursts (some with and some without clear precipitants) ever since the age of 9. He was also depressed, withdrawn, and suicidal. The product of a prolonged breech delivery, he was raised on a large estate in Peru owned by his multimillionaire family. He was reported to be "late for dates," not speaking until age 3. When his parents divorced (he was 8 at the time), he was sent to a boarding school in another country where he was sodomized by some of the other students. These attacks provoked counterattacks of violence on his part: He struck them, but later he struck his teachers and other pupils seemingly at random. He was then returned to Peru to undergo therapy with a psychiatrist, whom he smashed with a chair after the latter told him he was "brain-damaged." (It is not clear whether the psychiatrist regarded this outburst as a vindication of his original diagnosis.) The patient's education was then entrusted to male tutors residing on the family's *hacienda*. They also sodomized the patient, who by now was setting fires following these incidents of sexual assault. Eventually he was flown to the United States to receive residential treatment.

On the unit at PI, the patient was usually submissive and depressed, but occasionally became panicky (e.g., upon seeing the other male patients' genitals in the shower room), and sometimes struck out at these patients or at the staff. He was noted to appear "glazed over" for some minutes before these outbursts. This was taken as a sign of probable seizure disorder, although conventional electroencephalography (EEG) was unrevealing (nasopharyngeal leads were not used). The patient was treated with neuroleptics and Ritalin®. He became clingingly attached to his therapist; therapy was predominantly supportive.

After a year on the unit (during which time he remained indifferent to the milieu activities), one of the patient's relatives rather capriciously removed him to another facility. The family members considered him a bother and were motivated mostly by the desire to have him installed permanently in a locked facility. His was not a story that inspired optimism, so it was with considerable (and pleasant) surprise that I learned 18 years later, having traced his family through a very circuitous route, that the patient was now married and able to work productively (i.e., at a position that was not a sinecure) within his family's business empire.

FACTITIOUS ILLNESS
(MUNCHAUSEN SYNDROME)

Because of our fascination with those who attempt to deceive us, patients with factitious illness are overrepresented in the literature, in proportion to their actual number. Many fanciful terms adorn this literature. The most popular is "Munchausen syndrome," in honor of Raspe's tall tales ascribed (falsely) to an actual Baron von Munchausen (Asher,

1951; Raspe, 1785; Spiro, 1968). Several recent articles suggest that patients who repeatedly feign illness harbor primitive personalities. Sometimes they resemble border-lines (Nadelson, 1979); sometimes they are antisocial or else not easily classified (Reich, 1983). The five such patients known to me personally all mutilated themselves. One bled herself down to a hemoglobin level of 3; another injected *Staphyloccus aureus* into her skin; a third enucleated one eye. All showed serious disturbances in sense of identity, as well as manifest hostility to one or both parents. The typical patient is a single woman in her 20s who works in a profession ancillary to medicine (e.g., nursing, laboratory technician), acquiring as a result firsthand knowledge of various obscure ailments (Stone, 1977). Although some "Munchausen" patients do not exhibit the features of DSM-defined borderline personality disorder (BPD), their denial of illness and their general untreatability place them in a category apart. They almost never respond favorably to psychotherapy.

Pope, Jonas, and Jones (1982), for example, found that outcome measures, 4–7 years after discharge, of nine hospitalized patients with factitious illness closely resembled those noted in their schizophrenic patients and were well below scores obtained by their manic and schizoaffective comparison groups. Seven of these nine patients met DSM criteria for BPD; only one was currently well. More recently, Pessar (1988) has presented a less gloomy picture, having had better success in her series of "Munchausen" patients. Hers may, however, have been a less severely ill group at the outset, since her patients were borderline in functioning but did not as often have BPD.

The one case of factitious illness in the PI-500 was that of a girl of 16, who had entered the hospital on an internal medical unit because of unexplained fainting spells. Although a cardiac workup revealed mild mitral insufficiency stemming presumably from rheumatic fever, her physicians felt that her spells could not be explained solely on this basis. While on the unit, she began to tell lurid and seemingly far-fetched stories about incest, first with her father, then with various cousins; later, she claimed that these stories were all lies invented to elicit sympathy from those around her. A psychiatric consultant concluded that hers was a case of "pseudologia fantastica" (see below), set in motion by loneliness, deteriorating schoolwork, and family strife. She came from a large and chaotic family whose function was under considerable strain from parental alcoholism and unevenness of income. Upon transfer to our unit, it emerged that she had induced her syncopal attacks with drugs. She had also made a number of suicide attempts. Though preoccupied with sex, highly seductive, and exhibiting many of the features of the "incest profile" (see Stone, 1990), she remained elusive throughout her stay.

We still do not know what fires (if any) lay underneath this thick symptomatic smoke. Her progress, at all events, was most encouraging. She was readmitted briefly 5 years later for depression; however, she never made further suicide gestures nor feigned illness in the 23 years prior to follow-up. Married in her mid-20s, she went on to have four children. She described her husband as warmly supportive and her life as fulfilling. She expressed gratitude to the hospital staff in helping her over the "pains of adolescence." Her GAS score at follow-up was 82.

GLOBUS HYSTERICUS

A hysterical condition characterized by constriction of the throat, brought about by psychological complexes rather than by disease in the upper gastrointestinal tract, has been known usually under its late-19th-century label "globus hystericus." Even earlier, references to what is probably the same condition went under the name "epigastralgia" or "esophagism." There is passing mention in Willis (1668, p. 163) of a hysterical affliction causing abrupt vomiting after meals, itself an allusion to the ancient literature on hysteria. The condition appears to affect women much more often than men. Whytt (1765) described several cases, including that of an "unmarried gentlewoman aged 44, irregular as to the menses, [who] was seized with a pain in her stomach, and soon after every meal became sick, and vomited what she had eaten" (p. 479). Briquet (1859), the originator of the eponymous "Briquet syndrome," claimed that "epigastralgia" with vomiting was one of the commonest manifestations of hysteria, occurring in 317 of 358 hysterical women (p. 216). Briquet cited as contributory factors hereditary predisposition to hysteria, menstrual irregularities (especially in girls of 15 or 16), and various nervous tendencies. LeGrand Du Saulle (1891) described, under the heading "oesophagisme," several hysterical women in their 20s and 30s with "irregular menses" and abrupt tightening in the throat and vomiting after meals. LeGrand Du Saulle commented that "whereas hysterics often seem able to fast for prodigious periods—weeks or even months—without losing their strength, those given to repetitive vomiting are vulnerable to severe weakness" (1891, p. 109; my translation).

These earlier accounts make no observations about the general psychological problems that may have been present in the women they describe, let alone any speculations about specific dynamics. Hypotheses concerning these issues appear first in Freud's (1905b) *Three Essays on the Theory of Sexuality,* where he stated (in the section on the oral erotogenic zone and on thumbsucking) that "many of my women patients who suffer from disturbances of eating, *globus hystericus,* constriction of the throat and vomiting, have indulged energetically in sucking during their childhood" (p. 182). In the generation of psychoanalytic pioneers, most theories concerning the unconscious symbolism of globus hystericus centered around instinctual aims of incorporation (see Ferenczi, 1923). Fenichel (1945) mentions, for example, that "The fellatio idea is extraordinarily common in the unconscious fantasies of hysterical women (globus hystericus). Analysis shows that this idea is a distorted expression for the wish to bite off and incorporate the penis" (p. 229).

In the PI-500 only one patient, a borderline woman of 20 with hysterical, masochistic, and narcissistic features, complained of the "ball in the throat" and inability to get food down characteristic of globus hystericus. Far from having had a seductive father, as many such patients had had in the early psychoanalytic accounts, she had almost no relationship with her father at all. Many interpretations regarding supposed fellatio fantasies were made during the 2-year course of her inpatient treatment, without alleviation of her symptom. An attractive woman with artistic talent in a number of areas, she was (while at PI) considered to have a poor prognosis, largely because of her tendency to ally herself with men who abused her physically and because of her lack of goal-directedness. Twenty-two years later, however, there were surprises on two fronts. She had, after 10 years of sporadic work and doomed love affairs, married a most suitable man and opened a large clothing establishment, which earned her both high respect in her field and a high income. Her "globus" disappeared after it was finally discovered to be, rather than the sequel of an unresolved incorporation complex, the mere accompaniment of an achalasia. After the latter was corrected by esophageal surgery, she was asymptomatic. I include this vignette as a cautionary note, reminding us of the need to look hard for possible physical causes in certain erstwhile and rather exotic psychological conditions.

HYPERACTIVITY

Childhood hyperactivity is etiologically diverse and therefore to be noted as a nonspecific trait in a number of (adult) conditions. This hyperkinetic syndrome is seen with greater than expected frequency in children of manic–depressive parents (Kron et al., 1982) and in adolescent borderlines. Similar correlations exist between borderline conditions and (looking backward) family pedigrees containing MDP, or (looking forward) future development of MDP (see Stone, Kahn, & Flye, 1981). Elsewhere in this book, I discuss in some detail the controversy regarding possible connections between MDP and borderline psychopathology, as highlighted by outcomes in the PI-500 (see Chapter Five).

As with the many traits that have correlative though not necessarily causal connection to borderline conditions (some of which are outlined in Table 5.2, Chapter Five), a problem in Bayseian algebra always arises: If "borderline," what is the conditional probability of X? If X (in this case, hyperactivity), what is the conditional probability of (being or becoming) borderline? These questions usually hang in the air, because we scarcely know the incidence of BPD in the population as a whole (recent estimates suggest 2%), let alone the incidence of less well-studied entities such as "hyperactivity," "tantrums," "separation anxiety," and the like. Nor do we usually know the degrees of overlap: What percentage of hyperactive children go on, as they reach adulthood, to exhibit a borderline disorder? Obviously, if all hyperactive children became borderline and only borderline, and if 90% of borderlines had been hyperactive children, so powerful a correlation might entitle us to claim that hyperactivity "causes" borderline conditions, or that whatever antecedent factors cause hyperactivity are also responsible later on for borderline conditions. Equally obvious: The connection between hyperactivity and borderline conditions is not nearly of this order. So we are left with clinical hunches, hypotheses to test, and so on.

The situation is further complicated by the fact that some pedigrees are replete with father–son or other combinations (usually of males) with hyperactivity, but no varieties of MDP (Morrison & Minkoff, 1975). In other families, hyperactivity (in male children especially) and MDP are fellow-travelers; some of the children eventually become "borderline."

In the PI-500, there were several borderlines who had been markedly hyperkinetic/ hyperactive as children. One was a male admitted when he was 13, both of whose parents appeared to have risk genes for MDP. Both were irascible and violent. The patient eventually became a murderer and is described in the section on "Gradations of Antisociality" (see Chapter Six). Another, admitted when he was 14, had an irascible, withdrawn father and a depressed, agoraphobic mother. The family was not chaotic (as the family of the boy who murdered had been). From age 8, the second boy was described as violent, explosive, uncontrollable, demanding, and friendless. He would occasionally threaten to harm his parents. His IQ was 135, but his condition impaired his concentration and his academic performance. While he was at PI, group pressure and the emotional distance from home had an ameliorative effect, but he did not appear to benefit much from dyadic psychotherapy. At follow-up 23 years later, he was still hyperactive, volatile, and somewhat abrasive in personality. But he now had a circle of friends, was not violent, and derived much satisfaction (and a modest income) from fishing—an interesting transformation, considering that as a youngster he used to torture pet fish. It is not clear whether he ever had a trial of Ritalin® or Cylert®.

One of the female patients (neurotic-level) with hyperactivity responded well to Cylert®; like the preceding patient, she was exceptionally bright. She was eventually able to complete graduate school and to function socially and occupationally at a high level.

HYPOGLYCEMIA

As Foster and Rubinstein (1983) assert, "[Hypoglycemia] is often self-diagnosed by those who have read the lay-oriented literature that describes hypoglycemia as a common cause of ill health" (p. 683). True alimentary hypoglycemia in the absence of gastrointestinal surgery, according to these authors, is rare. Central nervous system (CNS) symptoms such as dizziness, headache, blunted mental acuity, and abnormal (including hostile) behavior are nonetheless often ascribed to hypoglycemia. Abnormal glucose tolerance tests are sometimes recorded in these cases, although as Gorman and Liebowitz (1985) point out, "there is no scientific proof at present that 'reactive hypoglycemia' is ever a cause of any psychiatric disturbance" (p. 10). False positives are quite common in glucose tolerance tests; one would need to document a low blood sugar level at the time the patient was symptomatic. Documented cases are most exceptional.

Foster and Rubinstein (1983) recommend substitution of the term "idiopathic postprandial syndrome" for the older label "idiopathic postabsorptive hypoglycemia," especially because patients with this condition usually have slightly *elevated* glucose concentrations during spontaneous attacks "because of the hyperglycemic actions of epinephrine and cortisol, the stress hormones that induce the symptoms" (p. 686). Hall and Beresford (1985), though acknowledging the controversy that surrounds this topic, allow as how "unprovoked outbursts of anger or violence, periods of aloofness, episodic confusion, etc." (p. 12) may, in certain patients, be the manifestations of postprandial hypoglycemia. One can appreciate that an organic condition (if it could be substantiated) characterized by angry outbursts and strange behavior might be confused with a borderline disorder.

Two young borderline women in the PI-500 were admitted because of such symptoms as moodiness, depression, outbursts of temper and screaming (in one instance), or headaches and stomachaches after breakfast, violent arguments, and rebelliousness (in the other). They failed to improve while at PI, but were given the diagnosis of hypoglycemia several years later by consultants to whom the parents turned in desperation. Both patients improved after they "got off sugar" and had been asymptomatic for years at follow-up. One became a mathematics teacher; the other, a lawyer. The latter sometimes got "almost suicidal" after eating foods high in sugar content, or else would lose control of her temper. She was also dyslexic (see above) until late adolescence. Neither patient had had blood glucose levels drawn at the time of attacks, and thus may have fallen into the category of "idiopathic postprandial syndrome." Their cures may be have been the results more of placebo effects than of appropriate medical intervention. One of the patients came from a home where the parents got along quite well; the other came from a disturbed family (alcoholic relatives, frequent parental separations and reconciliations). The cases are puzzling from whichever angle they are viewed, though informative to the extent that they demonstrate that borderline patients sometimes become ill for no obvious reason (the girl with the normal family) and sometimes get better for reasons that are equally mysterious.

THE CASE OF THE IMPOSTER

Imposters have been known since just after the beginning of time; they never fail to fascinate, and often earn the grudging admiration even of those they have fooled. The famous novels about "confidence men" by Melville (1857) and Mann (1955) are built around such characters. Celebrated imposters (such as Frank Demara in the 1940s, who impersonated surgeons and professors) are usually so clever as to inspire the comment, "If he had just used his talents in conventional ways, he could have gone far." Obviously, there are forces at work that make conventional society and the conventional path to success abhorrent to the imposter.

In the case of the one imposter in the PI-500, those forces consisted mainly of an abusive father who lost no opportunity to belittle his son through withering verbal humiliation and frequent physical assaults, and of a predisposition to MDP (manifest also in the father) that seemed to cause drivenness and Wanderlust. When the patient was in his early 20s, he began to impersonate men in positions of authority—presumably, his way of compensating for his shattered self-esteem. His IQ was 140; he had little difficulty in performing the jobs of those he impersonated as well as (or better than) they could. At one point he became a "Navy officer," but was found out. His superiors, in a burst of leniency, concluded that "anyone crazy enough to impersonate a Navy officer was more of a psychiatric case than a criminal," and thus remanded him to residential treatment.

At PI this patient was considered "borderline," mainly from the standpoint of identity disturbance, though he satisfied DSM criteria for BPD as well. He charmed his therapist, appeared to mend his ways, and was released (after a year) when a job became available in a laboratory. There he distinguished himself by making a substantial improvement in one of the standard medical tests. Success, however, led to boredom: He moved on to a company that pirated records. Afterwards he remained on the other side of the law, became involved in illegal drugs, was jailed on a number of occasions, and ultimately died (in prison) of a heart attack in his 40s. He was likeable and flamboyant; everyone in his family respected his mind, but no one knew when he was telling the truth. His life, in their eyes, was a "total waste"; it is not clear that the psychiatric community could have done a better job with such a patient nowadays than we were able to do at PI in the 1960s. To the extent that individuals with antisocial personality (ASP)— of whom imposters are a subset—can be treated at all, recourse to special group technics might prove more effective than would the dyadic psychotherapy upon which we relied in our work with this man.

MULTIPLE PERSONALITY

Even more popular than imposters, in the domain of psychiatric oddities, are cases of "multiple personality." The diagnosis depends upon the discovery within one person of two or more distinct personalities, each dominant at a particular time, each controlling the person's behavior at that time, and each endowed with its own complexity and unique pattern of behavior and social relationships (Gilmore & Kaufman, 1985, p. 8). Depending upon whom one reads, cases are either very rare (Gilmore & Kaufman, 1985), rather rare (Bliss, 1986), or not so rare (Kluft, 1985, 1987). Celebrated cases have been the subjects of several books (Schreiber, 1973; Thigpen & Cleckley, 1957). Bliss mentions that many purported cases have been viewed with skepticism as instances of histrionic patients' fooling or pleasing their therapists. Nevertheless, in Bliss's experience and also in Kluft's, many cases of multiple personality seem genuine. It is also becoming clear that the crucial etiological factor is severe trauma during childhood, of a sort that exceeds the capacity of a young person to integrate. Usually the trauma consists of extreme physical abuse or frank incest at the hands of a parent (i.e., someone the child has been raised to love and trust). The "alternate" personalities are, indeed, generally the repositories of the unassimilable emotions generated by these dismal experiences. One alternate self may be whorish; another, prudish, a third, rageful. Most cases are female, in part because most victims of incest are girls (see Chapter Seven).

In the PI-500, there was no classical case of multiple personality satisfying the criteria of DSM-III or the more complex criteria of Greaves (1980). The closest approximation was found in a woman of 20 who had become ill shortly after menarche: She developed eating disorders, dysmorphophobia (see above), delusional ideas about food, and ideas of being controlled by other people's thoughts. In time, she felt that various thoughts belonged to 12 different personalities. Her (main) personality was described as infantile and demanding. Some senior consultants felt that she was not truly delusional, but merely emotionally labile and "borderline" (whereas initially she was considered "schizophrenic"). Trials of neuroleptics and of lithium were of no benefit. Her subsequent course was erratic: She worked only sporadically, married (impulsively) an inappropriate man, made a suicide attempt necessitating a brief rehospitalization, and in general showed only marginal adjustment. Of interest was the fact that she had not been the victim of abuse or molestation as a child, but decompensated following a sexual relationship with a previous therapist. Her "dozen personalities," however, antedated this experience.

In cases of more genuine "multiple personality," the prognosis is usually a function of the nature and severity of the antecedent traumata. The presence or absence of genetic vulnerability to a psychosis will render the outcome less or more favorable, respectively. Cases of multiple personality are often confused with borderline conditions, or else viewed as an unusual variant. By Kernberg criteria such patients show a psychotic structure, technically speaking, because the main "self" denies totally the existence of the alternate(s). Each "self," taken one at a time, may show the features of a borderline (or of any other) personality. As such, these cases do not fit neatly into our taxonomy and usually defy our glib assumptions about their being "borderline."

A number of the patients with BPD showed distinct but less extreme forms of dissociation than those associated with "multiple personality." Some, for example, exhibited severe premenstrual personality changes (see Chapter Eight)—becoming irritable, depressed, even suicidal—only to recoup their more customary, placid selves several days later. One of these women, who also had pseudocyesis (see below), tended to oscillate between two markedly different states. At times, she was cooperative, compliant, and docile; at others (especially when under stress), she was angry and grandiose. But these dissociative tendencies, though they left her with a marked identity disorder, never progressed to the point of compartmentalization into two "selves" with two different names and lack of awareness of one another. She was rehospitalized for a few days, several years after leaving PI, because of a manic episode. Though on lithium after this incident, she was never well; she remained unable to work with any consistency and led a reclusive life. Her GAS score at follow-up was 52.

NARCOLEPSY

A familial syndrome characterized by (1) rapid eye movement (REM) sleep attacks during wakefulness, (2) cataplexy, (3) sleep paralysis, and (4) hypnagogic hallucinations, "narcolepsy" is said to occur in about 5 persons out of 10,000 and to become clinically apparent during early adolescence (Keener & Anders, 1985; Schulz & Reynolds, 1985). The daytime REM intrusions into consciousness account for the hypnagogic hallucinations, which may lead to a misdiagnosis of schizophrenia. Such was the case with one of the patients in the PI-500, admitted at 18 because of "delusions and hallucinations" and erratic behavior. He was shown to have the narcoleptic tetrad outlined above. This patient also had features of ASP: He ran away from home, was violent toward his parents, and abused psychoactive drugs. He eloped from PI, though he later returned. In retrospect, he was "borderline" by Kernberg criteria, but not by those of DSM-III. His life course was consistent with that of narcoleptic patients not optimally responsive to medication (e.g., methylphenidate) and of persons with mild sociopathic tendencies. He never worked consistently, had rather exploitative relationships with others, lacked ambition, and at follow-up was still subject to sleep attacks.

Two other PI-500 patients had narcolepsy. One, a borderline (BPD) woman, had concomitant bipolar illness (diagnosed after discharge). She responded well to Dexedrine® and was asymptomatic in later years. The other patient, a male, functioned at the borderline level but did not have BPD. Instead he had an anxiety disorder and mixed personality traits, with narcissistic and passive–aggressive features predominating. His narcolepsy began shortly after a fall from a horse at age 11, and was accompanied by nonspecific dysrhythmia on EEG. Amphetamines gave him some symptomatic relief but made him more anxious; he discontinued taking them. Mildly alcoholic when hospitalized at age 30, he became more severely so after discharge. His course was determined not by his narcolepsy, but by his severe personality disorder and his alcoholism. Several years later—alone, and on the "outs" with his family—he ended his life with an overdose of barbiturates.

NEUROLEPTIC MALIGNANT SYNDROME

Neuroleptic malignant syndrome (NMS) differs from the other conditions mentioned in this appendix by virtue of its being iatrogenic. The possibility of this adverse reaction, some 200 cases of which have been reported in the literature, was not widely appreciated in the mid-1960s (when the one case occurred among the PI-500), although Ayd (1956) had described it and Delay (1968) had given a name to it some years earlier.

Our example is of interest because of its surprise value—an excellent recovery occurring in someone who appeared hopeless while on our unit. When first admitted, our patient, a young man of 20 who had dropped out of college, was diagnosed as "schizophrenic." We gave him modest doses of chlorpromazine, but as he became more delusional with each succeeding day, we rapidly increased the dose until, 10 days later, he was taking 2,000 mg/day. By then he was drooling, diaphoretic, and rigid. In our insouciance (about NMS), we considered him the most severely schizophrenic patient we had ever seen. Luckily, he also became febrile (the one feature that was universal in Shalev & Munitz's [1986] review of the syndrome). This alerted us to the probability that something medical rather than merely psychological was wrong with this man. We discontinued all medications; within a few weeks his psychosis and loss of contact were much less pronounced. Eight months later he left the unit rather the worse for wear—awkward-appearing, embittered, and prognostically unpromising. He went into therapy with a private psychiatrist, with whom he remained about 8 years. He got well enough to finish college and to do graduate work in engineering. He married, took a responsible position with a large firm, and raised a family. In retrospect, he did not have DSM-defined SZ to begin with, but had instead an acute schizophreniform illness (precipitated by medications for a different condition), onto which we superimposed NMS via the chlorpromazine. At follow-up 19 years later, as his family mentioned, no one would know he was ever ill. His GAS score was 78.

OBSESSIVE HANDWASHING

Compulsive handwashing seemed to be a fairly common symptom in Freud's time. Symbolically, this compulsion was often linked with masturbatory guilt (Freud, 1905a; Goldman, 1938). As guilt over sexual themes has lessened over the course of the century (partly through the impact of psychoanalysis), the syndrome has become less common among more integrated persons; cases are still to be found either in neurotic persons from primitive cultures (Stone, 1970), in schizophrenics from more sophisticated cultures, or in persons with obsessive–compulsive disorder (OCD). Guilt over real crimes rather than over sexual indiscretions may also figure in the dynamics (as in the case of Lady Macbeth!).

There were 10 cases of obsessive handwashing in the PI-500; 5 of these were in borderline patients. Masturbatory guilt was an important factor in these patients, though in several instances extreme perfectionism (with a sense of having "failed" to live up to parental expectations) also played a role. The five borderline patients did surprisingly well; their average follow-up GAS score was 71 (range = 61–84). Two obtained doctorates; one of these was married with two children. Two others were working and able to maintain a circle of friends, though they remained sexually inhibited. The remaining patient had been doing well at work until he suffered severe injuries during an accident, from which he never fully recovered. The patient with the best outcome in this group was the one who appeared sickest when first seen (he had made a number of severe suicide attempts and self-mutilative gestures with knives before coming to PI).

The one schizoaffective handwasher was married at follow-up, doing well, and no longer under the care of a psychiatrist, though she had been rehospitalized several times shortly after leaving PI. The two who were schizophrenic have committed suicide. One had prominent "negative signs" of schizophrenia (see Chapter Twelve); she also had delusional preoccupations about germs and was unable to lick stamps or envelopes. One of the two schizophreniform patients, who showed referential and paranoid ideation in addition to the handwashing symptom, made an excellent adjustment with his new family (wife and two children), though relations were still strained with his parents.

The borderline patients with this syndrome improved with psychotherapy alone; the others, with a combination of behavioral and supportive therapy. Given the general stubbornness of compulsive handwashing, one may wonder how it is that the majority of these patients (especially the borderlines) did so well. (Currently, many—but not all—patients with OCD are responding favorably to serotonergic drugs like clomipramine or fluoxetine.) I believe that the answer lies in the relative absence, in this group, of hostility toward others: They were, if anything, *intro*punitive and afflicted with an ego-dystonic symptom that kept up their motivation for change through therapy.

PATHOLOGICAL JEALOUSY

Freud (1922) described three degrees of jealousy: "normal" jealousy, engendered, for example, by spouses who flaunt their infidelity; "projected" jealousy, in which one's own impulses toward infidelity are experienced as residing in one's mate; and "delusional" jealousy. The last-mentioned, also known as "pathological" jealousy, Freud understood as a (paranoid) defense against homosexual strivings. Several contemporary authors have speculated on the underlying dynamics, including Pao (1969a), who emphasized "narcissistic unrelatedness" and the interweaving of Oedipal and pre-Oedipal issues; Frosch (1981), who drew attention to humiliations in early life; and Coen (1987), who noted the tendency to become attracted to persons similar, in gender as well as in personality, to oneself. According to Coen, the homosexual aspects of this are simultaneously denied and acted out (e.g., in minute inquiry about the same-sex third person whom one's mate supposedly "loves"). Males who demonstrate this condition sometimes show intense fixation on their mothers (Freud, 1922).

One would expect to see examples of pathological jealousy in any large population of borderline and psychotic patients, many of whom are inordinately insecure about their attractiveness, correspondingly possessive, and thus prone to jealous discomfort over the real or imagined attention of their sexual partners toward other persons. In the PI-500, however, I could only identify one such patient. Possibly this may relate to the relative youthfulness of the patients; many of them were adolescents who had not as yet developed the kind of intimacy that, in poorly integrated persons, can so readily become tainted with jealousy.

The one patient in question, who had BPD, was hospitalized when he was 22 because of aggressive behavior toward his fiancée. He would constantly see her in his mind's eye making love with her previous boyfriend. Accusing her of preferring that man to himself, he would become enraged to the point of combativeness. Throughout his life, his mother had behaved seductively toward him (walking into his room naked, making disparaging remarks about his father, etc.). He found her behavior both exciting and repellent. His jealousy became less intense by the end of his 6-month hospital stay. Eventually he married his fiancée, but after several years they divorced. He continued to work with a therapist for many years, took an advanced degree, and began a successful professional career; his jealous symptoms gradually abated. At follow-up, he had been essentially well throughout the past 24 years, and had grown more compassionate and mellow toward both family and friends. His GAS score was 86.

Despite isolated reports of successful outcome (such as this one; see also Pao, 1969a), pathological jealousy usually presents the same enormous difficulties to the therapist as does any entrenched paranoid mind-set. The dynamics are deceptively straightforward; however, as with the Hydra's head, each doubt put to rest by the therapist causes 10 new ones to sprout in the mind of the patient. Why, then, did this man do so well? I have no answer, other than to suggest that pathological jealousy might be easier to resolve when a parent has been merely seductive but not frankly incestuous. Hospitalized borderline females, for example, have often been incest victims. They have witnessed *real* betrayal, *real* infidelity (especially in cases of father–daughter incest), and thus have had their capacity to trust undermined not just by innuendo but by actual experience. Crowe, Clarkson, Tsai, and Wilson (1988) found recently that pathological (delusional) jealousy, though it tended not to change over the course of time, had a more benign evolution (less rehospitalization) than nonjealous delusional disorder. Neither type of delusional disorder was associated with a family history of schizophrenia.

PSEUDOCYESIS

Pseudocyesis has a long tradition in medicine: Mary Tudor believed herself pregnant when she was not for many years.[2] The syndrome is nonspecific in regard both to underlying diagnosis and to psychodynamic underpinnings. In some patients, sexual guilt may predominate; in others, envy of pregnancy in a relative or close friend is the chief conflict. Fear about the possibility of being pregnant is paramount in a few patients; still others develop the symptom primarily to win attention (Bivin & Klinger, 1937; Hofstätter, 1924). In the PI-500, two patients maintained false beliefs of being pregnant. One was a borderline woman; the other a schizophrenic.

The borderline woman had showed severe separation anxiety as a young child. During adolescence, a number of symptoms developed in rapid succession. These included fluctuations in mood and in weight, agoraphobia, and a fear that she was pregnant. The patient herself had had no sexual contact. A cousin had recently given birth; this seemed to serve as the trigger for the pseudocyesis. The symptom gradually subsided, but was replaced by several others that, in the aggregate, were enough to establish a diagnosis of BPD with concomitant major affective disorder (MAD). Panic attacks, associated with the latter, were what led to her hospitalization on our unit. The clinical picture evolved, in the 14 years after discharge, along the lines of a bipolar II illness, responsive to lithium. Her recovery was only partial (GAS score at follow-up = 58): She did well academically and socially, but fatigued easily, to the point where sustained work was difficult. On two occasions of unusual stress, she expressed unrealistic ideas (not related to the theme of pregnancy) that persisted for a day or two.

The schizophrenic patient was 22 when admitted to our unit, having been hospitalized because of a delusional psychosis that occurred after the sudden death of a family member. The delusions, which shifted in content from time to time, first took the form of pseudocyesis: She believed that she was pregnant with the just-deceased relative, who was now alive again inside her. Though she rather quickly relinquished the convictions associated with her pseudocyesis, she remained ill and was still seriously handicapped (follow-up GAS score = 25) 20 years later.

One might suppose that a symptom with delusory overtones, such as pseudocyesis, might be associated with the more severe forms of emotional illness; given the rarity of the disorder, it is hard to be certain. I do not think that such a correlation exists, however. I have recently had the experience of working with a well-integrated, ambulatory patient who had pseudocyesis briefly during adolescence, in a setting of emotional deprivation.

PSEUDOLOGIA FANTASTICA

Pseudologia fantastica was mentioned rather often in the psychiatric literature at the turn of the century; by contrast, it has been described only rarely in our era (Fenichel, 1939;

[2]She maintained this belief despite being married to Philip II of Spain, who was seldom with her even geographically. "Bloody Mary" had a tumor, whose bulk she misinterpreted as a pregnancy.

Hoyer, 1959; Wendt, 1911). This should not be attributed to any diminution in the level of mendacity in present times, but merely to the changes in terminology over the decades. Fenichel (1939) spoke of compulsive lying in certain persons given to overconscientiousness in small details but to falsifications of the grosser facts about their everyday lives. I have seen pseudologia in men ashamed over their lack of competence in the sexual arena, who boast to their fellow employees of "conquests and exploits" fabricated out of whole cloth. One, for example, who seemed unable to tell the truth even about the correct time, told his friends that he was en route (in tuxedo and top hat) to a party where his engagement to the daughter of a European baron was to be announced. Secretly followed by his friends, he got no farther than a pool hall two blocks away, having jettisoned a dozen roses for his "fiancée" in a litter basket along the way. Certain patients with painful secrets are susceptible to this sort of flamboyant lying. For example, two incest victims made up incredible stories of terrible things that did not happen, which were nevertheless closely related symbolically to still worse things that *did* happen. One woman told of a dark stranger having repeatedly run over her pet cat in the driveway of her home—a fanciful tale, yet one closely related to her father's incestuous advances throughout her adolescence. A similar case in which a borderline woman with pseudologia had been an incest victim was reported by Snyder (1986).

One borderline and dysthymic patient in the PI-500 with pseudologia first began her compulsive lying following the death of her mother when she was 16. The year before, her alcoholic father had left the family. Though most people would be moved by the already tragic story of her actual life, she made up even more pitiful stories, as though to remove the last vestiges of doubt as to whether her listeners would react sympathetically. She was quite unreachable in psychotherapy while at PI, because no one could get through the thicket of her distortions. Fifteen years later, however, the picture was much more encouraging. She was working full-time and getting a bachelor's degree in English at night school. She was still single, but had a number of close friends and was active in church affairs. As her self-sufficiency increased in the years just after leaving PI, her need for pity diminished, and with it the pseudologia. She was never rehospitalized. The nonamenability of the pseudologia to psychotherapy is reminiscent of another syndrome in which prevarication is a central feature: factitious illness.

The only other patient with this syndrome happened also to present with factitious illness and is mentioned above under that heading.

TRICHOTILLOMANIA

"Trichotillomania" represents another attempt (along with "strephosymbolia" and "dysmorphophobia") to give scientific cachet to a humble act by translating it into ancient Greek. The compulsive pulling out of one's hair (which is all that the term signifies) is not specific to any diagnostic entity (though, in comtemporary thought, many cases may be manifestations of OCD); many persons (usually young women) resort to it at moments of great stress. Extreme examples of the phenomenon do attract attention, of course (both public and medical), and may constitute one symptom of a more generalized impulse disorder, including a borderline condition. There is a small literature devoted to the syndrome (see Greenberg & Sarner, 1965). Like many other self-damaging acts committed within an atmosphere of desperation and frenzy, (extreme) trichotillomania is often the accompaniment of bipolar MDP, or a borderline ("subaffective"; Akiskal et al., 1978) variant thereof.

This was the case with the one patient among the PI-500 who pulled out her hair to a marked degree (necessitating a wig). Aged 25 when admitted, she had frequent oscillations between hypomania and severe depression, and was volatile, angry, and chaotic in her relationships with men. This patient became notable on our unit for her (unwitting) demonstration of the overlap among various diagnostic categories. Having been referred to our service by Philip Polatin as a case of "pseudoneurotic schizophrenia," she was diagnosed as "borderline" (in her level of personality organization) by Kernberg; as having "BPD" by Gunderson (then an occasional consultant to our unit); and, several months later, as "hysteroid dysphoric" by Donald Klein when he assumed directorship of the service. Since each of these men is the originator of one of the four terms, respectively, the diagnoses (1) cannot be challenged and (2) therefore must overlap conceptually to a degree that would permit all four to be correct. "Pseudoneurotic schizophrenia" is the least felicitous of these labels, by the way, inasmuch as few of Polatin's original cases would conform to the more stringent criteria for schizophrenia employed nowadays (Stone, 1980a).

This patient responded only modestly to psychotherapy, partly because of the drivenness of her (hypomanic) personality. She responded well to monoamine oxidase inhibitors (which she was still taking at follow-up 12 years later). She now had "beautiful hair," which she no longer tugged at, and was content with her life. She worked until her marriage a few years ago.

Selected Topics Pertaining to the Posthospitalization Period

DEATHS OTHER THAN BY SUICIDE

The death rate for the entire PI-500, as I have gone about tracing the last few patients, hovers between 11% and 12%. As of this writing, 62 are dead (12%). Statisticians at Metropolitan Life Insurance (Kranzer, 1986) inform me that, actuarially speaking, only about 10 deaths would have occurred in a group of 507 people of this era, moving from an average age of 22 to an average of 38½ and composed of men and women in the particular ratio found in this sample. Men in this age range show a higher death rate than women, in part because of the greater likelihood of their having fatal accidents.

Of the 62 already dead, only 13 died of causes other than suicide. One borderline woman weighed over 350 pounds when admitted and died in her late 30s from the cardiac complications of obesity. Two died of cancer; another of an aneurysm. Two males died in car accidents; a third was killed when his motorcycle went out of control as he swerved to avoid hitting a dog. A schizophrenic man imprisoned for murder died of the hepatotoxic effects of chlorpromazine; the borderline "imposter" (see Appendix A) died in prison of heart disease. Schizophrenic patients are said to be vulnerable to "weird deaths" (Endicott, 1985). There were two such in the PI-500. One woman fell down some stairs, developed a blood clot, and died of a pulmonary embolus. Another schizophrenic woman was cachectic from severe anorexia, and her inanition left her vulnerable to "opportunistic" infections; she died of Legionnaire's disease. A male homosexual patient with borderline personality disorder (BPD) died of opportunistic infection as a sequela of acquired immune deficiency syndrome (AIDS). Finally, one (schizophrenic) man was shot to death while in the act of committing a crime.

The numbers, by diagnostic group, are too small to permit meaningful comparisons. It may be of some significance, however, that these nonsuicide deaths occurred in 1 out of 100 borderlines, but in 6 out of 100 schizophrenics.

LOBOTOMY

One of the darker chapters in the history of psychiatry, lobotomy enjoyed a brief spasm of popularity in the 1940s and 1950s, whereafter its practitioners fell into oblivion, their instruments into desuetude—apart, that is, from the originator of this procedure, which in its heydey so captivated the attention of the scientific world that the Nobel committee saw fit to award Egaz Moniz the prize they denied Freud. So much for history (see Valenstein, 1986).

There was one patient among the PI-500 who underwent prefrontal lobotomy. Originally, we diagnosed her as suffering from a "schizophrenic" illness (for which the operation was usually reserved); shortly after the death of her father, she had developed an erotomanic psychosis (see Appendix A) vis-à-vis her therapist. She became labile in mood, alternating between crying spells and outbursts of rage, in which she tended to break crockery and furniture. She made a suicide attempt, but also attacked one of her brothers. Ideas of reference and obsessional rituals were prominent symptoms on admission; there were no hallucinations. Her delusions were partly mood-congruent (centered around feelings of responsibility for her father's death), partly not (the erotomania). Perhaps her clinical picture equated better with the notion of a psychotic depression (in a patient with mixed borderline features and schizotypal personality [STP]) than with DSM-defined SZ. Others might now call her condition "obsessive–compulsive disorder."

The patient spent over a year in the hospital, without much improvement. We then entrusted her care to a female therapist, in hopes of reducing the likelihood of her again getting mired in erotomanic attachments. Her franticness continued, however, and she became convinced that only a lobotomy could cure her. Eventually she found someone willing to perform one.

The trail went cold for over a year at this point; the posthospital therapist, when contacted, knew only that the lobotomy had been done about 15 years earlier. We assumed that hers was a bad outcome: Perhaps she was now languishing in some institution or, at best, rocking on the porch of a nursing home.

After much difficulty, I finally succeeded in tracing her. The search had taken me on a circuitous path that led me past former doormen of her old apartment and a family physician alluded to parenthetically in her chart. The facts overturned our assumptions completely. Far from languishing in a nursing home, the patient was now self-supporting, working every day at a travel agency, and managing her own apartment. She had required neither rehospitalization nor therapy in recent years and was no longer subject to rage attacks.

Although psychosurgery has been discredited as a treatment for cases such as this one, perhaps there are after all, as Bartlett, Bridges, and Kelly (1981) suggest, isolated instances where it has proven distinctly beneficial. Jenike, Baer, and Minichello (1987), reviewing the psychosurgery literature in relation to severe obsessive–compulsive disorder, concluded that even when lobotomy was popular (1940s through the 1950s), obsessive–compulsive patients did substantially better than did those with schizophrenia. Apathy and lethargy were common side effects in half the cases. Untoward effects with the less drastic procedures (modified leucotomy, cingulotomy) appeared to be even less frequent. Since psychodynamic therapies are often unavailing (despite the obviousness of the symbolism) in severe obsessive–compulsive disorder, and electroconvulsive therapy (ECT) is also usually ineffective, Jenike et al. argue for behavior modification technics or, failing these, some limited form of psychosurgery. Perhaps our patient was a case in point.

As for the more drastic methods of leucotomy and their (3-year) follow-up, the reader should familiarize himself with the singular case reported by Solyom (1987)—that of a 19-year-old man driven by his obsessions to commit suicide by shooting a gun into his mouth. Miraculously, he survived. The resulting damage to the left frontal lobe apparently reduced the level of his obsessions, and was confined largely to the same fronto-orbital cortex and cingulum targeted in the less unconventional forms of psychosurgery.

MISSING PERSONS, VAGRANTS, AND THE HOMELESS

A total of 10 patients left hospital, home, and every other potential source of shelter to take their chances on the open road. They became—some briefly, others for years on end—missing persons, vagrants, and homeless persons. Of the 10, 9 were male. Six were borderline; the others had SZ. Eight came from intact homes, though the parents' relationship was more often strained than not. Only two could be said to have unsafe homes: One borderline woman was an incest victim, and one borderline man had been physically abused by his stepmother. The woman was missing for 10 years and became alcoholic, but eventually joined Alcoholics Anonymous and made a recovery as dramatic as her disappearance.

One borderline man deserted his wife and three children; at follow-up, his parents had lost touch with him for over 15 years. He was often in trouble with the law for passing bad checks before coming to PI, and showed other features of antisocial personality (ASP) as well. One of the younger borderline men disappeared the day he was discharged from the hospital and has never been found, despite intensive efforts spanning 19 years. At this writing, his family still entertains hopes that he is alive; it is much more likely that he met with foul play at some point.

One of the schizophrenic men disappeared for over a decade. When the family ultimately located him, he had changed occupations, married and divorced, and become involved in arcane religious/philosophical abstractions. Yet in later years he functioned reasonably well and effected a rapprochement with his parents. In fact, he became of the most successful of the schizophrenic patients—an outcome no one was prepared to forecast during the years of his absence. As such, his was another "counterintuitive result" (see Chapter Fifteen), of the sort that justifies the extensive efforts necessary in tracing some of the families (including his).

Another schizophrenic man wandered over the country for the better part of a year. In later years he held a number of fairly steady jobs, preferring those that required little interaction with others. This hermit-like quality was characteristic of all the patients in this section, except for the (rather gregarious) borderline woman mentioned above.

Three of the borderline males lived for several years apiece as vagrants. Two became homosexual prostitutes. All three came from severely disturbed homes where alcoholic fathers had abused them. Two had spent brief periods in jail for vagrancy, rape, and drunkenness. At follow-up, they no longer lived on the streets but led a marginal and asocial existence, surviving on public assistance and odd jobs.

One of the schizophrenics ended up in the ranks of New York City's homeless. Having become delusional after a mugging, he spent several years at PI, with no improvement even after seemingly appropriate amounts of neuroleptics. He remained markedly suspicious and was on occasion assaultive. Later, he went to a less conservative institution and was soon released. Still disorganized and unable to work, but with his "civil rights" respected, he roamed the streets of the city. Surviving on money from his family or else from begging, he slept under the cars in a parking lot. He repudiated more help from his family than he accepted; usually they had no idea where he was. The police would sometimes spot him as a vagrant, sense that he was mentally ill, and try to take him to a municipal hospital. But on most of these occasions he would refuse, citing his "right" not to be committed. More often than not, the police would acquiesce. At follow-up he was in a hospital, but only after considerable effort on the part of his parents, who finally located him and pleaded with the authorities to shelter him in a safe place. He was still disorganized, though less actively psychotic and less belligerent.

The plight of this man and many others with chronic schizophrenic, doomed by the now-prevailing treatment philosophy in our country to oscillate between brief hospitalizations and the streets (or "single-room occupancy" dwellings), bypassing any semblance of either rehabilitation or sanctuary, deserves more than a brief paragraph. I have also discussed the subject in the "Afterword" (see Chapter Sixteen).

Though the number of missing persons was small, there is one generalization that I feel I can broach. The schizophrenic patients who disappeared had families that were genuinely concerned about them. The parents were baffled, at times exasperated, as the illness unfolded, but they were not without love. The patients' dropping out of contact seemed mostly a function of their aberrant thinking, and of their inability to deal with the society around them or with the pressures inherent in a family network to "relate" to its other members. In order to preserve some sense of separate identity, they needed distance at any price. Of the borderline patients who disappeared, it usually seemed that their families did not care about them very much, or else had mistreated them. Parental indifference or cruelty had made them feel valueless. Bereft of the noninvasive parental love that makes us feel cherished members of our families, and ultimately of the human community, these patients became drifters, pariahs, and sociopaths. One of the homosexual men had endured, the whole length of his earlier years, his father's taunts about his "sissiness." The father was also alcoholic and abusive. He had deserted the family when the patient was 10 and died 4 years later. At about that time, the patient ran away from home. Haughty and inaccessible throughout his year and a half at PI, he "deserted" us as well; he then lived for a few months with a roommate who, when I phoned him, had no idea where he had gone or what had become of him. Past that point, my efforts to trace him have failed.

RELIGIOUS CULTS

After leaving the hospital, over two dozen of the PI-500 joined (either transitorily or permanently) various religious cults, or else religious groups other than the ones in which they were raised. Of these, the majority made such decisions almost immediately upon discharge.

The subject of religious sects and cults is as complex as their history is long. Halperin (1983) and Schwartz (1986) have discussed many aspects of cults, both historical and psychological. For a compassionate and more detailed discussion of cults and of how they achieve their effects (via group cohesiveness, shared beliefs, and altered consciousness), the reader should consult the recent book by Galanter (1989).

Cults may perform most if not all of the same functions as the major contemporary religions, some of which had their beginnings in millenarian or messianic cults centuries earlier. One important function of these groups is the reduction of despair (through group support and belief in an afterlife). Another is the provision (to those who lack one) or enhancement of a sense of identity. Some cults offer a "positive" sense of identity for those whose deficient identity stems from parental neglect or deprivation. Others offer an equally appealing "negative" identity (which is *experienced* as positive by the adherents, however) for those who have felt unduly intruded upon by their parents and caretakers.

Religious groups of all varieties serve to help their adherents contain socially unacceptable impulses. Many cults, because of their charismatic and pervervid nature, have the power to contain even the scarcely governable impulses of persons others might regard as "wild." Conversely, certain cults, unlike most major religions, sanction the gratification of ordinarily proscribed impulses (e.g., those that condone or encourage "free love," violence against the "majority," Satanic rites, and the like).

There are cults of many different types (with respect to the factors just outlined) that supply structure and a sense of purpose to those who lack these qualities inwardly. There is a long history—not just recently and in our country, but over millenia in almost all countries—of religious communes springing up that set useful tasks to its members, forcing them, as it were, to acquire a measure of discipline and goal-directedness that had often been nowhere in evidence before their joining. Related to this is the usefulness of certain cults in offering group-sanctioned alternatives to young persons whose aspirations about "making it big" in the established society grossly exceed their particular and rather limited resources and talents. In addition, when large segments of the so-called "Establishment" show themselves as corrupt or misdirected (as in prerevolutionary Russia or in our country during the Vietnam era), many "splinter groups" arise; though these are often of a primarily political nature, at times they take on the qualities of a religious sect or cult. Some of the peace movement groups that became popular here during the years the PI-500 patients were in, or just out of, the hospital (1963–1976) were expressions of an antiwar sentiment. Many were in fact cults—half religious, half political in their emphasis—based on Oriental religion and philosophy. Six patients joined communes emphasizing crafts, macrobiotic diet, and the like; religion and politics played only a secondary role.

The one function of cult membership that has a universal quality, regardless of the group's specific characteristics, is to curb feelings of loneliness and alienation. Any religious organization can serve effectively in this capacity, needless to say; however, because of their generally small size and intensely personal atmosphere, cults often prove even more powerful antidotes to these painful emotions. The same holds true for the related feelings of anomie and purposelessness, which formed the basis of many of our patients' "chief complaints."

With these thoughts in mind, we may look more closely at the nature of the cults joined by 14 borderline and 12 initially psychotic patients from among the PI-500. In some cases I have chosen to refrain from naming a particular cult, lest it reveal the identity of the patient. The cults are discussed here under a number of different headings; it should be noted that membership often served three or four functions at once, and thus the same patient may be alluded to in more than one section.

Containment

Containment was the most prevalent function I could discover among those who joined cults. Patients who had formerly struggled either with socially unacceptable impulses, or else with impulses condoned by society but condemned by the patient in question, gravitated toward cults that emphasized strict control. It is probably significant that only a few borderlines, despite their problems with impulsivity, immersed themselves in such cults, whereas the psychotic patients often joined for reasons of control. Three patients, of whom two were paranoid schizophrenics, became involved with the Hare Krishna sect. This group, known for its stress on self-denial, appeared to help one patient (a borderline who had lived for years as a petty thief, homosexual prostitute, and vagrant) gain mastery over his antisocial and sexual impulses and achieve some level of self-respect. For another patient, Hare Krishna became a refuge from drug abuse.

As one might have anticipated, there was a tendency for the more poorly integrated patients to seek out the more eccentric and intrusive cults. By "intrusive," I refer to the manner in which certain cults and their charismatic leaders "invade"—and demand total control over—a wide sector of an adherent's personality and life functioning. One example concerns a severely ill and sexually inhibited schizophrenic man, a Holocaust survivor; he had emigrated to South America (before coming to the United States and to PI), where he was attracted to the cult of Subud. Deeply ashamed of any erotic feelings, he found himself a comfortable haven in this cult. One of the group's rituals consisted of a dozen or so men and women standing in a circle naked; the mission was to gain such self-control as not to feel, let alone show bodily signs of, sexual arousal. This was an insuperable task for some of the initiates, so the patient once told me, but one he rather excelled at. The story did not end happily: After a year of thrice-weekly sessions during which he was scarcely able to say a word, let alone communicate to his therapist how attached he felt to her, he committed suicide before her vacation.

Another schizophrenic patient became a Jehovah's Witness; still another, a "born-again" Christian; and another, a monk. All of these represent choices less exotic than Subud.

Pathological Entitlement; Gratification of Unacceptable Impulses

The PI-500 patients rarely joined cults oriented toward license rather than restraint. None ended up in cults that expressed open contempt for or sanctioned violence toward other people or the surrounding society.

One borderline patient had practiced some form of witchcraft and Satanic rites as an adolescent before she ever came to PI. She had been sexually abused by her father, himself a severe alcoholic who ultimately abandoned the family. After leaving the hospital, she led a lonely and ungratifying life, for which she found some solace in two charismatic cults. The first of these was an ecstatic cult promising its members release from their earthly suffering, in exchange for release (to the leader) of their earthly savings. It was only with great difficulty that her family was able to extricate her from this organization. She then joined a fundamentalist sect to which several of her siblings also belonged—a sect that allowed more personal freedom than the one in which she had earlier been entrapped.

Normal Entitlement; Gratification of Socially Acceptable Impulses

A few of the PI-500 borderlines sought membership in cults sanctioning impulses that most of Western society regards as quite within bounds, but that were condemned within the oppressive environment of their original families. Not finding the strength within themselves to stand up for what they felt was reasonable and morally proper, they gained this strength through merger with the group.

One young woman grew up in a severely moralistic family, among whose articles of faith were the condemnation of physical attractiveness and sex; she felt torn apart by the conflict between her natural desires and her loyalty to her family. The psychotherapy she was offered while at PI dislodged her only a little from her immobilized position. Toward the end of her stay, however, abetted as much by the mere distance from her parents as by the differing values of her therapist and fellow-patients, she felt emboldened to join a sect that practiced glossolalia (speaking in tongues).

The ritual of speaking in tongues (see Acts of the Apostles, 10:46, 19:6; Walsh, 1986) depends on developing a freedom to say whatever word-like sounds (foreign to the speaker's mother tongue and often enough to any recognized language) occur spontaneously at the moment of utterance. This is one of many practices that have the effect of lifting the participant out of everyday, logical reality (literally, "ec-static") into the reality of the spirit (as through meditation or yoga) or of the unconscious (as through free association). In time this patient went on to develop a comfortable set of internal standards, became less inhibited about sex, and came to occupy a position equidistant from both license and repression. In due course she no longer felt the need of this cult and joined a more conventional religious organization (though a less repressive one than that of her parents). By the time I had traced her, she had finished college, worked, married, raised three children, and found considerable contentment.

Identity

Although a serious disturbance in identity sense is often present in BPD (see Chapter Five), patients with STP also routinely exhibit this disturbance. In fact, very few of the

PI-500 (apart from the handful of neurotic-level patients) had anything like a firmly established sense of identity or cohesive "self."

The religious organizations offered many of our patients a more sharply delineated sense of who they were, particularly because in the adolescents and young adults who made up the ranks of the PI-500, there were only two "burning issues" that bedeviled them concerning their identity: group allegiance and gender. Occupational identity was of course of critical importance to the older patients; for the younger ones, however, this was a problem that, like the iceberg awaiting the *Titanic,* was actually almost upon them yet seemed still far away.

For several of the borderline patients, the philosophy of the religious groups to which they attached themselves might be seen as the crystallization of many hitherto inchoate and disconnected ideas concerning "Who am I?" and "What should I be like?" If a religious group represented a compromise solution not too distant from the value system of the parents, the resulting identity, though still uncomfortably dependent upon external (rather than truly internalized) sources of validation, could be seen as positive. This was true of the young woman mentioned above, whose temporary allegiance to a group that spoke in tongues was still well within the Christian fold in which she was raised.

A small number of our borderline patients latched onto an identity that felt "real and right" specifically because it represented a 180-degree turn from the cherished beliefs of their parents. We encountered this situation in several instances where the families had been experienced as unusually intrusive (such that the patients had been unable to distinguish what they really wanted to be from what the parents *told* them they ought to be). We witnessed a similar evolution in cases where the families had so grievously hurt or rejected the patients as to make *any* other choice—especially a choice clearly *opposite* to the parents' values—seem far more attractive. One of the Jewish women who had felt swamped by her parents' exhortations to live according to their prearranged plans repudiated her background altogether and ended up in a commune, as a Buddhist. Another Jewish patient—a borderline man who felt unable to compete with the more successful members of his family, and who felt himself the object of their condescension—found contentment and a more comfortable sense of self in Christianity. Ten years or so after PI, he began studying for the ministry. One of the Protestant women turned to a Hindu sect; a Protestant man, who had had a very strained and distant relationship with his father, joined a Hindu sect that practiced yoga.

Olsson (1983) has drawn attention to the increasing numbers of adolescents in our generation who are at risk for "malevolent surrender" to perverse, supernatural cults, which constitute a whole cafeteria to choose from: the traditional, the nontraditional, the meditative, the secular/occult, and the antireligious (pp. 254–255). Borderline-level young persons, including those with narcissistic character structure, seem particularly vulnerable to the more perverse, mind-controlling cults. The all-or-none, good-or-bad thinking prevalent in such cults makes borderlines, because of their own primitive, polarized thought patterns, feel very much at home. Luckily, few of the PI-500 borderlines were snared by brainwashing cults. There was one still enmeshed in Scientology at follow-up; none became a "Moonie."

One might predict that the schizophrenic (and schizoaffective) patients, with their often fragmented sense of identity, would be even more vulnerable to "love bombardment" and to some of the other technics and blandishments used by the "strong-arm" cults. The PI-500, however, did not show such a trend: The percentage of borderlines who joined a cult (13 of 275, or 5%) did not differ significantly from that noted among the combined schizophrenic and schizoaffective patients (11 of 157, or 7%).

Sexual identity was more problematic an issue for the schizophrenic patients than group identity. Besides profound worry about being homosexual, the males (who were, if anything, asexual in practice and mixed in their fantasy life) experienced intense guilt over masturbation. Cultural factors obviously play a role in shaping the "typical" symptoms: In the current generation, masturbatory guilt—which had often been the precipitating factor in hospitalization for the PI-500 schizophrenics—is encountered far less often. At all events, the cults adopted by the PI-500 schizophrenic patients emphasized *asceticsm,* thereby creating out of the patients' inhibitions and personal handicaps (which had led to feelings of worthlessness) a sense of belonging to a higher moral order (which led to feelings of superiority). Three became Hare Krishna devotees. Besides the patient who joined Subud, another joined an ashram; another, as noted earlier became a monk.

Structure

A predominant characteristic of borderline patients, whatever descriptive system one employs, is their lack of internal structure. What is meant by "lack of structure" in this context is a combination of qualities that are not all necessarily present in any one patient: a serious deficiency in self-discipline; franticness when alone; and an inability to channel anxieties into crafts, hobbies, sports, or other useful social outlets. Life, for the borderline, often lacks a sense of purpose: Choice of friends or sexual partners is often a decision made on the spur of the moment, lacking commitment and appropriateness.

Patients with manic–depressive psychosis (MDP) tend to oscillate from one extreme to another in their attitudes and enthusiasms; the periodic changes of mood may put an abrupt halt to the pursuit of a certain activity or to the continuity of a love relationship. Some borderline conditions are *formes frustes* of MDP and show similar qualities (experienced by others as "storminess" or "fickleness"). Borderline women with affective comorbidity are susceptible to severe premenstrual tension. When the latter is present, some course of action (some new study, etc.) that has been embarked upon in midcycle is abandoned during the premenstrual affective upheaval. Borderlines and manic–depressive are often sensation-seeking: They are highly dependent upon strong external stimuli as antidotes to the uncomfortable void within. Lack of inner structure was noted in most of our schizophrenic patients as well; in them, we found not so much the shifting enthusiasms of the mood-disordered patients, but rather an inability to define themselves in any coherent manner, with the result that no project seemed worth pursuing. Instead of frantic or inconsistent activity, there was often paralysis.

Borderline and psychotic patients alike were attracted to cults that "took over" every aspect of daily existence. Several of the schizophrenic patients who joined cults lived for many years in communes that took their inspiration from Eastern religion. Some were still residing in these communes at follow-up and would have been untraceable except through their relatives. The eccentric and grandiose thinking typical of certain schizophrenic patients found a comfortable haven in messianic cults, the adoption of whose beliefs also liberated them from the humiliation of confronting their failures in everyday life. Even the schizophrenic patient who made the best adjustment, from the standpoint of conventional society, had not only found structure and meaning in the cabalistic cult he joined shortly after leaving PI; even much later, as a successful businessman and father, he reverted in moments of stress to immersing himself in the Zohar and other cabalistic writings. He was able to retain a measure of objectivity during these episodes, which spared him engulfment in the psychosis that had precipitated his initial hospitalization. "Whenever I notice myself getting preoccupied with gematria," he told me, "I know it's time to check in with my shrink again."[1] Another schizophrenic man, at follow-up a successful manufacturer raising two children, disappeared for many years after leaving PI; found a sense of structure in a cult/commune (where he was assigned various tasks); and retained, even after rejoining his family, bizarre ideas about religion and nutrition.

Self-Esteem

In the preceding section, I have alluded to problems in self-esteem posed by the difficulty in measuring up to peers in a highly competitive environment. For a number of patients, both borderline and psychotic, cults provided a solution: They elevated self-esteem either through self-laudatory, propagandistic technics (of the sort used by certain political groups) or through the more reality-oriented technic of teaching new skills, helping the adherents learn useful crafts, and so on. Some of these organizations succeeded where PI had failed.

Emotionally handicapped offspring of enormously successful parents suffered some of the severest problems in self-esteem, since nothing they could do in everyday society could approach even remotely the levels achieved by the parents. Many of the PI-500 patients caught in this situation committed suicide, as happened with one schizophrenic man whose father was a famous writer, and with another whose father was a wealthy entrepreneur and industrialist. Both had IQs of 135. To convince either of these young men—neither of whom had ever worked, and both of whom were chronically delusional—that it was a far better and much worthier life selling behind a counter or washing cars (which they could easily have managed) than vegetating in a state hospital required salesmanship beyond the powers of the best therapists we had available. But several other schizophrenics left PI neither worse nor better than when they arrived, and earned both self-support and self-respect in some of the more benign communes.

[1] "Gematria" refers to the mystical numerology based on the numerical values of the Hebrew letters. For example, words whose letters add up to the number value of the letters of God's name were thought by the cabalistic writers to have special significance.

Some of the borderlines also developed a more realistic self-esteem through hard work and group support in communities based on Eastern religious cults. The best of these tended to be monetarily exploitative, but at least allowed (as did the Maharishi Mahesh Yogi) some personal freedom and training in useful occupations. One borderline woman worked with the poor in the SIDDHA foundation in India; another, a devotee of Maha Baba, became a successful ceramist. Both women dropped out of conventional urban life altogether and, at follow-up, were performing their useful work in tropical settings on the other side of the globe.

Hope and the Alleviation of Despair

Last but not least of the topics relevant to the religious cults is hope. The capacity of the cults to provide hope in a positive sense, or to alleviate feelings of despair, purposelessness, and nihilism, figured as an attractive element (though not always the crucial element) for all the PI-500 patients who ultimately joined a cult. Which particular cult they chose and how the cult worked as an anodyne for despair depended upon the main sources of despair in the patients, and these were by no means uniform.

For two patients—one borderline, the other schizophrenic—the theme of reincarnation was the key element. The borderline woman had lost several members of her immediate family through suicide; several others had long been incapacitated because of mental illness. The belief that death was not final, and that one might even be happier in another life than in the life one had just quit, was immensely soothing to this woman. One might have thought that she would turn to a religious group that carried out séances (where one spoke with one's dead relatives), such as were popular some years ago. But neither she nor any of the other PI-500 patients sought contact with lost loved ones in this way. Analytic psychotherapy while this patient was at PI had made her feel worse—pouring salt, as it seemed to her, on old wounds. The schizophrenic man whose hopelessness was assuaged through belief in reincarnation was one of the four or five PI-500 patients who had had a near-death experience. While at PI, he had tried to hang himself. The staff resuscitated him after he lost both consciousness and heartbeat. Twenty years later he remained within his reincarnation sect, committed to the idea that he would come back as some other person in return for leading a morally correct life in the here-and-now. He sold newspapers in a kiosk and lived alone, apart from meetings with other members of his religious group. Having been raised a Catholic, he felt remorseful over the suicide attempt, which he regarded as sinful. The Hindu sect of which he was a member at follow-up largely relieved this guilt through emphasis on upright behavior and on *chakra*—the wheel of reincarnation, which might allot him a better fate the next time around.

There were three psychotic patients (two schizophrenic, the other manic–depressive) who not only joined messianic sects but, while in the hospital, fought off despair through the delusional conviction that they were themselves the messiah. As such, they became the butt of pathetic humor while at PI (they were all there at the same time), in that each believed the other two to be "false messiahs" (and thus remained unruffled at the multiplicity of their number).

In a related phenomenon, two of the PI-500 patients became "born-again" Christians—a choice that afforded them a feeling not only of rebirth but, more importantly for them, of starting life over with a new set of chances and with the old mistakes erased.

Those who feel baffled by the powerful appeal of cults, especially the charismatic cults, will perhaps be instructed (as I was) by the following example. The brother of the borderline patient described above under "Pathological Entitlement" had, of course, also been abandoned by his father. Far more successful than his sister in overcoming the disadvantages of his upbringing, he completed professional training and went on to achieve pre-eminence in his field. During his adolescence and early 20s, he too had struggled with feelings of emptiness and despair, despising the father who had left them and longing for some idealized father to love and take care of him. He found this idealized father in Christ, within the context of a cult—charismatic in nature but not extreme and "presumptuous" (as he viewed it), like the one his sister joined. We spoke for an hour on the phone, and as the conversational focus shifted from his sister to his own life, he told me, "You need a close relationship with the Lord—a personal and very real relationship, not a distant one. We've lost what family is all about. If you're not a member of a family, you're *nothing!*"

It became clear to me that for many lonely and suffering persons, the trinitarian deity in Christianity, one of whose aspects is the man Jesus, can offer the solace of a *personal* relationship as compensation for what may be missing in one's actual family. This kind of relationship is much less readily achieved through a religion that remains purely abstract. As psychoanalysts we tend to reduce all this to a matter of "transitional objects," "symbolic replacement," and the like. But for this fatherless but religious man, too poor in his younger days even to think of getting "realistic" help from a psychiatrist, Christ was *there* for him, more palpable despite His invisibility than the biological father who had deserted him. Sitting in my small cell in the megalopolitan honeycomb of New York, I think of the telephone company's ad urging us to "reach out and touch someone." It was one of the great rewards for me in carrying out this study to be able to "touch" people from 40 states and a few foreign countries, and to be touched by them in return, as I was by this man. His reminiscences and personal philosophy made it possible for me to understand the forces that led many of our former patients to ally themselves with the nontraditional groups mentioned throughout this section.

References

Abraham, S., Mira, M., and Llewellyn-Jones, D. (1983) Bulimia: A study of outcome. *Int. J. Eating Disord.* 2: 175–180.

Achté, K. A. (1961) Der Verlauf der Schizophrenien und der schizophreniformen Psychosen. *Acta Psychiatr. Neurol. Scand.* (Suppl. 155): (1–273.

Adam, K. S., Bouckoms, A., and Streiner, D. (1982) Parental loss and family stability in attempted suicide. *Arch. Gen. Psychiatry 39:* 1081–1085.

Akiskal, H. S. (1981) Subaffective disorders: Dysthymic, cyclothymic and bipolar II disorders in the "borderline" realm. *Psychiatr. Clin. N. Am.* 4(1): 25–46.

Akiskal, H. S., Chen, S.E., Davis, G.C., Puzantian, V.R., Kashgarian, M., and Belinger, J. M. (1985) Borderline: An adjective in search of a noun. *J. Clin. Psychiatry 46:* 41–48.

Akiskal, H. S., Djenderedjian, A. H., Bolinger, J. M., Bitar, A. H., Khani, M. K., and Haykal, R. F. (1978) The joint use of clinical and biological criteria for psychiatric diagnosis: II. Their application in identifying subaffective forms of bipolar illness. In Akiskal, H. S., and Webb, W. L. (Eds.), *Psychiatric Diagnosis: Exploration of Biological Predictors.* New York: Spectrum, pp. 133–145.

Aldrich, C. K. (1986) The clouded crystal ball: A thirty-five year follow-up of psychiatrists' predictions. *Am. J. Psychiatry 143:* 45–49.

Allebeck, P., Varla, A., and Wistedt, B. (1986) Suicide and violent death among patients with schizophrenia. *Acta Psychiatr. Scand. 74:* 43–49.

Allen, J. G., Colson, D. B., Coyne, L., Dexter, N., Jehl, N., Mayer, C. A., and Spohn, H. (1986) Problems to anticipate in treating difficult patients in a long-term psychiatric hospital. *Psychiatry 49:* 350–358.

Allen, J. G., Tarnoff, G., Kearns, N.W., and Coyne, L. (1986) Paranoid versus nonparanoid schizophrenia and long-term hospital treatment outcome. *Bull. Menninger Clin. 50:* 341–350.

Alpert, A. (1954) Observations on the treatment of emotionally disturbed children in a therapeutic center. *Psychoanal. Study Child 9:* 334–343.

Alpert, A. (1959) Reversibility of pathological fixations associated with maternal deprivation in infancy. *Psychoanal. Study Child 14:* 169–185.

Alter-Reid, K., Gibbs, M. S., Lachenmeyer, J. R., Sigal, J., and Massoth, N. A. (1986) Sexual abuse of children: A review of the empirical findings. *Clin. Psychol. Rev. 6:* 249–266.

Ambelas, A. (1987) Life events and mania: A special relationship? *Br. J. Psychiatry 150:* 235–240.

Andreasen, N. C., and Olsen, S. (1982) Negative vs. positive schizophrenia: Definition and validation. *Arch. Gen. Psychiatyry 39:* 789–794.

Andrulonis, P. A., Glueck, B. C., Stroebel, C. F., and Vogel, N. G. (1982) Borderline personality subcategories. *J. Nerv. Ment. Dis. 170:* 670–679.

Andrulonis, P. A., Glueck, B. C., Stroebel, C. F., Vogel, N. G., Shapiro, A. L., and Aldridge, D. M. (1981) Organic brain dysfunction and the borderline syndrome. *Psychiatr. Clin. N. Am. 4*(1): 47–66.

Angst, J. (1986a) The course of affective disorders. *Psychopathologie 19*(Suppl. 1): 47–52.

Angst, J. (1986b) European long-term follow-up studies of schizophrenia. Unpublished manuscript, Psychiatric University Hospital, Zürich.

Angst, J. (1988) Personal communication.

Angst, J., and Clayton, P. (1986) Premorbid personality of depressive, bipolar and schizophrenic patients with special reference to suicidal issues. *Compr. Psychiatry 27:* 511–532.

Angst, J., Felder, W., and Frey, R. (1979) The course of unipolar and bipolar affective disorders. In Schou, M., and Strömgren, E. (Eds.), *Origin, Prevention and Treatment of Affective Disorders.* London: Academic Press, pp. 215–226.

Angst, J., Felder, W., and Lohmeyer, B. (1979) Are schizoaffective psychoses heterogeneous? *J. Affective Disord. 1:* 155–165.

Angst, J., Felder, W., and Lohmeyer, B. (1980) Course of schizoaffective psychoses: Results of a follow-up study. *Schizophr. Bull. 6:* 579–585.

Angst, J., Scharfetter, C., and Stassen, H. H. (1983) Classification of schizoaffective patients by multidimensional scaling and cluster analysis. *Psychiatr. Clin. 16:* 254–265.

Angst, J., and Stassen, H. H. (1986) Verlaufsaspekte affektiver Psychosen: Suizide, Rückfallrisiko im alter. In G. Huber (Ed.), *Fortschritte in der Psychosenforschung?* (Proceedings of the Seventh Weissnauer Schizophrenia Symposium, Bonn, 1986). Stuttgart: Schattauer, pp. 145–164.

Arieti, S. (1977) Parents of the schizophrenic patient: A reconsideration. *J. Am. Acad. Psychoanal. 5:* 347–358.

Åsberg, M., Nordström, P., and Traskman-Bendz, L. (1989) Biological factors in suicide. In Roy, A. (Ed.), *Suicide.* Baltimore: Williams & Wilkins, pp. 47–71.

Åsberg, M., Traskman, L., and Thorén, P. (1976) 5-HIAA in the cerebrospinal fluid: A biochemical suicide predictor? *Arch. Gen. Psychiatry 33:* 1193–1197.

Asher, R. (1951) Munchausen's syndrome. *Lancet i:* 339–341.

Ayd, F. J. (1956) Fatal hyperpyrexia during chlorpromazine therapy. *J. Clin. Psychiatry 22:* 189–192.

Barasch, A., Frances, A., Hurt, S., Clarkin, J., and Cohen, S. (1985) Stability and distinctness of borderline personality disorder. *Am. J. Psychiatry 142:* 1484–1486.

Bardenstein, K.K., and McGlashan, T.H. (1988) The natural history of a residentially treated borderline sample: Gender differences. *J. Pers. Disord. 2:* 69–83.

Barnard, C. P., and Hirsch, C. (1985) Borderline personality and victims of incest. *Psychol. Rep. 57:* 715–718.

Bartlett, J., Bridges, P., and Kelly, D. (1981) Contemporary indications for psychosurgery. *Br. J. Psychiatry 138:* 507–511.

Bech, P., Allerup, P., and Rosenberg, R. (1978) The Marke–Nyman temperament scale. *Acta Psychiatr. Scand. 57:* 49–58.

Beck, S. (1959) Schizophrenia without psychosis. *Arch. Neurol. Psychiatry 8:* 85–96.

Benjaminsen, S. (1985) Coping with precipitating life stress of primarily depressed inpatients. *Compr. Psychiatry 21:* 71–79.

Beres, D., Eissler, R., Freud, A., and Glover, E. (1951) Vicissitudes of superego function and superego precursors in childhood. *Psychoanal. Study Child 13:* 324–351.

Bergeret, J. (1984) *La Violence Fondamentale.* Paris: Dunod.

Bergler, E. (1957) *Homosexuality: Disease or Way of Life?* New York: Hill & Wang.

Bick, P. A. (1986) Seasonal affective disorder. *Am. J. Psychiatry 143:* 90–91.

Bieber, I. (1962) *Homosexuality: A Psychoanalytic Study.* New York: Basic Books.

Biondi, R., and Hecox, W. (1987) *All His Father's Sins: Inside the Gerald Gallego Sex-Slave Murders.* Rocklin, Calif.: Prima.

Bivin, G. D., and Klinger, M. P. (1937) *Pseudocyesis.* Bloomington, Ind.: Principia Press.

Blackburn, R. (1988) On moral judgments and personality disorders: The myth of psychopathic personality revisited. *Br. J. Psychiatry 153:* 505–512.

Bleuler, E. (1911) *Dementia Praecox oder Gruppe der Schizophrenien.* Leipzig: Franz Deuticke.

Bleuler, M. (1972) *Die Schizophrenen Geistesstörungen.* Stuttgart: Thieme Verlag.

Bliss, E. L. (1986) *Multiple Personality, Allied Disorders and Hypnosis.* New York: Oxford University Press.

Blumenthal, S. J., and Kupfer, D. J. (1986) Generalizable treatment strategies for suicidal behavior. *Ann. NY Acad. Sci. 487:* 327–340.

Brandon, C. (1986) *Murder in the Adirondacks: An American Tragedy Revisited.* Utica, N. Y.: North Country Books.

Brassard, M. R., Germain, R., and Hart, S. N. (Eds.). (1987) *Psychological Maltreatment of Children and Youth.* New York: Pergamon Press.

Brent, D. A., Perper, J. A., Goldstein, C. E., Kolko, D. J., Allan, M. J., Allman, C. J., and Zelenak, J. P. (1988) Risk factors in adolescent suicide. *Arch. Gen. Psychiatry 45:* 581–588.

Breslau, N., and Davis, G. C. (1987) Posttraumatic stress disorder: The stressor criterion. *J. Nerv. Ment. Dis. 175*(5): 255–264.

Bridge, T. P., Cannon, E., and Wyatt, R. J. (1978) Burned-out schizophrenia: Evidence for age effects on schizophrenic symptomatology. *J. Gerontol. 33:* 835–839.

Briquet, P. (1859) *Traité Clinique et de l'Hystérie.* Paris: Baillière.

Brockington, I. F., and Meltzer, H. Y. (1983) The nosology of schizoaffective psychosis. *Psychiatr. Dev. 4:* 317–338.

Brotman, A. W., Herzog, D. B., and Hamburg, P. (1988) Long-term course in 14 bulimics treated with psychotherapy. *J. Clin. Psychiatry 49:* 157–160.

Brown, G. L., Ebert, M. H., Goyer, P. F., Jimerson, D. C., Klein, W. J., Bunney, W. E., and Goodwin, F. K. (1982) Aggression, suicide and serotonin: Relationships to CSF amine metabolites. *Am. J. Psychiatry 139:* 741–746.

Bruch, H. (1978) *The Golden Cage: The Enigma of Anorexia Nervosa.* New York: Vintage Books.

Bugliosi, V. (1978) *Till Death Do Us Part.* New York: Norton.

Cadoret, R., Troughton, E., O'Gorman, T. W., and Heywood, E. (1986) An adoption study of genetic and environmental factors in drug abuse. *Arch. Gen. Psychiatry 43:* 1131–1136.

Cahill, T. (1986) *Buried Dreams: Inside the Mind of a Serial Killer.* New York: Bantam Books.

Canton, G., and Fraccon, I. G. (1985) Life events and schizophrenia. *Acta Psychiatr. Scand. 71:* 211–216.

Cantwell, D. P., Sturzenburger, S., Burroughs, J., Salkin, B., and Green, J. K. (1977) Anorexia nervosa: An affective disorder. *Arch. Gen. Psychiatry 34:* 1087–1093.

Capgras, J., and Reboul-Lachaux, J. (1923) L'illusion des "sosies" dans un délire systematisé. *Bull. Soc. Clin. Med. Ment. 11:* 6–16.

Carey, G., and Gottesman, I. (1981) Twin and family studies of anxiety, phobic and obsessive disorders. In Klein, D.F., and Rabkin, J.G. (Eds.), *Anxiety: New Research and Changing Concepts.* New York: Raven Press, pp. 117–136.

Carpenter, W. T., Jr., and Gunderson, J. G. (1977) Five year follow-up comparison of borderline and schizophrenic patients. *Compr. Psychiatry 18:* 567–571.

Carpenter, W. T., Jr., Gunderson, J. G., and Strauss, J. S. (1977) Considerations of the borderline syndrome: Longitudinal and comparative study of borderline and schizophrenic patients. In Hartocollis, P. (Ed.), *Borderline Personality Disorders.* New York: International Universities Press, pp. 231–253.

Carpenter, W. T., Jr., Strauss, J. S., and Bartko, J. (1973) Flexible system for the diagnosis of schizophrenia. *Science 182:* 1275–1278.

Chase, L. S., and Silverman, S. (1941) Prognostic criteria in schizophrenia. *Am. J. Psychiatry 98:* 360–368.

Ciompi, L., and Müller, C. (1976) *Lebensweg und Alter der Schizophrenen.* Berlin: Springer-Verlag.

Claridge, G. (1987) "The schizophrenias as nervous types" revisited. *Br. J. Psychiatry 151:* 735–743.

Clarkin, J. F., Widiger, T. A., Frances, A., Hurt, S., and Gilmore, M. (1983) Prototypic typology and the borderline personality disorder. *J. Abnorm. Psychol. 92:* 263–275.

Clayton, P., Rodin, L., and Winokur, G. (1968) Family history studies: III. Schizoaffective disorder, clinical and genetic factors including a one to two year follow-up. *Compr. Psychiatry 9:* 31–49.

Cleckley, H. (1976) *The Mask of Sanity* (5th ed.). St. Louis: C. V. Mosby.

Cloninger, C. R. (1986) A unified biosocial theory of personality and its role in the development of anxiety states. *Psychiatr. Dev. 3:* 167–226.

Coen, S. J. (1987) Pathological jealousy. *Int. J. Psychoanal. 68:* 99–108.

Coid, J., Allolio, B., and Rees, L. H. (1983) Raised plasma metenkephalin in patients who habitually mutilate themselves. *Lancet ii:* 545–546.

Colson, D. B., Allen, J. G., Ceyne, L., Deering, D., Jehl, N., Kearns, W., and Spohn, H. (1986) Profiles of difficult psychiatric hospital patients. *Hosp. Community Psychiatry 37:* 720–724.

Crook, T., and Raskin, A. (1975) Association of childhood parental loss with attempted suicide and depression. *J. Consult. Clin. Psychol. 43:* 277.

Cross, C. K., and Hirschfeld, R. M. A. (1986) Psychosocial factors and suicidal behavior: Life events, early loss and personality. *Ann. NY Acad. Sci. 487:* 77–89.

Crow, T. (1980) Molecular pathology of schizophrenia. *Br. Med. J. 280:* 1–9.

Crowe, R. R., Clarkson, C., Tsai, M., and Wilson, R. (1988) Delusional disorder: Jealous and non-jealous types. *Eur. Arch. Psychiatr. Neurol. Sci. 237:* 179–183.

Crumley, F. E. (1981) Adolescent suicide attempts and borderline personality disorder. *South. Med. J. 74:* 546–549.

Dawkins, R. (1976) *The Selfish Gene.* New York: Oxford University Press.

De Clérambault, G. (1942) *Oeuvre Psychiatrique.* Paris: Presse Universitaire Française.

DeJong, R., Rabinow, D. R., Roy-Byrne, P., Hoban, C., Grover, G. N., and Post, R. M. (1985) Premenstrual mood disorder and psychiatric illness. *Am. J. Psychiatry* *142:* 1359–1361.

Delay, J. (1968) Drug induced extrapyramidal syndrome. In Vinken, D., and Bruyen, G. (Eds.), *Handbook of Clinical Neurology* (Vol. 6). New York: Elsevier, pp. 248–266.

Delpirou, A., and Labrousse, A. (1986) *Coca Coke.* Paris: Editions La Découverte.

DeRosa, P. (1988) *The Vicars of Christ.* New York: Crown.

Deutsch, H. (1942) Some forms of emotional disturbance and their relationships to schizophrenia. *Psychoanal. Q. 11:* 301–321.

Diagnostic and Statistical Manual of Mental Disorders (3rd ed.; DSM-III). (1980) Washington, D. C.: American Psychiatric Association.

Diagnostic and Statistical Manual of Mental Disorders (3rd ed., rev.; DSM-III-R). (1987) Washington, D. C.: American Psychiatric Association.

Diekstra, R. F. W. (1987) Renée, or the complex psychodynamics of adolescent suicide. In Diekstra, R. F. W., and Hawton, K. (Eds.), *Suicide in Adolescence.* Dordrecht, The Netherlands: Martinus Nijhoff, pp. 43–75.

Diekstra, R. F. W. (1988) *Prevention of Suicide.* Kinderhook, N.Y.: Brill.

Diekstra, R. F. W., and Moritz, B. J. M. (1987) Suicidal behavior among adolescents: An overview. In Diekstra, R. F. W., and Hawton, K. (Eds.), *Suicide in Adolescence.* Dordrecht, The Netherlands: Martinus Nijhoff, pp. 7–24.

Dillmann, J. (1986) *Unholy Matrimony: A True Story of Murder and Obsession.* New York: Macmillan.

Dorpat, T. L., Jackson, J. K., and Ripley, H. S. (1965) Broken home and attempted and completed suicide. *Arch. Gen. Psychiatry 12:* 213–216.

Drewnowski, A., Yee, D. K., and Krahn, D. D. (1988) Bulimia in college women: Incidence and recovery rates. *Am. J. Psychiatry 145:* 753–755.

Dunner, D. L., Gershon, E. S., and Goodwin, F. K. (1976) Heritable factors in the severity of affective illness. *Biol. Psychiatry 11:* 31–42.

Dunner, D. L., Patrick, V., and Fieve, R. R. (1979) Life events at onset of bipolar affective illness. *Am. J. Psychiatry 136:* 508–511.

Easser, R.-R., and Lesser, S. (1965) Hysterical personality: A reevaluation. *Psychoanal. Q. 34:* 390–402.

Eckert, E. D., Bouchart, T. J., Bohlen, J., and Heston, L. L. (1986) Homosexuality in monozygotic twins reared apart. *Br. J. Psychiatry 148:* 421–425.

Edelberg, S., and Tange, M. (1987) Incest problemes et ambulant bjørnepsykiatrisk klientel, Københavns Kommune 1982–1984. *Månedsakr. Prakt. Laegegern.* (Feb): 129–137.

Ellis, L., and Ames, M. A. (1987) Neurohormonal functioning and sexual orientation: A theory of homosexuality–heterosexuality. *Psychol. Bull. 101*(2): 233–258.

Ellis, P., and Mellsop, G. (1985) De Clérambault's syndrome. *Br. J. Psychiatry 140:* 90–95.

Endicott, J. (1985) Personal communication.

Endicott, J., Halbreich, U., and Schacht, S. (1981) Premenstrual changes and affective disorders. *Psychosom. Med. 43:* 519–529.

Endicott, J., Spitzer, R. L., Fleiss, J. L., & Cohen, J. (1967) The Global Assessment Scale. *Arch. Gen. Psychiatry 33:* 766–771.

Erikson, E. H. (1956) The problem of ego identity. *J. Am. Psychoanal. Assoc. 4:* 56–121.

Erlenmeyer-Kimling, L. (1966) Current reproductive trends in schizophrenia. In Hoch,

P.H., and Zubin, J. (Eds.), *Psychopathology of Schizophrenia*. New York: Grune & Stratton, pp. 252–276.

Esquirol, E. (1838) *Des Maladies Mentales*. (Vol. 2) Paris: Baillière.

Faravelli, C. (1986) Early life events and affective disorder revisited. *Br. J. Psychiatry 148:* 288–295.

Feighner, J., Robins, E., Guze, S. B., Woodruff, R. A., Jr., Winokur, G., and Munoz, R. (1972) Diagnostic criteria for use in psychiatric research. *Arch. Gen. Psychiatry 26:* 57–63.

Felthous, A., and Bernard, H. (1979) Enuresis, fire-setting and cruelty to animals: The significance of two-thirds of this triad. *J. Forensic Sci. 24:* 240–246.

Felthous, A. R., and Kellert, S. R. (1987) Childhood cruelty to animals and later aggression against people: A review. *Am. J. Psychiatry 144:* 710–716.

Fenichel, O. (1939) Zur Oekonomik der Pseudologia Phantastica. *Int. Z. Psychoanal. 24:* 21–32.

Fenichel, O. (1945) *The Psychoanalytic Theory of Neurosis*. New York: Norton.

Ferenczi, S. (1923) Die 'Materialisation' bei Globus hystericus. *Int. Z. Psychoanal. 9:* 68.

Fine, A. (1986) *The Shaky Game: Einstein, Realism and the Quantum Theory*. Chicago: University of Chicago Press.

Finkelhor, D. (1984) *Child Sexual Abuse*. New York: Free Press.

Finstad, S. (1987) *Ulterior Motives: The Killing and Dark Legacy of Tycoon Henry Kyle*. New York: William Morrow.

Foon, A. F. (1987) Locus of control as a predictor of outcome of psychotherapy. *Br. J. Med. Psychol. 60:* 99–107.

Forward, S., and Buck, C. (1979) *Betrayal of Innocence*. Harmondsworth, England: Penguin Books.

Foster, D. W., and Rubinstein, A. H. (1983) Hypoglycemia, insulinoma, and other hormone-secreting tumors of the pancreas. In Petersdorf, R. G., Adams, R. D., Braunwald, E., Isselbacher, K. J., Martin, J. B., and Wilson, J. D. (Eds.), *Harrison's Principles of Internal Medicine* (10th ed.). New York: McGraw-Hill, pp. 682–689.

Frances, A., Clarkin, J., Gilmore, M., Hurt, S., and Brown, R. (1984) Reliability of criteria for borderline personality disorder: A comparison study of DSM-III and the D.I.B. (Diagnostic Interview for Borderline Patients). *Am. J. Psychiatry 141:* 1080–1084.

Frank, J. D. (1988) Specific and non-specific factors in psychotherapy. *Curr. Opin. Psychiatry 1:* 289–292.

Freud, S. (1905a) Fragment of an analysis of a case of hysteria. *Standard Edition 7:* 1–122.

Freud, S. (1905b) Three essays on the theory of sexuality. *Standard Edition 7:* 123–245.

Freud, S. (1911) Psycho-analytic notes on an autobiographical account of a case of paranoia (dementia paranoides). *Standard Edition 12:* 1–82.

Freud, S. (1922) Some neurotic mechanisms in jealousy, paranoia and homosexuality. *Standard Edition 18:* 22–232.

Friedman, R. C. (1988) *Male Homosexuality*. New Haven, Conn.: Yale University Press.

Frosch, J. (1981) The role of unconscious homosexuality in the paranoid constellation. *Psychoanal. Q. 50:* 587–613.

Fyer, A. J., and Klein, D. F. (1985) Agoraphobia, social phobia and simple phobia. In Michels, R., Cavenar, J. O., Brodie, H. K. H., Cooper, A. M., Guze, S. B., Judd, L. L., Klerman, G. L., and Solnit, A. J. (Eds.), *Psychiatry* (Vol. 1). Philadelphia: J. B. Lippincott, Chapter 33.

Galanter, M. (1989) *Cults*. New York: Oxford University Press.

Gallwey, P. L. G. (1985) The psychodynamics of borderline personality. In Farrington, D. P., and Dunn, J. G. (Eds.), *Aggression and Dangerousness*. New York: Wiley, pp. 127–152.

Gardiner, M. (Ed.). (1971) *The Wolf Man by the Wolf Man*. New York: Basic Books.

Gardner, D. L., and Cowdry, R. W. (1985) Suicidal and parasuicidal behavior in borderline personality disorder. *Psychiatr. Clin. N. Am. 8:* 389–403.

Garfinkel, P. E., and Garner, D. M. (1982) *Anorexia Nervosa: A Multidimensional Perspective*. New York: Brunner/Mazel.

Garfinkel, P. E., Moldofsky, H., and Garner, D. M. (1977) The outcome in anorexia nervosa. In Vigersky, R. (Ed.), *Anorexia Nervosa*. New York: Raven Press, pp. 315–329.

Geller, J. L. (1987) Firesetting in the adult psychiatric population. *Hosp. Community Psychiatry 38:* 501–506.

Gelles, R. J., and Straus, M. A. (1988) *Intimate Violence*. New York: Simon & Schuster.

Gidro-Frank, L., Peretz, D., Spitzer, R., and Winikus, W. (1967) A five year follow-up of male patients hospitalized at Psychiatric Institute. *Psychiatr. Q. 41:* 1–35.

Gilmore, M. M., and Kaufman, C. (1985) Dissociative disorders. In Michels, R., Cavenar, J. O., Brodie, H. K. H., Cooper, A. M., Guze, S. B., Judd, L. L., Klerman, G. L., and Solnit, A. J. (Eds.), *Psychiatry* (Vol. 1). Philadelphia: J. B. Lippincott, Chapter 39.

Giovacchini, P. L. (1982) Structural progression and vicissitudes in the treatment of severely disturbed patients. In Giovacchini, P. L., and Boyer, L. B. (Eds.), *Technical Factors in the Treatment of the Severely Disturbed Patient*. New York: Jason Aronson, pp. 3–64.

Gleick, J. (1987) *Chaos*. New York: Viking Press.

Goldman, G. (1938) An act of compulsive handwashing. *Psychoanal. Q. 7:* 96–121.

Golub, S. (1985) Menstrual cycle symptoms from a developmental perspective. In DeFries, Z., Friedman, R. C., and Corn, R. (Eds.), *Sexuality: New Perspectives*. Westport, Conn. Greenwood Press, pp. 251–270.

Goodman, R. (1983) Biology of sexuality: Inborn determinants of human sexual response. *Br. J. Psychiatry 143:* 216–255.

Goodwin, J. (1982) *Sexual Abuse: Incest Victims and Their Families*. Littleton, Mass.: PSG.

Goodwin, J., Cheeves, K., and Connell, V. (1988) Defining a syndrome of severe symptoms in survivors of extreme incestuous abuse. *Dissociation 1:* 11–16.

Gorman, J. M., and Liebowitz, M. R. (1985) Panic and anxiety disorders. In Michels, R., Cavenar, J. O., Brodie, H. K. H., Cooper, A. M., Guze, S. B., Judd, L. L., Klerman, G. L., and Solnit, A. J. (Eds.), *Psychiatry* (Vol. 1). Philadelphia: J. B. Lippincott, Chapter 32.

Graff, H., and Mallin, R. (1967) The syndrome of the wrist cutter. *Am. J. Psychiatry. 124:* 74–80.

Grafton, S. (1987) *"D" is for Deadbeat*. New York: Henry Holt.

Graves, P. (1988) Suicide risk assessment and the Habits-of-Nervous-Tension Survey: A 40-year follow-up on medical students. Paper presented at the Barnard Institute for Medical Research: Symposium on College Student Suicide, Columbia University, New York, June 16.

Greaves, G. (1980) Multiple personality: 165 years after Mary Reynolds. *J. Nerv. Ment. Dis. 168:* 577–596.

Greenberg, H., and Sarner, C. H. (1965) Trichotillomania. *Arch. Gen. Psychiatry 12:* 482–489.

Grinker, R. R., Sr., and Werble, B. (1977) *The Borderline Patient.* New York Jason Aronson.

Grinker, R. R., Sr., Werble, B., and Drye, R. C. (1968) *The Borderline Syndrome.* New York: Basic Books.

Gross, G., and Huber, G. (1973) Zur Prognose der Schizophrenien. *Psychiatr. Clin. 6:* 1–16.

Grove, W. M., Andreasen, N. C., Winokur, G., Clayton, P. J., Endicott, J., and Coryell, W. H. (1987) Primary and secondary affective disorders: Unipolar patients compared on familial aggregation. *Compr. Psychiatry 28:* 113–126.

Grunebaum, H. U., and Klerman, G. L. (1967) Wrist slashing. *Am. J. Psychiatry 124:* 113–120.

Guelfi, J. D. (1982) Paranoia et délires paranoiaques. In Koupernik, C., Loo, H., and Zarifian, E. (Eds.), *Précis de Psychiatrie.* Paris: Flammarion, pp. 162–169.

Gunderson, J. G. (1977) Characteristics of borderlines. In Hartocollis, P. (Ed.), *Borderline Personality Disorders.* New York: International Universities Press, pp. 173–192.

Gunderson, J. G., Carpenter, W. T., Jr., and Strauss, J. S. (1975) Borderline and schizophrenic patients: A comparative study. *Am. J. Psychiatry 132:* 1257–1264.

Gunderson, J. G., Frank, A. F., Katz, H. M., Vannicelli, M. L., Frosch, J. P., and Knapp, P. H. (1984) Effects of psychotherapy in schizophrenia: II. Comparative outcome of two forms of treatment. *Schizophr. Bull. 10:* 564–598.

Gunderson, J. G., and Singer, M. T. (1975) Defining borderline patients: An overview. *Am. J. Psychiatry 132:* 1–10.

Guze, S. B., and Robins, E. (1970) Suicide and primary affective disorders. *Br. J. Psychiatry 117:* 437–438.

Gyllenhammer, C., and Wistedt, B. (1987) Life events and psychiatric disorders. *Stress Med. 3:* 239–245.

Hall, R. C. W., and Beresford, T. P. (1985) Psychiatric manifestations of physical illness. In Michels, R., Cavenar, J. O., Brodie, H. K. H., Cooper, A. M., Guze, S. B., Judd, L. L., Klerman, G. L., and Solnit, A. J. (Eds.), *Psychiatry* (Vol. 2). Philadelphia: J. B. Lippincott, Chapter 88.

Hallman, J. (1986) The premenstrual syndrome—an equivalent of depression? *Acta Psychiatr. Scand. 73:* 403–411.

Hällström, T. (1987) Major depression, parental mental disorder and early family relationships. *Acta Psychiatr. Scand. 75:* 259–263.

Halperin, D. A. (Ed.). (1983) *Psychodynamic Perspectives on Religion, Sect and Cult.* Boston: John Wright/PSG.

Hankoff, L. (1980) Suicidal behavior in the institutional setting. *J. Psychiatr. Treat. Eval. 2:* 19–24.

Harding, C. M., Brooks, G. W., Ashikaga, T., Strauss, J. S., and Breier, A. (1987) The Vermont longitudinal study of persons with severe mental illness: II. Long-term outcome of subjects who retrospectively met DSM-III criteria for schizophrenia. *Am. J. Psychiatry 144:* 727–735.

Harding, C. M., and Strauss, J. S. (1985) The course of schizophrenia: An evolving concept. In Alpert, M. (Ed.), *Controversies in Schizophrenia.* New York: Guilford Press, pp. 339–353.

Harris, T., Brown, G. W., and Bifulco, A. (1987) Loss of parent in childhood and adult psychiatric disorder: The rôle of social class position and premarital pregnancy. *Psychol. Med. 17:* 163–183.

Haskett, R. F., Steiner, M. Osmun, J.N., and Carroll, B. J. (1980) Severe premenstrual tension: Delineation of the syndrome. *Biol. Psychiatry 15:* 121–139.

Haslam, J. (1809) *Observations in Madness and Melancholy.* London: J. Callow.

Hawton, K. (1987) Assessment of suicide risk. *Br. J. Psychiatry 150:* 145–153.

Hay, G. G. (1970) Dysmorphophobia. *Br. J. Psychiatry 116:* 399–406.

Heller, S. (1986) Personal communication.

Hellman, D. S., and Blackman, N. (1966) Enuresis, firesetting and cruelty to animals: A triad predictive of adult crime. *Am. J. Psychiatry 122:* 1431–1435.

Herman, J. L. (1981) *Father–Daughter Incest.* Cambridge, Mass.: Harvard University Press.

Herzog, D. B., Keller, M. B., and Lavori, P. W. (1988) Outcome in anorexia nervosa and bulimia nervosa: A review of the literature. *J. Nerv. Ment. Dis. 176:* 131–143.

Herzog, D. B., Norman, D. K., Rigotti, N. A., and Pepose, M. (1986) Frequency of bulimic behaviors and associated social maladjustment in female graduate students. *J. Psychiatr. Res.* 20(4): 355–361.

Hirschfeld, R. M. A., and Davidson, L. (1988) Clinical risk factors for suicide. *Psychiatr. Ann. 18:* 628–635.

Hoch, P. H., Cattell, J. P., Strahl, M.D., and Penness, H. H. (1962) The course and outcome of pseudoneurotic schizophrenia. *Am. J. Psychiatry 119:* 106–115.

Hofstätter, P. R. (1924) *Über eingebildete Schwangerschaft.* Vienna: Urban & Schwarzenberg.

Holinger, P. C., Offer, D., and Zola, M. A. (1988) A prediction model of suicide among youth. *J. Nerv. Ment. Dis. 176:* 275–279.

Hollingshead, A. B., and Redlich, F. C. (1958) *Social Class and Mental Illness.* New York: Wiley.

Holm, K., and Hundevadt, E. (1976) Psykiatrisk pasient—episode eller livsform? En etterundersøkelse. *Tidsskr. Norske Laegeforen. 96:* 1131–1135.

Holm, K., and Hundevadt, E. (1981) Borderline states: Prognosis and psychotherapy. *Br. J. Med. Psychol. 54:* 335–340.

Holmboe, R., & Astrup, C. (1957) A follow-up study of 255 patients with acute schizophrenia and schizophreniform psychoses. *Acta Psychiatr. Neurol. Scand.* (Suppl. 115): 1–61.

Holmes, J. (1988) Transference and countertransference. *Curr. Opin. Psychiatry 1:* 277–283.

Hooker, E. (1969) Parental relations and male homosexuality in patient and non-patient samples. *J. Consult. Clin. Psychol. 33:* 140–142.

Hoyer, T. V. (1959) Pseudologia fantastica: A consideration of "the lie" and a case presentation. *Psychiatr. Q. 33:* 203–220.

Hsu, L. K. G., Crisp, A. H., and Harding, B. (1979) Outcome of anorexia nervosa. *Lancet i:* 61–65.

Huber, G. (1983) Der Konzept substratnaher Basissymptome und seine Bedeutung für Theorie and Therapie schizophrener Erkrankungen. *Nervenarzt 54:* 23–32.

Huber, G., Gross, G., Schüttler, R., and Linz, M. (1980) Longitudinal studies of schizophrenic patients. *Schizophr. Bull. 6:* 592–605.

Hudgens, R. W., Morrison, J. R., and Barchha, R. G. (1967) Life events and onset of primary affective disorders: A study of 40 hospitalized patients and 40 controls. *Arch. Gen. Psychiatry 16:* 134–145.

Hurt, S., Clarkin, J., Widiger, T., Eyer, M., Sullivan, T., Stone, M. H., and Frances, A. (1988) DSM-III and borderline personality disorder: Decision rules and their implications. Paper presented at the First International Congress on the Disorders of Personality, Copenhagen, August 4.

Hyler, S. E., and Lyons, M. (1988) Factor analysis of the DSM-III personality disorder clusters: A replication. *Compr. Psychiatry 29*(3): 304–308.

Hynd, G. W., and Cohen, M. (1983) *Dyslexia: Neuropsychological Theory, Research and Clinical Differentiation.* New York: Grune & Stratton.

International Classification of Diseases (9th ed.; ICD-9). (1977) Geneva: World Health Organization.

Isager, T., Brinch, M., Kreiner, S., and Tolstrup, K. (1985) Death and relapse in anorexia nervosa: Survival analysis of 151 cases. *J. Psychiatry. Res. 19:* 515–521.

Jacobson, A., Koehler, J. E., and Jones-Brown, C. (1987) The failure of routine assessment to detect histories of assault experienced by psychiatric patients. *Hosp. Community Psychiatry 38:* 386–389.

Jacobson, B., Eklund, G., Hamberger, L., Linnarsson, D., Sedvall, G., and Valerius, M. (1987) Perinatal origin of adult self-destructive behavior. *Acta Psychiatr. Scand. 76:* 364–371.

Jaffe, P., Wolfe, D., Wilson, S. K., and Zak, L. (1986) Family violence and child adjustment: A comparative analysis of girls' and boys' behavioral symptoms. *Am. J. Psychiatry 143:* 74–77.

Jeammet, P., Jayle, D., Terrasse-Brechon, G., and Gorge, A. (1984) Le devenir de l'anorexie mentale. *Neuropsychiatr. de l'Enf. 32:* 97–113.

Jenike, M. A., Baer, L., and Minichiello, W. E. (1987) Somatic treatments for obsessive–compulsive disorder. *Compr. Psychiatry 28:* 250–263.

Jenkins, M. E. (1987) An outcome study on anorexia nervosa in an adolescent unit. *J. Adolesc. 10:* 71–81.

Johnstone, E. C., Crow, T., Frith, C. D., Husband, J., and Kreel, L. (1976) Cerebral ventricular size and cognitive impairment in chronic schizophrenia. *Lancet ii:* 924–926.

Johnstone, E. C., Owens, D. G. C., Frith, C. D., and Crow, T. C. (1986) The relative stability of positive and negative features in chronic schizophrenia. *Br. J. Psychiatry 150:* 60–64.

Jørgensen, P. (1986) Delusional psychosis: Hospital incidence, symptoms and classification. *Acta Psychiatr. Scand. 74:* 18–23.

Jørgensen, P. (1987) Clinical course and outcome of delusional psychoses. *Acta Psychiatr. Scand. 76:* 317–323.

Jung, C. (1921) *Psychologische Typen.* Zürich: Rascher.

Justice, B., and Justice, R. (1979) *The Broken Taboo.* New York: Human Sciences Press.

Kardiner, A., and Spiegel, H. (1947) *The Traumatic Neuroses of War.* New York: Hoeber.

Kasanin, J. (1933) Acute schizoaffective psychosis. *Am. J. Psychiatry 97:* 97–120.

Kashiwagi, T., McClure, J. N., and Wetzel, R. D. (1976) Premenstrual affective syndrome and psychiatric disorder. *Dis. Nerv. Syst. 37:* 116–119.

Kay, S. R., Opler, L. A., and Fiszbein, A. (1986) Significant positive and negative syndromes in chronic schizophrenia. *Br. J. Psychiatry 149:* 439–448.

Keener, M. A., and Anders, T. F. (1985) New frontiers of sleep disorders. In Michels,

R., Cavenar, J. O., Brodie, H-K. H., Cooper, A. M., Guze, S. B., Judd, L. L., Kierman, G. L., and Solnit, A. J. (Eds.), *Psychiatry* (Vol. 2). Philadelphia: J.B. Lippincott, Chapter 52.

Kempe, R. S., and Kempe, C. H. (1984) *The Common Secret: Sexual Abuse of Children and Adolescents*. New York: W. H. Freeman.

Kernberg, O. F. (1967) Borderline personality organization. *J. Am. Psychoanal. Assoc. 15:* 641–685.

Kernberg, O. F. (1975) *Borderline Conditions and Pathological Narcissism*. New York: Jason Aronson.

Kernberg, O. F. (1987) The differential diagnosis of antisocial behavior. Paper presented at the 140th Annual meeting of the American Psychiatric Association, Chicago, May 11.

Kestenbaum, C. J. (1982) Children and adolescents at risk for manic–depressive illness. In Feinstein, S. C., Looney, J. G., Schwartzberg, A. Z., and Sorosky, A. D. (Eds.), *Adolescent Psychiatry* (Vol. 10). Chicago: University of Chicago Press, pp. 245–255.

Kety, S. S. (1979) Disorders of the human brain. *Sci. Am. 241:* 202–214.

Kety, S. S. (1989) Genetic factors in suicide. In Roy, A. (Ed.), *Suicide*. Baltimore: Williams & Wilkins, pp. 41–45.

Kety, S. S., Rosenthal, D., Wender, P. H., and Schulsinger, F. (1968) Mental illness in the biological and adoptive families of adopted schizophrenics. In Rosenthal, D., and Kety, S. (Eds.), *Transmission of Schizophrenia*. Oxford: Pergamon Press, pp. 345–362.

Kinsey, A. C., Pomeroy, W. B., and Martin, C. I. (1948) *Sexual Behavior in the Human Male*. Philadelphia: W. B. Saunders.

Klein, D. (1977) Psychopharmacological treatment and delineation of borderline disorders. In Hartocollis, P. (Ed.), *Borderline Personality Disorders*. New York: International Universities Press, pp. 365–383.

Klein, D., and Davis, J. (1969) *Drug Treatment and Psychodiagnosis*. Baltimore: Williams & Wilkins.

Klein, H. (1980) Personal communication.

Klerman, G. L., Lavori, P. W., and Rice, J. (1985) Birth cohort trends in rates of major depressive disorder among relatives of patients with affective disorder. *Arch. Gen. Psychiatry 42:* 689–693.

Kluft, R. P. (1985) *Childhood Antecedents of Multiple Personality*. Washington, D.C.: American Psychiatric Press.

Kluft, R. (1987) An update on multiple personality. *Hosp. Community Psychiatry 38:* 363–373.

Knight, R. P. (1953) Borderline states. *Bull. Menninger Clin. 17:* 1–12.

Knutson, J. F., and Mehm, J. G. (1988) Transgenerational patterns of coercion in families and intimate relationships. In Russell, G.W. (Ed.), *Violence in Intimate Relationships*. New York: PMA, pp. 67–90.

Koehler, K., Vartzopoulos, D., and Ebel, H. (1986) Agoraphobia and depression: Relationships and severity in hospitalized women. *Compr. Psychiatry 27:* 533–539.

Kohut, H. (1971) *Analysis of the Self*. New York: International Universities Press.

Kolb, J. E., and Gunderson, J. G. (1980) Diagnosing borderline patients with a semi-structured interview. *Arch. Gen. Psychiatry 37:* 37–41.

Kolb, L. C. (1982) Assertive traits fostering social adaptation and creativity. *Psychiatr. J. Univ. of Ottawa, 7:* 219–225.

Kolb, L. C. (1987) A neuropsychological hypothesis explaining post-traumatic stress disorders. *Am. J. Psychiatry 144:* 989–995.

Kotila, L., and Lönnqvist, J. (1987) Adolescents who make suicide attempts repeatedly. *Acta Psychiatr. Scand. 76:* 386–393.

Koupernik, C. (1982) Psychopathologie de l'adolescence. In Koupernik, C., Loo, H., and Zarifian, E. (Eds.), *Précis de Psychiatrie.* Paris: Flammarion, pp. 305–307.

Kraepelin, E. (1913) *Dementia Praecox and Paraphrenia* (Barclay, R., and Robertson, G., Trans.). New York: Krieger, 1971.

Kraepelin, E. (1921) *Manic–Depressive Insanity and Paranoia.* Edinburgh: Livingstone.

Kranzer, S. (1986) Personal communication.

Kreitman, N. (Ed.). (1977) *Parasuicide.* Chichester, England: Wiley.

Kröber, H.-L. (1988) Die Persönlichkeit bipolar manisch–depressiv Erkrankender. *Nervenarzt 59:* 319–329.

Kroll, J. L. (1988) *The Challenge of the Borderline Patient.* New York: Norton.

Kroll, J. L., Carey, K. S., and Sines, L. K. (1985) Twenty year follow-up of borderline personality disorder: A pilot study. In Shagass, C. (Ed.), *IV World Congress of Biological Psychiatry* (Vol. 7). New York: Elsevier, pp. 577–579.

Kron, L., Decina, P., Kestenbaum, C., Farber, S., Gargan, M., and Fieve, R. (1982) The offspring of bipolar manic–depressives: Clinical features. In Feinstein, S. C., Looney, J. G., Schwartzberg, A. Z., and Sorosky, A. D. (Eds.), *Adolescent Psychiatry* (Vol. 10). Chicago: University of Chicago Press, pp. 273–291.

Kulhara, P., and Chadda, R. (1987) A study of negative symptoms in schizophrenia and depression. *Compr. Psychiatry 28:* 229–235.

Kullgren, G. (1988) Factors associated with completed suicide in borderline personality disorder. *J. Nerv. Ment. Dis. 176:* 40–44.

Kullgren, G., Renberg, E., and Jacobsson, L. (1986) An empirical study of borderline personality disorder and psychiatric suicides. *J. Nerv. Ment. Dis. 174:* 328–331.

Kundera, M. (1980) *The Book of Laughter and Forgetting.* New York: Knopf.

Kurz, A., Moller, J. H., Baindl, G., Burk, F., Torhort, A., Wachtler, C., and Lauter, H. (1987) Classification of parasuicide by cluster analysis: Types of suicidal behaviour, therapeutic and prognostic implications. *Br. J. Psychiatry 150:* 520–525.

Ladurie, E. L. (1978) *Montaillou.* New York: George Braziller.

Laessle, R. G., Kittl, S., Fichter, M. M., Wittchen, H.-V., and Pirke, K. M. (1987) Major affective disorder in anorexia nervosa and bulimia. *Br. J. Psychiatry 151:* 785–789.

Langfeldt, G. (1937) The prognosis is schizophrenia and the factors influencing the course of the disease. *Acta Psychiatr. Neurol. Scand.* (Suppl. 13): 1–228.

Langfeldt, G. (1956) The prognosis in schizophrenia. *Acta Psychiatr. Neurol. Scand.* (Suppl. 110): 1–66.

Leff, J., and Vaughn, C. (1980) The interaction of life events and relatives' expressed emotion in schizophrenia and depressive neurosis. *Br. J. Psychiatry 136:* 146–153.

LeGrand Du Saulle, A. (1891) *Les Hystériques: État Physique et État Mental.* Paris: Baillière.

Léon, C. A. (1989) Clinical course and outcome of schizophrenia in Cali, Colombia: A 10-year follow-up study. *J. Nerv. Ment. Dis. 177:* 593–606.

Leuner, H. (1962) *Die experimentelle Psychose.* Berlin: Springer-Verlag.

Levine, R. M. (1982) *Bad Blood: A Family Murder in Marin County.* New York: New American Library.

Leyton, E. (1986) *Compulsive Killers: The Story of Modern Multiple Murder.* New York: New York University Press.

Liddle, P. F. (1987) The symptoms of chronic schizophrenia: A re-examination of the positive–negative dichotomy. *Br. J. Psychiatry 151:* 145–151.

Lindenmayer, J. P., Kay, S. R., and Friedman, C. (1986) Negative and positive schizophrenic syndromes after the acute phase: A prospective follow-up. *Compr. Psychiatry 27:* 276–286.

Lindesay, J. (1987) Laterality shift in homosexual men. *Neuropsychologia 25:* 965–969.

Lindy, J. D., & Titchener, J. (1983) Acts of God and man. *Behav. Sci. Law 1:* 85–96.

Linehan, M. M. (1986) Suicidal people: One population or two? *Ann. NY Acad. Sci. 487:* 16–33.

Links, P. S., Steiner, M., and Huxley, G. (1988) The occurrence of borderline personality disorder in the families of borderline patients. *J. Pers. Disord. 2:* 14–20.

Livesley, W. J., Reiffer, L. I., Sheldon, A. E. R., and West, M. (1987) Prototypicality ratings of DSM-III criteria for personality disorders. *J. Nerv. Ment. Dis. 175:* 395–401.

Loranger, A. W., Oldham, J. M., and Tulis, E. H. (1982) Familial transmission of DSM-III borderline personality disorder. *Arch. Gen. Psychiatry 39:* 795–799.

Loranger, A. W., Susman, V.L., Oldham, J., and Russakoff, L. M. (1987) The Personality Disorder Examination: A preliminary report. *J. Pers. Disord. 1:* 1–13.

Luborsky, L. (1963) Clinicians' judgment of mental health. *Arch. Gen. Psychiatry 9:* 407–417.

Mailer, N. (1979) *The Executioner's Song.* Boston: Little, Brown.

Malmquist, C. P. (1986) Children who witness parental murder: Post-traumatic aspects. *Acad. Child Psychiatry 25:* 320–325.

Mann, J. (1987) Biological aspects of suicide. Grand Rounds, New York Hospital, Westchester Division, March 13.

Mann, T. (1955) *Confessions of Felix Krull, Confidence Man* (Lindley, D. Trans.). New York: Knopf.

Manos, N., Vasilopoulous, E., and Sotiriou, M. (1987) DSM-III diagnosed borderline personality disorder and depression. *J. Pers. Disord. 1:* 263–268.

Maqueda, F. (1988) Coups de fil pour coups de fils: Rencontres dans une permanence avec des mères battues par leurs enfants adolescents. *L'Inform. Psychiatr. 64:* 909–915.

Marneros, A., Rohde, A., Deister, A., Fimmers, R., and Jüremann, H. (1988) Long-term course of schizoaffective disorders: III. Onset, types of episodes and syndrome shift, precipitating factors, suicidality, seasonality, inactivity of illness and outcome. *Eur. Arch. Psychiatr. Neurol. Sci. 237:* 283–290.

Masters, B. (1985) *Killing for Company: The Case of Dennis Nilsen.* New York: Stein & Day.

Masterson, J. (1981) *Borderline and Narcissistic Disorders.* New York: Brunner/Mazel.

Masterson, J., and Costello, J. (1980) *From Borderline Adolescent to Functioning Adult.* New York: Brunner/Mazel.

May, P. R. A. (1968) *Treatment of Schizophrenia.* New York: Science House.

McClure, J. N., Reich, T., and Wetzel, R. D. (1971) Premenstrual symptoms as an indicator of bipolar affective disorder. *Br. J. Psychiatry 119:* 527–528.

McGlashan, T. H. (1984a) The Chestnut Lodge follow-up study: I. Follow-up methodology and study sample. *Arch. Gen. Psychiatry 41:* 573–585.

McGlashan, T. H. (1984b) The Chestnut Lodge follow-up study: II. Long-term outcome of schizophrenia and the affective disorders. *Arch. Gen. Psychiatry 41:* 586–601.

McGlashan, T. H. (1985) The prediction of outcome in borderline personality disorder: Part V of the Chestnut Lodge follow-up study. In McGlashan, T.H. (Ed.), *The Borderline: Current Empirical Research.* Washington, D.C.: American Psychiatric Press, pp. 63–98.

McGlashan, T. H. (1986a) The Chestnut Lodge follow-up study: III. Long-term outcome of borderline personalities. *Arch. Gen. Psychiatry 43:* 20–30.

McGlashan, T. H. (1986b) The prediction of outcome in chronic schizophrenia: IV. The Chestnut Lodge follow-up study. *Arch. Gen. Psychiatry 43:* 167–176.

McGlashan, T. H. (1986c) Schizotypal personality disorder: Long-term follow-up perspectives. VI: Chestnut Lodge follow-up study. *Arch. Gen. Psychiatry 43:* 329–334.

McGlashan, T. H. (1987) Borderline personality disorder and unipolar affective disorder. *J. Nerv. Ment. Dis. 175:* 467–473.

McGlashan, T. H. (1988) Prognostic factors in borderline patients. Paper presented at the 141st Annual Meeting of the American Psychiatric Association, Montreal, May 11.

McGlashan, T. H., Levy, S. T., and Carpenter, W. T., Jr. (1975) Integration and sealing over. *Arch. Gen. Psychiatry 32:* 1269–1272.

McGuire, C., and Norton, C. (1988) *Perfect Victim.* New York: Arbor House/William Morrow.

Melville, H. (1857) *The Confidence-Man.* New York: Hendrick House, 1954.

Menninger, K. A. (1935) A psychoanalytic study of the significance of self-mutilations. *Psychoanal. Q. 4:* 408–466.

Mewshaw, M. (1980) *Life for Death.* New York: Doubleday.

Michel, K. (1987) Suicide risk factors. *Br. J. Psychiatry 150:* 78–82.

Michels, R. (1988) The borderline patient: Shifts in theoretical emphasis; implications for treatment. Lecture given at the Clinical Symposium on the Borderline Patient, Mt. Sinai Hospital, Toronto, October 15.

Mihalik, G. J. (1988) Sexuality and gender: An evolutionary perspective. *Psychiatr. Ann. 18:* 40–42.

Modestin, J., and Villiger, C. (1989) Follow-up study on borderline versus nonborderline personality disorders. *Compr. Psychiatry 30:* 236–244.

Mogul, H. (1988) Suicide attempters: Their identification by survey instruments and their relationship to suicide completers. Paper presented at the Barnard Institute for Medical Research: Symposium on College Student Suicide, Columbia University, New York, June 16.

Molnar, G., and Cameron, P. (1975) Incest syndromes: Observations in a general psychiatric unit. *Can. J. Psychiatry 20:* 373–377.

Money, J. (1980) Genetic and chromosomal aspects of homosexual etiology. In Marmor, J. (Ed.), *Homosexual Behavior.* New York: Basic Books, pp. 59–72.

Morgan, H. G., Burns-Cox, C. J., Pocock, H., and Pottles, S. (1975) Deliberate self harm. *Br. J. Psychiatry 127:* 564–574.

Morgan, H. G., and Russell, G. F. M. (1975) Value of family background and clinical features as predictors of long-term outcome in anorexia nervosa: Four year follow-up of 41 patients. *Psychol. Med. 5:* 355–371.

Morris, H., Gunderson, J. G., and Zanarini, M. C. (1986) Transitional object use and borderline psychopathology. *Am. J. Psychiatry 143:* 1534–1538.

Morrison, J. R., Hudgens, R. W., and Barchha, R. G. (1968) Life events and psychiatric illness: A study of 100 patients and 100 controls. *Br. J. Psychiatry 114:* 423–432.

Morrison, J. R., and Minkoff, K. (1975) Explosive personality as a sequel to the hyperactive-child syndrome. *Compr. Psychiatry 16:* 343–348.

Morselli, E. (1866) Sulla dismorfofobia e sulla tafefobia. *Boll. Acad. Sci. Med. Genova 6:* 110.

Munk-Jørgensen, P., and Mortensen, P. B. (1989) Schizophrenia: A 13-year follow-up. *Acta Psychiatr. Scand. 79:* 391–399.

Murphy, E., and Brown, G. W. (1980) Life events, psychiatric disturbance and physical illness. *Br. J. Psychiatry 136:* 326–338.

Murphy, G. E. (1988) Suicide and substance abuse. *Arch. Gen. Psychiatry 45:* 593–594.

Nadelson, T. (1979) The Munchausen spectrum. *Gen. Hosp. Psychiatry 1:* 11–17.

New York Post. (1987) Mass murder suspect: "No one left to kill." December 30, p. 17.

Niederland, W. G. (1984) *The Schreber Case: Psychoanalytic Profile of a Paranoid Personality.* Hillsdale, N.J.: Analytic Press.

Norris, J. (1988) *Serial Killers.* Garden City, N.Y.: Doubleday.

Nyman, A. K. (1978) Nonregressive schizophrenia: Clinical course and outcome. *Acta Psychiatr. Scand.* (Suppl. 272): 1–143.

O'Connor, A., and Daly, J. (1986) The problems of tracing. *Bull. Roy. Coll. Psychiatrists 10:* 51–52.

Ogawa, K., Miya, M., Watarai, A., Nakazawa, M., Yuasa, S., and Utena, H. (1987) A long-term follow-up study of schizophrenia in Japan—with special reference to the course of social adjustment. *Br. J. Psychiatry 151:* 758–765.

Oliver, J. E. (1988) Successive generations of child maltreatment: The children. *Br. J. Psychiatry 153:* 543–553.

Olsen, J. (1972) *Son: A Psychopath and His Victims.* New York: Dell.

Olsson, P. A. (1983) Adolescent involvement with the supernatural and cults. In Halperin, D. A. (Ed.), *Psychodynamic Perspectives on Religion, Sect and Cult.* Boston: John Wright/PSG, pp. 235–256.

Opjørdsmoen, S. (1989) Long-term course and outcome in unipolar affective and schizoaffective psychoses. *Acta Psychiatr. Scand. 79:* 317–326.

Opler, L. A., Kay, S. R., and Rosado, V. (1984) Positive and negative syndromes in chronic schizophrenic inpatients. *J. Nerv. Ment. Dis. 172:* 317–325.

O'Reilly, R., and Malhotra, L. (1987) Capgras syndrome: An unusual case and discussion of psychodynamic factors. *Br. J. Psychiatry 151:* 263–265.

O'Sullivan, G. H., and Kelleher, M. J. (1987) A study of firesetters in the south-west of Ireland. *Br. J. Psychiatry 151:* 818–823.

Ostwald, P. (1985) *Schumann: The Inner Voices of a Musical Genius.* Boston: Northeastern University Press.

Pallis, O. J., Barraclough, B. M., Levey, A. B., Jenkins, J. S., and Sainsbury, P. (1982) Estimating suicide risk among attempted suicides: I. The development of new scales. *Br. J. Psychiatry 141:* 37–44.

Pao, P. N. (1969a) Pathological jealousy. *Psychoanal. Q. 38:* 616–638.

Pao, P. (1969b) The syndrome of delicate cutting. *Br. J. Med. Psychol. 42:* 195–206.

Paris, J., Brown, R., and Nowlis, D. (1987) Long-term follow-up of borderline patients in a general hospital. *Compr. Psychiatry 28:* 530–535.

Parker, G. (1982) Re-searching the schizophrenic mother. *J. Nerv. Ment. Dis. 170:* 452–462.

Parlee, M. E. (1973) The premenstrual syndrome. *Psychol. Bull. 80:* 454–465.

Pattison, E. M., and Kahan, J. (1983) The deliberate self-harm syndrome. *Am. J. Psychiatry 140:* 867–872.

Paykel, E. S., Rao, B. M., and Taylor, C. N. (1984) Life stress and symptom patterns in outpatient depression. *Psychol. Med. 14:* 559–568.

Pearlson, G. D., Garbacz, D. M., Moberg, P. J., Ahn, H. S., and DePaulo, J. R. (1985) Symptomatic, familial, perinatal and social correlates of computerized axial tomography (CAT) changes in schizophrenics and bipolars. *J. Nerv. Ment. Dis. 173:* 42–50.

Perris, C. (1966) A study of bipolar and unipolar recurrent depressive psychoses. *Acta Psychiatry. Scand. 42*(Suppl. 194).

Pessar, L. (1988) Factitious illness. Grand Rounds, New York State Psychiatric Institute, February 12.

Pickar, D. (1986) Neuroleptics, dopamine and schizophrenia. *Psychiatr. Clin. N. Am. 9:* 35–48.

Pinel, P. (1799) *Nosographie Philosophique.* Paris: de Crapelet.

Plakun, E. M., Burkhardt, P. E., and Muller, J. P. (1985) 14 year follow-up of borderline and schizotypal personality disorders. *Compr. Psychiatry 26:* 448–455.

Pogue-Geile, M. F., and Harrow, M. (1984) Negative and positive symptoms in schizophrenia and depression: A follow-up. *Schizophr. Bull. 10:* 371–387.

Pogue-Geile, M. F., and Zubin, J. (1988) Negative symptomatology and schizophrenia: A conceptual and empirical review. *Int. J. Ment. Health 16:* 3–45.

Pokorny, A. (1983) Prediction of suicide in psychiatric patients. *Arch. Gen. Psychiatry 40:* 249–257.

Pope, H. G., Frankenburg, F. R., Hudson, J. I., Jonas, J. M., and Yurgelun-Todd, D. (1987) Is bulimia associated with borderline personality disorder? A controlled study. *J. Clin. Psychiatry 48:* 181–184.

Pope, H. G., Jonas, J. M., and Hudson, J. (1983) The validity of DSM-III borderline personality disorder. *Arch. Gen. Psychiatry 40:* 23–30.

Pope, H. G., Jonas, J. M., and Jones, B. (1982) Factitious psychosis: Phenomenology, family history and long-term outcome of nine patients. *Am. J. Psychiatry 139:* 1480–1483.

Pope, H. G., Lipinski, J. F., Cohen, B. M., and Axelrod, D. T. (1980) "Schizoaffective disorder": An invalid diagnosis? A comparison of schizoaffective disorder, schizophrenia, and affective disorder. *Am. J. Psychiatry 137*(8): 921–927.

Prudo, R., and Blum, H. M. (1987) Five-year outcome and prognosis in schizophrenia. *Br. J. Psychiatry 150:* 345–354.

Putnam, F. W. (1986) The scientific investigation of multiple personality disorder. In Quen, J. M. (Ed.), *Split Minds, Split Brains.* New York: New York University Press, pp. 109–125.

Rado, S. (1956) *The Psychoanalysis of Behavior.* New York: Grune & Stratton.

Raspe, R. E. (1785) *Baron Munchausen's Narrative of His Marvellous Travels and Campaigns in Russia. Singular Travels, Campaigns and Adventures of Baron Munchausen.* New York: Dover, 1960.

Ray, I. (1839) *A Treatise on the Medical Jurisprudence of Insanity.* London: G. Henderson.

Reich, P. (1983) Factitious disorders in a teaching hospital. *Ann. Intern. Med. 99:* 240–247.

Resnick, R. J., Goldberg, S. C., Schulz, S. C., Schulz, P. M., Hamer, R. M., and Friedel, R. O. (1988) Borderline personality disorder: Replication of MMPI profiles. *J. Clin. Psychol. 44:* 354–360.

Rich, C. L., Fowler, R. C., Fogarty, L. A., and Young, D. (1988) San Diego suicide study. *Arch. Gen. Psychiatry 45:* 589–592.

Rich, C. L., Ricketts, J. E., Fowler, R. C., and Young, D. (1988) Some differences between men and women who commit suicide. *Am. J. Psychiatry 145*(6): 718–722.

Rifkin, A., Quitkin, F., and Klein, D. (1975) Akinesia. *Arch. Gen. Psychiatry 32:* 672–674.

Ritzler, B. A. (1981) Paranoia: Prognosis and treatment. *Schizophr. Bull. 7:* 710–728.

Robins, E. (1989) Completed suicides. In Roy, A. (Ed.), *Suicide*. Baltimore: Williams & Wilkins, pp. 123–133.

Ronningstam, E., and Gunderson, J. G. (1989) Descriptive studies on narcissistic personality disorder. *Psychiatr. Clin. N. Am. 12:* 585–601.

Root, M. P., and Fallon, P. (1988) The incidence of victimization experiences in a bulimic sample. *J. Interpers. Violence 3*(2): 161–173.

Rosen, D. H. (1976) The serious suicide attempt: 5-year follow-up of 886 patients. *JAMA, 235:* 2105–2109.

Rosen, L. W., and Thomas, M. A. (1984) Treatment technique for chronic wrist cutters. *J. Behav. Ther. Exp. Psychiatry 15:* 33–36.

Rosenthal, N. E., and Wehr, T. A. (1987) Seasonal affective disorders. *Psychiatr. Ann. 17*(10): 670–674.

Rosenthal, R. J., Rinzler, C., Wallsh, R., and Klausner, E. (1972) Wrist-cutting syndrome: The meaning of a gesture. *Am. J. Psychiatry 128:* 47–52.

Ross, C., Heber, S., Anderson, G., Norton, R., Anderson, B. A., DelCampo, M., and Pillay, N. (1989) Differentiating multiple personality disorder and complex partial seizures. *Gen. Hosp. Psychiatry 11:* 54–58.

Rothschild, A. J., Schatzberg, A. F., Langlacs, P. J., Lerbinger, J. E., Miller, M. M., and Cole, J. O. (1987) Psychotic and nonpsychotic depressions: I. Comparison of plasma catecholamines and cortisol measures. *Psychiatry Res. 20:* 143–153.

Roy, A. (1985) Suicide: A multidetermined act. *Psychiatr. Clin. N. Am. 8:* 243–250.

Rubinow, D. R., Hoban, C., and Grover, G. N. (1987) Menstrually-related mood disorders. In Nerozzi, D., Goodwin, F. K., and Costa, E. (Eds.), *Hypothalamic Dysfunction in Neuropsychiatric Disorders*. New York: Raven Press, pp. 335–346.

Ruitenbeck, H. M. (1973) *Freud as We Knew Him*. Detroit: Wayne State University Press.

Rule, A. (1987) *Small Sacrifices: A True Story of Passion and Murder*. New York: New American Library.

Russell, D. E. (1986) *The Secret Trauma*. New York: Basic Books.

Russell, G. A. (1985) Narcissism and the narcissistic personality disorder: A comparison of the theories of Kernberg and Kohut. *Br. J. Med. Psychol. 58:* 137–148.

Rutter, M. (1986) Meyerian psychobiology, personality development and the role of life experiences. *Am. J. Psychiatry 143:* 1077–1087.

Rutter, M. (1987) Temperament, personality and personality disorder. *Br. J. Psychiatry 150:* 443–458.

Schaffer, C. B., Carroll, J., and Abramowitz, S.I. (1982) Self-mutilation and the borderline personality. *J. Nerv. Ment. Dis. 170:* 468–473.

Scharfetter, C., and Nüsperli, M. (1980) The group of schizophrenias, schizoaffective psychoses and affective disorders. *Schizophr. Bull. 6*(4): 586–591.

Schatzberg, A. F., Rothschild, A. J., Langlais, P. J., Lerbinger, J. E., Schildkraut, J. J., and Cole, J. O. (1987) Psychotic and nonpsychotic depressions: II. Platelet M.A.O. activity, plasma catecholamines, cortisol, and specific symptoms. *Psychiatry Res. 20:* 155–164.

Schneider, K. (1959) *Klinische Pathologie.* Stuttgart: Geo. Thieme Verlag.

Schreiber, F. R. (1973) *Sybil.* Chicago: Regnery.

Schulz, S. C., and Reynolds, C. F., III. Sleep disorders. In Michels, R., Cavenar, J. O., Brodie, H. K. H., Cooper, A. M., Guze, S. B., Judd, L. L., Klerman, G. L., and Solnit, A. J. (Eds.), *Psychiatry* (Vol. 2). Philadelphia: J. B. Lippincott, Chapter 59.

Schwartz, K. M. (1986) The meaning of cults in the treatment of late adolescent issues. In Feinstein, S. C., Looney, J. G., Schwartzberg, A. Z., and Sorosky, A. D. (Eds.), *Adolescent Psychiatry* (Vol. 13). Chicago: University of Chicago Press, pp. 188–200.

Searles, H. F. (1986) *My Work with Borderline Patients.* Northvale, N.J.: Jason Aronson.

Seivewright, N. (1987) Relationships between life events and personality in psychiatric disorder. *Stress Med. 3:* 163–168.

Seligman, R., Gleser, G., Rauh, J., and Harris, L. (1974) The effect of earlier parental loss in adolescence. *Arch. Gen. Psychiatry 31:* 475–481.

Serban, C., Conte, H. R., and Plutchik, R. (1987) Borderline and schizotypal personality disorders: Mutually exclusive or overlapping? *J. Pers. Assess. 51*(1): 15–22.

Shalev, A., and Munitz, H. (1986) The neuroleptic malignant syndrome: Agent and host interaction. *Acta Psychiatr. Scand. 73:* 337–347.

Sheard, M. H., Marini, J. L., Bridges, C. I., and Wagner, E. (1976) The effect of lithium on impulsive aggressive behavior in man. *Am. J. Psychiatry 133:* 1409–1413.

Showers, J., and Pickrell, E. (1987) Child firesetters: A study of three populations. *Hosp. Community Psychiatry 38:* 495–501.

Siegelman, M. (1974) Parental background of male homosexuals and heterosexuals. *Arch. Sex. Behav. 3:* 3–18.

Siever, L. J., and Coursey, R. D. (1985) Biological markers for schizophrenia and the biological high-risk approach. *J. Nerv. Ment. Dis. 173:* 4–16.

Signer, S. F. (1987) Capgras' syndrome: The delusion of substitution. *J. Clin. Psychiatry 48:* 147–150.

Signer, S. F., and Swinson, R. P. (1987) Two cases of erotomania (De Clérambault's syndrome) in bipolar affective illness. *Br. J. Psychiatry 151:* 853–855.

Sims, A. C. P. (1973) Importance of a high tracing rate in long-term medical follow-up studies. *Lancet ii:* 433–435.

Synder, S. (1986) Pseudologia fantastica in a borderline patient. *Am. J. Psychiatry 143:* 1287–1289.

Soloff, P., George, A., Nathan, S., and Schulz, P. M. (1987) Characterizing depression in borderline patients. *J. Clin. Psychiatry 48:* 155–157.

Solyom, L. (1987) A case of self-inflicted leucotomy. *Br. J. Psychiatry 151:* 855–857.

Spillane, R. (1987) Rhetoric as remedy: Some philosophical antecedents of psychotherapeutic ethics. *Br. J. Med. Psychol. 60:* 217–224.

Spiro, H. R. (1968) Chronic factitious illness: Munchausen's syndrome. *Arch. Gen. Psychiatry 18:* 569–578.

Spitz, R. (1970) Effects of mother's personality disturbances on her infant. In Anthony, E., and Benedek, T. (Eds.), *Parenthood.* Boston: Little, Brown, pp. 503–524.

Spitzer, R. L., Endicott, J., and Gibbon, M. (1979) Crossing the border into borderline. *Arch. Gen. Psychiatry 36:* 17–24.

Spitzer, R. L., and Williams, J. B. W. (1982) Hysteroid dysphoria: An unsuccessful attempt to demonstrate its syndromal validity. *Am. J. Psychiatry 139:* 1286–1291.

Spungen, D. (1983) *And I Don't Want to Live This Life.* New York: Random House.

Stassen, H. (1988) Personal communication.

Steer, R. A., Beck, A. T., Garrison, B., and Lester, D. (1988) Eventual suicide in interrupted and uninterrupted attempters: A challenge to the cry-for-help hypothesis. *Suicide Life-Threat. Behav. 18:* 119–128.

Stern, A. (1938) Psychoanalytic investigation and therapy in the borderline group of neuroses. *Psychoanal. Q. 7:* 467–489.

Stone, M. H. (1970) Cultural factors in the treatment of an obsessive handwasher. *Psychiatr. Q. 44:* 1–9.

Stone, M. H. (1976) Madness and the moon revisited: Possible influence of the full-moon in a case of atypical mania. *Psychiatr. Ann. 6:* 47–60.

Stone, M. H. (1977) Factitious illness. *Bull. Menninger Clin. 41:* 239–254.

Stone, M. H. (1980a) *The Borderline Syndromes.* New York: McGraw-Hill.

Stone, M. H. (1980b) Traditional psychoanalytic characterology reexamined in the light of constitutional and cognitive differences between the sexes. *J. Am. Acad. Psychoanal. 8:* 381–401.

Stone, M. H. (1982) Premenstrual tension in borderline and related disorders. In Friedman, R. C. (Ed.), *Behavior and the Menstrual Cycle.* New York: Marcel Dekker, pp. 317–344.

Stone, M. H. (1985a) Disturbances in sex and love in borderline patients. In DeFries, Z., Friedman, R. C., and Corn, R. (Eds.), *Sexuality: New Perspectives.* Westport, Conn.: Greenwood Press, pp. 159–186.

Stone, M. H. (1985b) *Essential Papers on the Borderline.* New York: New York University Press.

Stone, M. H. (1985c) Genetische Faktoren in schizotypen Patienten. In Huber, G. (Ed.), *Basisstadien endogener Psychosen und das Borderline-Problem.* Stuttgart: Schattauer, pp. 225–237.

Stone, M. H. (1985d) Schizotypal personality: Psychotherapeutic aspects. *Schizophr. Bull. 11:* 576–589.

Stone, M. H. (1987) Psychotherapy of borderline patients in light of long-term follow-up. *Bull. Menninger Clin. 51:* 231–247.

Stone, M. H. (1988a) The borderline domain: The "inner script" and other common psychodynamics. In Howells, J. (Ed.), *Modern Perspectives in Psychiatry.* New York: Brunner/Mazel, pp. 200–230.

Stone, M. H. (1988b) Toward a psychobiological theory of borderline personality disorder. *Dissociation 1:* 2–15.

Stone, M. H. (1989a) The course of borderline personality disorder. *Annual Rev. Psychiatry 8:* 103–122.

Stone, M. H. (1989b) Long-term follow-up of narcissistic borderline patients. *Psychiatr. Clin. N. Am. 12:* 621–641.

Stone, M. H. (1990) Incest in borderline patients. In Kluft, R. (Ed.), *Incest-Related Syndromes of Adult Psychopathology.* Washington, D.C.: American Psychiatric Press.

Stone, M. H., Hurt, S. W., and Stone, D. K. (1987) The P.I.-500: Long-term follow-up of borderline inpatients meeting DSM-III criteria. I. Global outcome. *J. Pers. Disord. 1:* 291–298.

Stone, M. H., Kahn, E., and Flye, B. (1981) Psychiatrically ill relatives of borderline patients: A family study. *Psychiatr. Q. 53:* 71–84.

Stone, M. H., Unwin, A., Beacham, B., and Swenson, C. (1988) Incest in female borderlines: Its frequency and impact. *Int. J. Fam. Psychiatry* 9(3): 277–293.

Strauss, J. S. (1983) Schizoaffective disorders: 'Just another illness' or key to understanding the psychoses? *Psychiatr. Clin. 16:* 286–296.

Strauss, J. S., Carpenter, W. T., Jr., and Bartko, J. J. (1974) Speculations on the processes that underlie schizophrenic symptoms and signs. *Schizophr. Bull. 11:* 61–69.

Straus, M. A., Gelles, R. J., and Steinmetz, S. K. (1980) *Behind closed doors: Violence in the American family.* Garden City, N.Y.: Doubleday/Anchor.

Summers, A. (1985) *Goddess: The Secret Lives of Marilyn Monroe.* New York: Macmillan.

Swift, W. J., Ritzholz, M., Kalin, N. H., and Kaslow, N. (1987) A follow-up study of 30 hospitalized bulimics. *Psychosom. Med. 49:* 45–55.

Thigpen, G. H., and Cleckley, H. M. (1957) *The Three Faces of Eve.* New York: McGraw-Hill.

Toffler, G., and Modestin, J. (1987) Are there differences between borderline and other personality disorders? *Eur. Arch. Psychiatr. Neurol. Sci. 236:* 276–280.

Toner, B. B., Garfinkel, P. E., and Garner, D. M. (1986) Long-term follow-up of anorexia nervosa. *Psychosom. Med. 48:* 520–529.

Torgersen, S. (1984) Genetic and nosological aspects of schizotypal and borderline personality disorders: A twin study. *Arch. Gen. Psychiatry 41:* 546–554.

Tsuang, M. T. (1978) Suicide in schizophrenics, manics, depressives and surgical controls. *Arch. Gen. Psychiatry 35:* 153–155.

Tsuang, M. T. (1986) Atypical psychosis. Grand Rounds, New York Hospital, Westchester Division, March 21.

Tsuang, M. T., and Dempsey, M. (1979) Long-term outcome of major psychoses: II. Schizoaffective disorder compared with schizophrenia, affective disorders, and a surgical control group. *Arch. Gen. Psychiatry 36:* 1302–1304.

Tsuang, M. T., Dempsey, G. M., and Rauscher, F. (1976) A study of "atypical schizophrenia": Comparison with schizophrenia and affective disorder by sex, age of admission, precipitant, outcome and family history. *Arch. Gen. Psychiatry 33:* 1157–1160.

Tsuang, M. T., and Winokur, G. (1975) The Iowa 500: Field work in a 35 year follow-up of depression, mania and schizophrenia. *Can. Psychiatr. Assoc. J. 20:* 359–365.

Vaillant, G. E. (1963) Manic–depressive heredity and remission in schizophrenia. *Br. J. Psychiatry 109:* 746–749.

Vaillant, G. E. (1978) Prognosis and the course of schizophrenia. *Schizophr. Bull. 4:* 20–24.

Valenstein, E. S. (1986) *Great and Desperate Cures: The Rise and Decline of Psychosurgery and Other Radical Treatments for Mental Illness.* New York: Basic Books.

Vandereycken, W. (1987) Are anorexia nervosa and bulimia variants of affective disorders? *Acta Psychiatr. Belg. 87:* 267–280.

Van Eerdewegh, M. M., Van Eerdewegh, P., Coryell, W., Clayton, P. J., Endicott, J., Koepke, J., and Rochberg, N. (1987) Schizoaffective disorders: Bipolar–unipolar subtyping. *J. Affective Disord. 12:* 223–232.

Van Hasselt, V. B., Morrison, R. L., Bellack, A. S., and Hersen, M. (Eds.). (1988) *Handbook of Family Violence.* New York: Plenum Press.

van Praag, H. M., and Nijo, L. (1984) About the course of schizoaffective psychoses. *Compr. Psychiatry 25:* 9–22.

Volkan, V. D. (1987) *Six Steps in the Treatment of Borderline Personality Organization*. Northvale, N.J.: Jason Aronson.

Wahl, C. W. (1954) Some antecedent factors in the family histories of 392 schizophrenics. *Am. J. Psychiatry 110:* 668–676.

Waldinger, R. J. (1987) Intensive dynamic therapy with borderline patients: An overview. *Am. J. Psychiatry 144:* 267–274.

Wallerstein, R. (1986) *Forty-Two Lives in Treatment*. New York: Guilford Press.

Walsh, M. (1986) *The Triumph of the Meek*. New York: Harper & Row.

Warheit, G. J., and Auth, J. B. (1985) Epidemiology of alcohol abuse in adulthood. In Michels, R., Cavenar, J. O., Brodie, H. K. H., Cooper, A. M., Guze, S. B., Judd, L. L., Klerman, G. L., and Solnit, A. J. (Eds.), *Psychiatry* (Vol. 3). Philadelphia: J. B. Lippincott, Chapter 18.

Wax, D. E., and Haddox, U. G. (1974) Enuresis, firesetting and animal cruelty: A useful danger signal in predicting vulnerability of adolescent males to assaultive behavior. *Child Psychiatr. Hum. Dev. 4:* 151–156.

Weeke, A., and Vaeth, M. (1986) Excess mortality of bipolar and unipolar manic–depressive patients. *J. Affective Disord. 11:* 227–234.

Wehr, T. A., Jacobsen, F. M., and Sack, D. A. (1986) Phototherapy in seasonal affective disorder. *Arch. Gen. Psychiatry 43:* 870–875.

Weissman, M. M., Fox, K., and Klerman, G. L. (1973) Hostility and depression associated with suicide attempts. *Am. J. Psychiatry 130:* 450–455.

Welner, A., Fishman, R., and Robins, E. (1977) The group of schizoaffective and related psychoses: A follow-up study. *Compr. Psychiat. 18:* 413–422.

Wendt, C. F. (1911) Ein Beitrag zur Kasuistik der Pseudologia phantastica. *Allgem. Z. Psychiatrie 64:* 4.

Werble, B. (1970) Second follow-up study of borderline patients. *Arch. Gen. Psychiatry 23:* 3–7.

Wetzel, R. D., and McClure, J. N. (1972) Suicide and the menstrual cycle. *Compr. Psychiatry 13:* 369–374.

Wetzel, R. D., Reich, T., Murphy, G. E., Province, M., and Miller, J. R. (1987) The changing relationship between age and suicide: Cohort effect, period effect or both? *Psychiatry. Dev. 3:* 179–218.

Whitam, F. L., and Zent, M. (1984) A cross-cultural assessment of early cross-gender behavior and familial factors in male homosexuality. *Arch. Sex. Behav. 13:* 427–439.

Whytt, R. (1765) *Observations on the Nature, Causes, and Cure of Those Disorders Which Have Been Commonly Called Nervous, Hypochondriac, or Hysteric*. Edinburgh: T. Becket.

Widom, C. S. (1989) The cycle of violence. *Science 244:* 160–166.

Willi, J., and Grossman, S. (1983) Epidemiology of anorexia nervosa in a defined region of Switzerland. *Am. J. Psychiatry 140:* 564–567.

Willis, T. (1668) *Pathologiae Cerebri et Nervosi Generis Specimen*. Amsterdam: Daniel Elzevir.

Wilson, E. (1975) *Sociobiology*. Cambridge, Mass.: Harvard University Press/Belknap Press.

Wilson, J. O., and Herrnstein, R. J. (1985) *Crime and Human Nature*. New York: Simon & Schuster.

Winnicott, D. (1965) *The Maturational Processes and the Facilitating Environment*. New York: International Universities Press.

Winokur, G. (1974) The use of genetic studies in clarifying clinical issues in schizophrenia. In Mitsuda, H., and Fukuda, T. (Eds.), *Biological Mechanisms of Schizophrenia and Schizophrenia-Like Psychoses*. Tokyo: Igaku-Shoin, pp. 241–274.

Winokur, G., Dennert, J., and Angst, J. (1986) Independent familial transmission of psychotic symptomatology in the affective disorders or does delusional depression breed true? *Psychiatr. Fenn.:* 9–16.

Woollcott, P. (1985) Prognostic indicators in the psychotherapy of borderline patients. *Am. J. Psychother. 39:* 17–29.

Yates, A. (1987) Psychological damage associated with extreme eroticism in young children. *Psychiatr. Ann. 17:* 257–261.

Zamyatin, Y. (1924) *We* (Guerney, B.G., Trans.). Harmondsworth, England: Penguin Books, 1972.

Zanarini, M. C., Gunderson, J. G., Marino, M. F., Schwartz, E. O., and Frankenburg, F. R. (1989) Childhood experiences of borderline patients. *Compr. Psychiatry 30:* 18–25.

Index

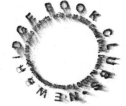